Biomaterials for Bone Tissue Engineering 2020

Biomaterials for Bone Tissue Engineering 2020

Editors

Nora Bloise
Lorenzo Fassina

MDPI • Basel • Beijing • Wuhan • Barcelona • Belgrade • Manchester • Tokyo • Cluj • Tianjin

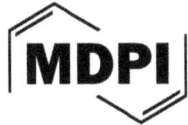

Editors
Nora Bloise
Dept. of Molecular Medicine
University of Pavia
Pavia
Italy

Lorenzo Fassina
Dept. of Electrical, Computer
and Biomedical Engineering
University of Pavia
Pavia
Italy

Editorial Office
MDPI
St. Alban-Anlage 66
4052 Basel, Switzerland

This is a reprint of articles from the Special Issue published online in the open access journal *Materials* (ISSN 1996-1944) (available at: www.mdpi.com/journal/materials/special_issues/Biomaterials_Bone_Tissue_Engineering).

For citation purposes, cite each article independently as indicated on the article page online and as indicated below:

LastName, A.A.; LastName, B.B.; LastName, C.C. Article Title. *Journal Name* **Year**, *Volume Number*, Page Range.

ISBN 978-3-0365-6104-2 (Hbk)
ISBN 978-3-0365-6103-5 (PDF)

© 2023 by the authors. Articles in this book are Open Access and distributed under the Creative Commons Attribution (CC BY) license, which allows users to download, copy and build upon published articles, as long as the author and publisher are properly credited, which ensures maximum dissemination and a wider impact of our publications.

The book as a whole is distributed by MDPI under the terms and conditions of the Creative Commons license CC BY-NC-ND.

Contents

Sara G. Pedrero, Pilar Llamas-Sillero and Juana Serrano-López
A Multidisciplinary Journey towards Bone Tissue Engineering
Reprinted from: *Materials* 2021, *14*, 4896, doi:10.3390/ma14174896 1

Laurens Parmentier, Mathieu Riffault and David A. Hoey
Utilizing Osteocyte Derived Factors to Enhance Cell Viability and Osteogenic Matrix Deposition within IPN Hydrogels
Reprinted from: *Materials* 2020, *13*, 1690, doi:10.3390/ma13071690 31

Sara Simorgh, Peiman Brouki Milan, Maryam Saadatmand, Zohreh Bagher, Mazaher Gholipourmalekabadi and Rafieh Alizadeh et al.
Human Olfactory Mucosa Stem Cells Delivery Using a Collagen Hydrogel: As a Potential Candidate for Bone Tissue Engineering
Reprinted from: *Materials* 2021, *14*, 3909, doi:10.3390/ma14143909 45

Nora Bloise, Alessia Patrucco, Giovanna Bruni, Giulia Montagna, Rosalinda Caringella and Lorenzo Fassina et al.
In Vitro Production of Calcified Bone Matrix onto Wool Keratin Scaffolds via Osteogenic Factors and Electromagnetic Stimulus
Reprinted from: *Materials* 2020, *13*, 3052, doi:10.3390/ma13143052 63

Gissur Örlygsson, Elín H. Laxdal, Sigurbergur Kárason, Atli Dagbjartsson, Eggert Gunnarsson and Chuen-How Ng et al.
Mineralization in a Critical Size Bone-Gap in Sheep Tibia Improved by a Chitosan Calcium Phosphate-Based Composite as Compared to Predicate Device
Reprinted from: *Materials* 2022, *15*, 838, doi:10.3390/ma15030838 85

Luis Carlos de Almeida Pires, Rodrigo Capalbo da Silva, Pier Paolo Poli, Fernando Ruas Esgalha, Henrique Hadad and Leticia Pitol Palin et al.
Evaluation of Osteoconduction of a Synthetic Hydroxyapatite/-Tricalcium Phosphate Block Fixed in Rabbit Mandibles
Reprinted from: *Materials* 2020, *13*, 4902, doi:10.3390/ma13214902 103

Ricardo Bento, Anuraag Gaddam and José M. F. Ferreira
Sol–Gel Synthesis and Characterization of a Quaternary Bioglass for Bone Regeneration and Tissue Engineering
Reprinted from: *Materials* 2021, *14*, 4515, doi:10.3390/ma14164515 119

Jacopo Barberi and Silvia Spriano
Titanium and Protein Adsorption: An Overview of Mechanisms and Effects of Surface Features
Reprinted from: *Materials* 2021, *14*, 1590, doi:10.3390/ma14071590 131

Elisabet Roca-Millan, Enric Jané-Salas, Albert Estrugo-Devesa and José López-López
Evaluation of Bone Gain and Complication Rates after Guided Bone Regeneration with Titanium Foils: A Systematic Review
Reprinted from: *Materials* 2020, *13*, 5346, doi:10.3390/ma13235346 173

Maria Laura Gatto, Riccardo Groppo, Nora Bloise, Lorenzo Fassina, Livia Visai and Manuela Galati et al.
Topological, Mechanical and Biological Properties of Ti6Al4V Scaffolds for Bone Tissue Regeneration Fabricated with Reused Powders via Electron Beam Melting
Reprinted from: *Materials* 2021, *14*, 224, doi:10.3390/ma14010224 185

Amani M. Basudan, Marwa Y. Shaheen, Abdurahman A. Niazy, Jeroen J. J. P. van den Beucken, John A. Jansen and Hamdan S. Alghamdi
Histomorphometric Evaluation of Peri-Implant Bone Response to Intravenous Administration of Zoledronate (Zometa®) in an Osteoporotic Rat Model
Reprinted from: *Materials* **2020**, *13*, 5248, doi:10.3390/ma13225248 205

Marwa Y. Shaheen, Amani M. Basudan, Abdurahman A. Niazy, Jeroen J. J. P. van den Beucken, John A. Jansen and Hamdan S. Alghamdi
Histological and Histomorphometric Analyses of Bone Regeneration in Osteoporotic Rats Using a Xenograft Material
Reprinted from: *Materials* **2021**, *14*, 222, doi:10.3390/ma14010222 219

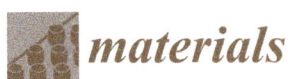

Review

A Multidisciplinary Journey towards Bone Tissue Engineering

Sara G. Pedrero [1], Pilar Llamas-Sillero [1,2] and Juana Serrano-López [1,*]

[1] Experimental Hematology Lab, IIS-Fundación Jiménez Díaz, UAM, 28040 Madrid, Spain; sara.gpedrero@quironsalud.es (S.G.P.); pllamas@fjd.es (P.L.-S.)
[2] Hematology Department, Fundación Jiménez Díaz University Hospital, 28040 Madrid, Spain
[*] Correspondence: juana.serrano@quironsalud.es; Tel.: +34-660141450

Abstract: Millions of patients suffer yearly from bone fractures and disorders such as osteoporosis or cancer, which constitute the most common causes of severe long-term pain and physical disabilities. The intrinsic capacity of bone to repair the damaged bone allows normal healing of most small bone injuries. However, larger bone defects or more complex diseases require additional stimulation to fully heal. In this context, the traditional routes to address bone disorders present several associated drawbacks concerning their efficacy and cost-effectiveness. Thus, alternative therapies become necessary to overcome these limitations. In recent decades, bone tissue engineering has emerged as a promising interdisciplinary strategy to mimic environments specifically designed to facilitate bone tissue regeneration. Approaches developed to date aim at three essential factors: osteoconductive scaffolds, osteoinduction through growth factors, and cells with osteogenic capability. This review addresses the biological basis of bone and its remodeling process, providing an overview of the bone tissue engineering strategies developed to date and describing the mechanisms that underlie cell–biomaterial interactions.

Keywords: bone tissue engineering; bone remodeling; bone disorders; biomechanics; scaffolds; microenvironment; 3D bioprinting; computational modeling

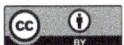

1. Introduction

Bone is a dynamic connective tissue that plays a crucial role in locomotion, mechanical support and protection of soft tissues, calcium and phosphate storage, and harboring of bone marrow [1,2].

Bone presents the intrinsic capacity for modeling and remodeling in order to preserve skeletal size, shape, and structural integrity [3]. Bone modeling involves the coordination of bone formation and resorption, being related to bone growth and mechanical adaption. Bone remodeling is responsible for removal and repair of damaged bone, necessary for fracture healing, stimuli adaptation, and homeostasis [1,4]. The proper coupling of these two processes allows normal healing of most small bone injuries [2]. However, larger bone defects and diseases require additional stimulation to fully regenerate and heal. In this context, millions of patients suffer yearly from bone fractures, mainly caused by accidental fractures, aging-related disorders, and autoimmune diseases [5]. Indeed, due to the growing prolonged life expectancy, there has been a rapid increase in musculoskeletal pathologies such as scoliosis, osteoporosis, bone tumors, congenital defects, and rheumatic diseases such as osteoarthritis [6].

The existing routes to address bone disorders include medical procedures, transplantation, and medication [5]. Among them, gold standard grafting methods and drugs present drawbacks concerning their efficacy and cost-effectiveness [4], and numerous side effects and long-term consequences in the normal bone remodeling [7], respectively. Thus, alternative therapies become necessary to overcome these limitations.

In this context, bone tissue engineering (BTE) emerged in recent decades as a promising strategy for treatment of bone pathologies. BTE aims to combine engineering and biological properties to generate temporary artificial environments specifically designed to facilitate bone tissue growth [8,9]. The principal strategies developed to date include bioactive scaffolds, nanomedicine, cell-based combination products, and 3D printed bioceramics, among others [10]. Overall, great efforts have been made towards tissue engineering strategies that can meet three essential factors: osteoconductive scaffolds, osteoinduction through growth factors, and cells with osteogenic capability [11].

Regulation of 3D scaffold properties allow the selective guidance of cell development and differentiation in bone tissue. Moreover, computational modeling has emerged as an excellent tool to predict and optimize the clinical potential in terms of cell proliferation and differentiation, tissue growth, adaptation, and maintenance [12]. Thus, a proper understanding of the molecular mechanisms involved in cell–biomaterial interactions will allow one step forward in the achievement of functional advanced biomaterials for tissue engineering (Figure 1).

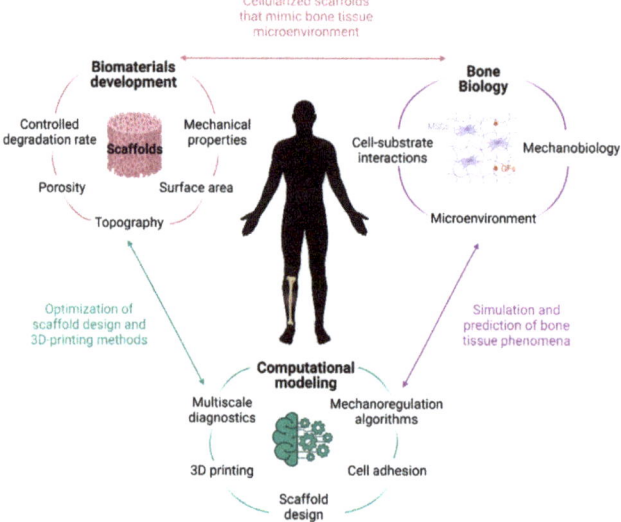

Figure 1. Integration of biomaterials development, bone biology, and computational modeling towards bone tissue engineering.

Herein, the basis of bone biology and the remodeling process are examined, providing an overview of the BTE strategies developed to date and the biological phenomena that underlie cell–biomaterial interactions. Moreover, computational modeling approaches for BTE are examined as a potential tool to help design better biomimetic materials.

2. Bone Biology
2.1. Bone Composition

Bone is a dynamic tissue that plays multiple functions in the body, including mechanical (structural support, locomotion, and protection of vital structures), and metabolic functions (mineral and acid–base homeostasis, calcium and phosphate storage, and harboring of bone marrow) [1,10,13]. Bone consists of a biomineral medium where four types of living bone cells are embedded: osteoblasts, osteocytes, osteoclasts, and bone-lining cells, which together constitute the basic multicellular unit (BMU) [1].

2.1.1. Osteoblasts

Osteoblasts are specialized bone-forming cells that exert an important role in bone remodeling through the synthesis, deposition, and mineralization of the bone matrix [3,10].

They create an extensive network of intercellular communication together with their progenitors, which play a functional role in beginning and directing new bone formation [13,14]. Moreover, numerous transmembrane proteins such as integrins, connexins, and cadherins and specific receptors are responsible of anchorage regulation, which has a direct impact on cellular function in their response to metabolic and mechanical stimuli [14].

Osteoblasts develop from mesenchymal cells (MSCs) in bone marrow and other connective tissues. These cells can differentiate through different pathways, leading to adipocytes, myocytes, chondrocytes, and osteoblasts, depending on regulatory transcription factors [3,15]. Particularly, synthesis of bone morphogenetic proteins (BMPs) and Wnt signaling pathways are crucial in regulating osteoblast differentiation and function [15,16]. When activated, they can follow different paths: remain quiescent osteoblasts or bone-lining cells, become osteocytes, or return to the osteoprogenitor cell line [13].

2.1.2. Osteocytes

Osteocytes constitute 90–95% of total bone cells; they are terminally differentiated osteoblasts embedded and immersed in the bone matrix [3,17]. They acquire dendritic morphology [1,15], which results in an elaborate osteocyte network that extends through the channels in the bone matrix, interacting with other osteocytes or osteoblasts from the bone surface [15,16]. This network allows osteocyte vascular supply, intercellular transport of small signaling molecules, and, in general, the communication among bone cells. Moreover, through this interconnected system, osteocytes act as mechanosensory cells, detecting mechanical strains and associated bone microdamage [3], thereby helping coordinate adaptive skeletal changes in response to mechanical loading [1,18]. For this reason, osteocytes are thought to initiate the bone remodeling process by a piezoelectric effect, which involves the conversion of mechanical stimuli into biochemical signals [1,19].

2.1.3. Osteoclasts

Osteoclasts are terminally differentiated myeloid cells that are located in shallow depressions on bone surfaces called Howship's lacunae [13]. Osteoclasts are highly migratory, multinucleated, and polarized cells, which make them uniquely adapted to bone resorption [14].

A disruption in osteoclast formation and activity leads to bone disorders such as osteoporosis, where resorption exceeds formation and causes decreased bone density and increased bone fractures. Furthermore, osteoclasts have been associated with several other functions, including regulation of the hematopoietic stem cell niche through cytokine production [1].

2.1.4. Bone-Lining Cells

Bone-lining cells are quiescent osteoblasts that are found lining the bone surface, being responsible for coupling bone resorption to bone formation. They anchor hematopoietic stem cells and provide them with appropriate signals to keep them in an undifferentiated state [1,20]. Thus, they play a crucial role in bone remodeling by gap junction communication with osteocytes in the bone matrix [10,20]. Specifically, these cells promote osteoclast differentiation and prevent undesired bone resorption by hampering direct interaction between osteoclasts and bone matrix [1]. Moreover, bone-lining cells prepare the bone surface by cleaning unmineralized collagen fibrils using matrix metalloproteinases (MMPs) and they deposit a smooth layer of collagen after remodeling [20].

2.1.5. Bone Matrix

Bone matrix constitutes a complex and organized framework that plays a crucial role in mechanical strength and adhesive characteristics of the bone, consisting of an organic (30%) and an inorganic component (70%) [10,13]. The organic segment is mainly composed of collagenous proteins (90%) such as type I collagen, and 10% non-collagenous proteins (i.e., osteocalcin, osteonectin, osteopontin, fibronectin, and bone sialoprotein II), BMPs, and growth factors [1,10]. All these proteins have been shown to be crucial in relevant processes such as bone osteogenesis, mineralization, and remodeling [13].

The inorganic matrix consists predominantly of hexagonal hydroxyapatite (HA) crystals ($Ca_{10}(PO_4)_6(OH)_2$), making up 99% of the body's storage of calcium, 85% of the phosphorous, and 40–60% of the magnesium and sodium [13]. In addition, ions such as bicarbonate, potassium, citrate, carbonate, fluorite, zinc, barium, and strontium are also present [1]. Biomineralization consist of deposition of HA crystals in the voids of a non-collagen protein and collagen-based scaffold, and allows interaction of organic and inorganic matrix [21]. Indeed, bone matrix proteins vary their concentration with age, nutrition habits, disorders, and treatments, which may increase bone fracture risk if disrupted [1].

2.2. Bone Remodeling Process

Bone remodeling constitutes a lifelong process that guarantees bone tissue integrity and mineral homeostasis by a coupling mechanism consisting of old or damaged bone removal (resorption) and new bone deposition (formation) [16,22].

The bone remodeling cycle comprises five different stages, depicted in Figure 2: activation, resorption, reversal, formation, and termination, occurring over several weeks (around 120 and 200 days in cortical and trabecular bone, respectively) [15,23].

2.2.1. Activation

The bone remodeling process begins when bone in a quiescent state detects an initiating signal. This trigger can occur via different pathways, including mechanical forces, microscopic bone damage, and systemic hormones such as parathyroid hormone (PTH) [23,24]. The detection of the signal can result in osteocyte apoptosis [3,15], which involves the release of osteoclastogenic factors such as colony-stimulating factor 1 (CSF-1) and receptor activator of NF-κB ligand (RANKL) that favor osteoclast precursor recruitment and activation [1].

The bone-lining cells separate from underlying bone, exposing the bone surface and forming a canopy that can be resorbed. Thus, active BMU includes bone-resorbing osteoclasts which cover the newly exposed bone surface, preparing it for the deposition of replacement bone, and osteoblasts that secrete and deposit unmineralized bone osteoid [15].

2.2.2. Resorption

Osteoclasts attach to bone matrix through Arg-Gly-Asp (RGD) binding sites and release enzymes and acids that help dissolve the mineral content of the organic matrix, forming an isolated environment known as the "sealing zone" and a ruffled border that provides an enhanced secretory surface area [10,16,23]. The remaining organic bone matrix is subsequently degraded by cathepsin K and matrix metalloproteinases [15]. The resorption phase lasts approximately 2–4 weeks and is concluded by mononuclear cells after osteoclasts undergo apoptosis [25], ensuring that excess resorption does not occur [23].

In addition, osteoblasts secrete cytokines and MMPs in order to degrade the unmineralized osteoid in bone surface and expose RGD adhesion sites to help osteoclast attachment [3]. Osteoclast differentiation, expansion, and survival depend on many factors and cytokines, such as CSF-1, RANKL, osteoprotegerin (OPG), interleukin (IL)-1, IL-6, PTH, and calcitonin [13,15].

2.2.3. Reversal

Following the resorption phase, cells from an osteoblastic lineage, also called "reversal" cells, prepare the bone surface by removing unmineralized collagen matrix. Furthermore, they deposit a "cement line" of non-collagenous mineralized matrix to enhance osteoblastic adhesion [23]. The reversal cells are responsible for sending and receiving coupling signals, including bone matrix-derived factors such as transcription growth factor (TGF)-β, insulin-like growth factor, and BMPs [25,26]. Moreover, osteocytes up-regulate osteoblasts by the production of second messengers, such as nitric oxide and prostaglandins, which induce bone formation [15,16].

Osteoclasts are also thought to secrete cytokines such as IL-6 and to express a regulatory surface receptor called Ephrin receptor family [23]. Additionally, semaphorins comprise a large family of glycoproteins that are expressed by osteoclasts, and they have been proposed as inhibitors of bone formation during bone resorption [1]. The switch between resorption and formation has also been proposed to be triggered by a strain gradient within the lacunae, which may provoke sequential activation of osteoclasts (reduced strain) and osteoblasts (increased strain) [25]. Osteoclasts are then replaced by osteoblast-lineage cells, promoting the initiation of bone formation [15].

2.2.4. Formation

Once early osteoblast progenitors have replaced osteoclasts in the resorption lacunae, they differentiate and start new bone formation [3]. Osteoblasts first synthesize and secrete a type 1 collagen-rich organic matrix, in order to fill in the cavities generated by osteoclasts [15,23]. Secondly, osteoblasts regulate osteoid mineralization, which involves the deposition of HA crystals amongst collagen fibrils. This process is mainly regulated by calcium and phosphate concentrations within membrane-bound matrix vesicles, and by local mineralization inhibitors such as pyrophosphate or proteoglycans [23,25]. Bone formation lasts approximately 4 to 6 months, completed by the apoptosis of the rest of the osteoblasts, which constitutes 50–70% of total osteoblasts [23].

2.2.5. Termination

When the amount of bone formed equals the resorbed bone, the remodeling cycle terminates [15]. Osteocytes produce TGF-β and sclerostin, suppressing osteoclastogenesis and osteoblast differentiation through the Wnt pathway, respectively, which directly inhibits bone formation [17,23]. Osteoblasts form new bone until they revert to bone-lining cells that cover the bone surface [15,25]. Then, the resting bone surface environment is reestablished and preserved until the bone remodeling cycle is again initiated [3].

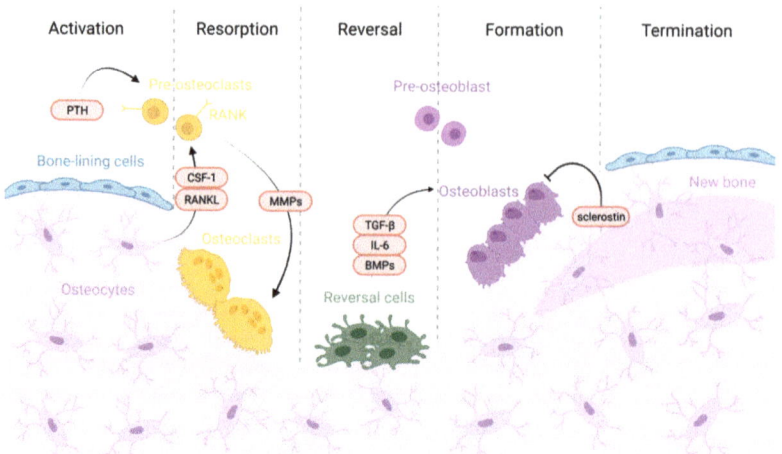

Figure 2. Bone remodeling process. Activation: Bone in quiescent state detects an initiating signal triggered by mechanical forces, microdamage, or systemic hormones such as PTH [23,24]. Osteocyte apoptosis is then induced [3,15], releasing osteoclastogenic factors such as colony-stimulating factor 1 (CSF-1) and receptor activator of NF-κB ligand (RANKL) that favor osteoclast precursor recruitment and activation [1]. Resorption: Osteoblasts secrete cytokines and matrix metalloproteinases (MMPs) in order to expose RGD adhesion sites to facilitate osteoclast attachment [3]. Osteoclasts dissolve mineralized matrix and organic bone matrix through hydrogen ions and MMP secretion, respectively [15]. Reversal: "reversal" cells remove unmineralized collagen matrix and deposit a "cement line" of non-collagenous mineralized matrix to enhance osteoblastic adhesion [23]. The reversal cells and the osteoclasts are responsible for sending and receiving coupling signals, including bone matrix-derived factors such as TGF-β, BMPs, and IL-6 [25,26]. Osteoclasts are then replaced by osteoblast-lineage cells, promoting the initiation of bone formation [15]. Formation: Osteoblast progenitors replace osteoclasts in the resorption lacunae, they differentiate and start new bone formation [3]. Osteoblasts continue to form new bone until they revert to bone-lining cells that cover the bone surface [15,25]. Termination: Osteocytes produce sclerostin, suppressing osteoblast differentiation and bone formation [17,23]. Then, the resting bone surface environment is reestablished and preserved until bone remodeling cycle is again initiated [3].

3. Bone Pathology

Bone disorders constitute the most common causes of severe long-term pain and physical disabilities [27]. They can result from several conditions, including tumors, genetic disorders, trauma, age-related disorders, and autoimmune diseases, among others [21,28]. In particular, disruptions in coupling bone resorption and formation during the bone remodeling cycle lead to loss of bone mass and skeletal integrity [29,30]. Among bone disorders, osteoporosis, Paget's disease, osteoarthritis, fractures, and bone metastasis are the most frequent, and will be briefly described in this section.

3.1. Osteoporosis

Osteoporosis is the most common metabolic disease, characterized by low bone mass and structural deterioration of bone, causing bone fragility and an increased fracture risk [31]. Three different types of osteoporosis can be distinguished: primary, secondary, and idiopathic.

Primary osteoporosis includes senile and postmenopausal varieties, both related to natural gradual loss of bone mass. In postmenopause, estrogen is responsible for inhibiting bone resorption. Secondary osteoporosis occurs in patients with chronic diseases that provoke loss of bone mass, such as nutritional deficiencies, anorexia, alcoholism, and chronic liver disease. Idiopathic osteoporosis occurs in young adults or children with no endocrine abnormality or risk factor [27].

3.2. Paget's Disease

Paget's disease is a metabolic bone disease with controversial etiology. Genetics factors have shown to affect Paget's development, specifically mutations that affect the RANK, OPG, and sequestosome 1. Paget's patients show increased bone metabolic activity and imbalance between bone formation and resorption. Serum alkaline phosphatase constitutes a bone formation marker that allows diagnosis and monitoring of patients [27]. Bone pain, osteoarthrosis, deformities, fractures, and hypercalcemia are complications in Paget's disease, among others [32].

3.3. Osteoarthritis

Osteoarthritis is the most common adult joint disease, appearing as a result from gradual loss of cartilage and development of bony spurs and synovial cysts at the ends of the joints [27]. It can be classified into primary osteoarthritis, which results from genetic causes and affects middle-aged people, and secondary osteoarthritis, related to metabolic diseases, endocrine disorders, etc. Risk factors for osteoarthritis include endogenous factors (age, obesity, sex, heredity, ethnic origin, and postmenopausal alterations), and exogenous factors (i.e., macrotrauma, prior joint surgery, and lifestyle factors) [27,33].

3.4. Autoinflammatory Diseases

Innate and acquired immunity disorders can cause autoinflammatory bone diseases by infiltrating innate cells into the bone with subsequent increased osteoclast activity, osteolysis, and bone remodeling [34]. Indeed, low-grade chronic inflammation leads to bone resorption in many rheumatic diseases, making up the link between the immune system and the bone. In autoimmune diseases, osteoclastogenesis might be triggered by autoreactive T cell-secreted IL-17 and RANKL. Moreover, Toll-like receptor signaling is thought to be involved in its modulation. The most common autoinflammatory bone diseases include chronic non-bacterial osteomyelitis; synovitis, acne, pustulosis, hyperostosis, and cherubism, among others [35].

3.5. Bone Metastasis

Bone metastasis constitutes a frequent consequence of many cancers and typically indicates a short-term prognosis in cancer patients [36]. Indeed, patients with bone metastasis have a higher mortality rate and suffer from pain and clinical complications such as fracture, spinal cord compression, and hypercalcemia, which seriously reduce the quality of life [37].

Bone metastases are classified as osteolytic, osteoblastic, or mixed, according to the interference with the bone remodeling cycle. Osteolytic metastasis is present in the great majority of bone cancers, destroying normal bone primarily mediated by osteoclasts, parathyroid hormone-related peptide (PTHrP) and RANKL. Osteoblastic metastasis is characterized by deposition of new bone, and occurs in prostate cancer and Hodgkin lymphoma, among others [36].

3.6. Therapeutics in Bone Disease

Broadly, most bone disease treatments only help to reduce the symptoms, but do not cause a total suppression of the disease. The mechanism of action for the majority of the drugs consists of disrupting the osteoclastic pathway and promoting the osteoblastic one [38]. Bisphosphonates constitute the most commonly used drugs in most bone treatments, mainly indicated for osteoporosis, Paget's disease, and bone tumors [7]. These agents bind to HA and block the bone resorption mediated by osteoclasts. Although they increase bone mineral density (BMD) and reduce serum PTH, long-term treatment causes inhibition of both bone resorption and formation markers. Moreover, they cause gastrointestinal and cardiovascular side effects [7]. To date, the Food and Drug Administration (FDA) has approved four different bisphosphonate-based drugs for the treatment of osteoporosis, including alendronate, risedronate, ibandronate, and zoledronic acid [27].

Calcitonin is used in the treatment of Paget's disease, binding to the calcitonin receptors located on the osteoclast surface. Calcitonin also presents analgesic properties that further help treat patients with bone pain [31]. However, it is only used in those patients with intolerance to bisphosphonate, since it shows a short duration of action, partial response, and acquired resistance. Denosumad, a monoclonal antibody, is an anti-resorptive pharmaceutical agent targeting RANKL signaling in osteoclast activation. It is indicated for anti-fracture in women with postmenopausal osteoporosis, and also in bone tumors [38]. It stimulates osteoclast differentiation and function and promotes osteoclast survival, increasing bone mineral density. In contrast, it causes hypercalcemia, nephrotoxicity, and seizures [7]. Raloxifene is approved for the treatment of osteoporosis and bone fracture. It is a selective estrogen receptor modulator that acts as an estrogen agonist on both bone and fat tissue, and as an estrogen antagonist on breast and uterine tissue. Raloxifene has been shown to cause cardiovascular events and venous thromboembolism [7].

Currently, bone metastasis can be treated by inhibiting cancer cell growth or by inhibiting the osteoclast activity. Chemotherapy is the most common approach to date to inhibit cancer cell growth, and efficient drug delivery to the bone metastasis is essential for success. Nevertheless, the skeleton presents significantly poorer blood supply than other tissues, decreasing the efficiency of drug delivery to bone and resulting in severe side effects caused by the lack of tissue specificity [37].

In the bone fracture framework, autologous bone grafting has been established as the gold standard technique for repairing bone tissue, consisting in bone harvested from the same individual receiving the treatment [21,28]. Autografts have been shown to be histocompatible and non-immunogenic, but they present significant limitations, such as donor site injury and morbidity, surgical risks (bleeding, inflammation, infection, and chronic pain), and resorption of the implanted bone [28]. Allografts provide an alternative method, particularly in areas with larger bone defects, based on transplanting donor bone tissue between genetically non-identical individuals of the same species [21,39]. However, they present reduced osteoinductive properties when compared to autografts [40], taking longer for a defect to be filled by native bone tissue [29], which leads to mechanical stress and immunogenesis [39].

Since no treatment option provides overall successful results in bone pathologies, recent research has been devoted to developing tissue engineering strategies that can overcome these issues. In this context, BTE has emerged as an excellent tool to design and implement new bone repair interventions. Fundamental notions behind this subject and the state of the art to date will be reviewed in the next section.

4. Scaffolds in Bone Tissue Engineering

BTE has arisen as a powerful tool for developing new bone treatment options to overcome shortages of existing bone graft materials and bone disease therapies. In recent decades, BTE strategies have been directed to produce bone constructs that mimic natural bone structure regarding mechanical strength and microstructure [41].

In this context, the design of accurate biomaterials for BTE should be broadly based on several components: (1) a biocompatible scaffold that resembles extracellular matrix (ECM), (2) osteogenic cells to build the bone tissue matrix, (3) morphogenic cues and growth factors to help guide osteogenic cells towards bone phenotype, and (4) material/host interactions mediated by immune cells that fulfill the bone healing process [39,40].

Ideally, the material should degrade following initial cellular colonization simultaneously to new bone formation. Then, the tissue will reestablish its function with no clinical intervention needed to remove the implant [42]. The key factors involved in the achievement of this smart biomaterial will be addressed in the following subsections, presenting the state of the art to date and the aspects to be considered in the material design.

4.1. Scaffold Composition

Scaffolds are temporary matrices built from biocompatible, bioactive, and biodegradable materials. An ideal scaffold should mimic the structure and function of the ECM of original bone, which will maintain a suitable environment and architecture for bone growth and development. Specifically, they should be based on a 3D structure that allows proliferation and homing, osteogenic differentiation, vascularization, host integration, and load bearing [6,43].

Since the different bone types present different remodeling period lengths, there is not one ideal scaffold material for all BTE purposes, being subject to the size, type, and location of the bone tissue to be regenerated [44]. First generation biomaterials include metals (mainly titanium derivates), synthetic polymers (such as Poly (methyl metacrylate) (PMMA) and Polyether Ether Ketone (PEEK)), and ceramics (such as alumina and zirconia), being bioinert and hardly interacting with host tissue. Second generation biomaterials stood out for their bioactive and biodegradable features, including synthetic and natural polymers, calcium compounds (phosphates, carbonates, and sulfates), and bioactive glasses. The third generation of biomaterials allow the addition of cells, biological factors, or external stimuli, among other instructive substances, to induce specific biological responses [45].

Most of the scaffolds that are currently used for BTE applications can be grouped into polymers, bioactive ceramics, composite materials, and nanomaterials.

4.1.1. Polymeric Scaffolds

Generally, polymeric materials present reproducible and adjustable physiochemical characteristics such as pore size, porosity, solubility, biocompatibility, and immune response [46]. Both natural and synthetic polymers are valuable materials for BTE.

Natural polymers include proteins (such as collagen, gelatin, fibrinogen, elastin, keratin, and silk); polysaccharides (chitosan, alginate, hyaluronic acid, and cellulose); and polynucleotides (DNA, RNA) [47,48]. ECM-based scaffolds have been also proposed due to their similarity to bone tissue. All of them have shown great biocompatibility, osteoconductivity, controlled biodegradation, and low immunogenicity [6,47]. However, they present poor mechanical properties, uncontrollable degradation rate, and reduced tunability [6,29].

Synthetic polymers consist of aliphatic polyesters such as poly(lactic-acid)(PLA), poly(glycolic-acid)(PGA), poly(caprolactone) (PCL), polypropylene fumarate (PPF), and PEEK and their copolymers [47]. They are biocompatible, biodegradable, and display a controlled degradation rate. Moreover, synthetic polymers offer tunable properties and structure, allowing a controllable degradation rate and mechanical properties [29]. These features guarantee predictable, reproducible, and cost-effective production of BTE scaffolds. However, they have shown reduced bioactivity and osteoconductivity when compared to natural polymers [48].

Hydrogels are hydrophilic polymeric 3D networks that constitute some of the most promising biomaterials in BTE applications, due to their flexibility and bioactivity. In contrast to rigid scaffolds, hydrogels can actively interact with the host tissue, allowing controlled release of cells and growth factors. Unfortunately, because of their low stiffness, they cannot be utilized in the repair of load-bearing lesions, such as large fractures of long bones [49].

4.1.2. Bioceramics

Bioceramics are inorganic biomaterials that almost mimic bone tissue composition, providing osteoconductive properties, nontoxic degradability, high compressive strength, and long shelf-life [38].

Most common bioceramics include coralline, HA, tricalcium phosphate (TCP), and calcium silicates [6]. Particularly, calcium phosphate ceramics (CPCs) have been extensively studied for bone tissue repair as tunable bioactive materials, providing the pores for tissue ingrowth and viability [50]. The capacity of these materials to elicit osteogenesis and angiogenesis effects through releasing biologically active ions has attracted great interest [46].

Bioactive glasses are usually composed of calcium-containing silicates. For instance, 45S5 Bioglass contains 45wt% SiO_2, 24.5wt% CaO, 24.5wt% Na_2O, and 6.0wt% P_2O_5, enabling an increased regeneration rate when compared with HA-based ceramics. Bioactive glasses are thought to create a bone-like apatite layer on the material surface, releasing ions such as Ca^{2+}, PO_4^{3-}, and Si^{4+} and hence promoting osteogenesis. Moreover, mesoporous bioactive glasses have emerged as an excellent tool for BTE, since they can be easily loaded with drugs or biomolecules, due to their large pore surface [46].

However, bioceramics are inherently brittle, making them difficult to handle in implantation. To overcome this issue, several strategies have been explored. For instance, coating bioceramics with polymers such as Poly Lactic-co-Glycolic Acid (PLGA), chitosan, or Polyethylene Glycol (PEG) has been shown to improve scaffold mechanical properties and also osteogenic capacity [50]. Furthermore, the composition of bioceramics can be altered to modulate the fracture toughness. In particular, doping β-TCP scaffolds with SiO2 (0.5%) and ZnO (0.25%) raised the compressive strength 2.5-fold and increased cell viability up to 92% [47].

4.1.3. Composite Materials

Composites combine two or more materials with different properties that may improve scaffold features when compared to their individual components, such as processability, printing performance, mechanical properties, or bioactivity [46]. They can be formed from co-polymers, polymer–polymer blends, or polymer–ceramic composites [6].

Composites can be based on co-polymers derived from two or more monomers, such as PLGA, which combines poly lactide and polyglycolide and shows adequate biodegradability and ease of fabrication. In this context, hydrogels seem to mimic ECM topography and hence they are ideal for cell adherence, proliferation, and differentiation. Hydrogels can be both natural (agarose, alginate, and gelatins) and synthetic (poly(vinyl alcohol) based) [6].

Polymer–ceramic composites resemble the natural bone, which is also a composite material made of inorganic HA crystals and collagen fibers. As has been previously mentioned, calcium phosphate (CP)–polymer composites show mechanical integrity and bioactivity, being successfully applied in bone regeneration. Moreover, the incorporation of bioceramic and bioglass particles, carbon nanotubes, or magnesium-based particles seems to improve scaffold mechanical properties [6].

4.1.4. Nanomaterials

In recent decades, nanosized materials have shown better bioactive properties than micro-sized ones, attracting much interest in BTE. In particular, nanoceramics appear to be promising biomimetic candidates, since bone can be considered a nanocomposite [6]. Specifically, the collagen fibers and HA crystals are nanosized in diameter, as well as all living molecular building blocks. Thus, bone cells are predisposed to interact at the nanoscale, enhancing adhesion, proliferation, and differentiation processes [40]. Indeed, changes at the nanoscale level of tissue hierarchy may have further effects on migration and cell signaling [42,51].

Furthermore, nanoparticles (NPs) can be incorporated into scaffolds, leading to superior mechanical properties, increased surface area, and roughness, as well as osteointegration, osteoconduction, and osteoinduction [40]. Consequently, biomaterial design has focused on the introduction of nanoparticles to elicit directed cellular behavior while imparting structural and mechanical advantages. Moreover, NPs can be applied as drug delivery and cell tracking systems, due to their functionalization versatility, allowing a significant improvement in prospective therapies.

For instance, HA–collagen nanocomposite systems, for example, are emerging rapidly and showing promise [52]. Yan et al. reported that the incorporation of calcium phosphate NPs into silk fibroin (SF)-based scaffolds induced increased bone formation after 3 weeks of implantation in rat femur, compared to bare SF scaffolds [53]. Wang et al. presented magnetic lanthanum (La)-doped HA NP/chitosan scaffolds (MLaHA/CS) that were able to recruit rat bone marrow MSCs and modulate host-to-scaffold immune responses via macrophage polarization [54].

In addition, multi-walled carbon nanotubes (MWCNTs) have been shown to improve the compressive strength and elastic modulus of 45S5 Bioglass® (Gainesville, FL, USA) scaffolds [55]. Mesoporous silica nanoparticles (MSNs) present high bioactivity and excellent biocompatibility, being also particularly suitable for loading bioactive agents due to their highly controllable morphology and structure [56]. Although nanosystems have not yet achieved clinical implementation, in vitro and in vivo studies have been performed in recent years, showing the great potential of this technology [9].

4.2. Scaffold Properties for BTE

The modulation of the scaffold characteristics is key in the final success of the biomaterial for clinical implementation (Table 1). In general terms, a scaffold must be biocompatible, not elicit an immune response, and be biodegradable into non-toxic components with a controllable degradation rate to match new bone formation [21,44]. Particularly, bioincompatibility could lead to immune system activation, tumor formation, and inflammation processes [6,40]. Recent research has been directed to immune-inert and immunomodulatory biomaterials that are potentially able to regulate host immune response [57].

Biodegradability of the material occurs through chemical or enzymatic breakdown of the material over time when introduced into living organisms [21]. Degradation products should be non-toxic components and they must be either recycled or excreted with negligible interference with other organs [6].

Scaffold bioactivity constitutes another key feature, comprising osteoconductivity and osteoinductivity processes [54]. Osteoconductive scaffolds facilitate bone deposition on the material surface by interacting with the surrounding living tissues. Bioactive scaffolds are hence designed to enhance cell migration, tissue formation, and integration, overcoming conventional passive biomaterial limitations [6]. Moreover, osteoinduction properties provide the scaffolds with the ability of promoting the differentiation of progenitor cells down an osteoblastic lineage [10,52].

Structurally, a scaffold must be a 3D network with highly interconnected pores that allow cell growth and mass transfer of nutrients and metabolic waste [44]. Moreover, a large surface area becomes crucial for vascularization and tissue infiltration [54]. Broadly, macroporosity might promote osteogenesis by facilitating cell and ion transport, while microporosity improves surface area for protein adsorption, increasing ionic solubility in the microenvironment, and providing attachment points for osteoblasts [58].

Typically, pores should be bigger than 300 µm to facilitate new bone formation and vascularization, since they provide enough space for oxygen and nutrient supply [54]. BTE scaffolds broadly range from 50 to 900 µm. Small pore sizes (75–100 µm) have shown successful bone regeneration in vitro and are thought to promote angiogenesis. On the other hand, macropores might promote osteoinductivity by mediating vascularization. A pore size range from 200 to 500 µm has shown the optimal tissue penetration vascularization in vivo [6,21].

Pore interconnectivity has been shown to positively influence bone deposition rate and depth of infiltration both in vitro and in vivo [58]. Percolation diameter is a key parameter in scaffold architecture, which defines the diameter of the largest tracer that can cross the interconnected pores of a scaffold. Thus, it determines the scaffold interconnectivity and hence the size of cells and nutrients that can pass through them. The bottleneck dimension describes the diameter of connections between pores, with it being established that the 700–1200 μm range is the optimal dimension for bone substitutes [54,59].

Other relevant surface features are surface roughness, surface free energy, surface charge, and surface topography, which can be easily tailored by chemical treatment or incorporation with bioactive molecules or artificial ECM [60]. Apparently, the biomaterial surface is the most critical aspect in the host immune response upon implantation and becomes responsible for avoiding macrophage adhesion and activation, as well as their fusion into foreign body giant cells [6]. Specifically, roughened surfaces have shown increased osteointegration by favoring epithelial attachment, when compared to smooth surfaces, improving implant durability and function [61].

Likewise, the scaffold is temporarily responsible for mechanical support and stability at the tissue formation site. Thus, mechanical properties are also considered crucial in BTE scaffolds and should be adapted to the site of implantation to minimize risk of stress shielding, implant-related osteopenia, and subsequent refracture [6]. In general terms, the scaffold material should be sufficiently robust to host cells and resist contraction forces during tissue healing [44].

Properties such as elastic modulus (a measure of the stiffness of a solid material), tensile strength (capacity of a scaffold to cope with loads tending to reduce size), and fatigue strength (the highest stress that a material can hold for a given number of cycles without breaking) should be similar to those of natural bone in order to ensure bone mechanical strength [62]. However, bone presents diverse and dynamic mechanical properties, tightly related to its complex hierarchical structure [63]. Specifically, the elastic moduli of human bone tissue usually varies between 1 and 20 GPa (around 2.0 GPa and 14-18 GPa for trabecular and cortical bone, respectively) [54,64], and the tensile strength of cortical and cancellous bones is 50–150 MPa and 10–100 MPa, respectively [65].

Table 1. Scaffold properties for design considerations.

Surface area	Crucial for cell–scaffold interactions, facilitating vascularization and tissue infiltration	[54]
	Macroporosity might promote osteogenesis by facilitating cell and ion transport	[58]

Table 1. *Cont.*

Pore size	Microporosity improves surface area for protein adsorption, increasing ionic solubility and attachment points for osteoblasts	[58]
	Pores > 300 μm facilitate new bone formation and vascularization	[54]
	75–100 μm pore size is thought to promote angiogenesis	[6]
	Pore size range from 200 to 500 μm results in optimal tissue penetration vascularization in vivo	[6,21]
Pore interconnectivity	Enhanced bone deposition rate and depth of infiltration	[58]
	Optimal diameter of connections between pores ranges from 700–1200 μm	[54,59]
Surface topology	Roughened surfaces promote osteointegration and favor epithelial attachment	[61]
Mechanical properties	Young's modulus should be close to 7–30 GPa and a tensile strength of 50–151 MPa	[62]
	Compressive strength should be comparable to cortical bone (100–230 MPa)	[62]
	Degradation rate should match the growth of native ECM to ensure scaffold mechanical support	[21,44]

Likewise, the mechanical strength can be weaken by high porosity and degradation rates [21]. Although higher porosity and pore size promote bone regeneration, both can impair the mechanical properties of the scaffold [54]. In addition, the degradation rate should match the growth of native ECM to ensure mechanical support throughout the lifecycle of the scaffold. This is also influenced by the porosity and pore size: if a scaffold degrades too quickly, it may lead to mechanical failure. In the same way, if the degradation rate is not sufficiently quick, an inflammatory process is triggered towards the foreign material, impairing tissue regeneration [62].

Therefore, a trade-off between biomechanical properties and degradation kinetics becomes necessary. Ideally, a scaffold material should provide sufficient mechanical stability while the newly formed bone tissue substitutes the scaffold matrix [44]. To achieve that, overall porosity can be tailored to adjust site-specific biomechanical requirements. Several studies claim that changes in macroporosity, and more specifically minimizing closed porosity, have shown a more significant effect in mechanical properties [58,66].

Considering all these scaffold requirements, the ideal scaffold is thought to have a compressive strength comparable to cortical bone (100–230 MPa), with a Young's modulus close to 7–30 GPa and a tensile strength of 50–151 MPa [62]. Scaffolds fabricated from biomaterials with a high degradation rate should avoid high porosities, whereas slowly degrading biomaterials can be highly porous and still present adequate mechanical integrity [44].

Furthermore, stimulus-responsive scaffolds have attracted much interest in terms of modulating their physicochemical and mechanical properties, as well as the degradation profile in response to stimuli (including photoirradiation, mechanical, magnetic, and electrical forces, and changes in pH or enzymatic reactions) [42]. For instance, thermoresponsive biomaterials based on different polymers are tailored to have transition temperatures to gelate when the temperature is elevated to physiologic temperature [67–69]. Recent studies have designed piezoelectric systems that might accelerate new tissue formation in response to mechanical loading. In addition, NP-reinforced polymers can offer better mechanical, electrical, and thermal properties [42]. The development of clear strategies for optimizing and balancing all these properties becomes crucial for BTE translation in clinics.

4.3. Scaffolds as Vehicles of Cells and Growth Factors

Although cell-free biomaterials have been used to stimulate bone regeneration, exogenous cells with osteoblast differentiation potential must be provided when osteoprogenitors are not available in the damaged tissue [49]. Thus, scaffolds can act as vehicles for different types of cells in order to promote bone formation in vivo by differentiating towards the osteogenic lineage [6]. These cells may be expanded ex vivo before the implant, and the most commonly utilized are embryonic stem cells, induced pluripotent stem cells, MSCs, and genetically modified cells [6].

Embryonic stem cells (ESCs) can differentiate into a number of specialized cells present in the bone, including MSCs, osteoblasts, chondrocytes, endothelial cells, etc. [70]. Moreover, ESCs show rapid proliferation and self-renewal over long periods of time, making them ideal tools in BTE. For instance, Tang et al. [71] described in 2012 how hESCd-MSC-encapsulating hydrogel microbeads in a macroporous CPC construct undergo osteogenic differentiation and bone mineral synthesis. However, ESCs have resulted in ethical concerns in various countries, as well as immunogenicity and tumorigenicity, which strongly hamper their clinical application [72].

In this context, induced pluripotent stem cells (iPSCs) show analogous advantages to ESCs, and they avoid the risk of immune rejection, since they derive from patient somatic cells. In many studies, iPSCs and MSC-like derived iPSCs cultured on an HA/TCP scaffold showed osteogenic differentiation both in vitro and in vivo [73]. However, incomplete or false reprogramming may result in teratomas, especially in the presence of oncogenes or reprogramming viral methods. Prior in vitro differentiation into MSCs and direct differentiation into osteoblasts, among other strategies, have been reported to avoid tumorigenicity associated with pluripotency [72].

MSCs are relevant in osteoblast differentiation and immunomodulatory capability, being critical for stimulating tissue regeneration. In particular, MSCs secrete immunosuppressive and anti-inflammatory cytokines, regulate T cells, and promote a local healing response by stimulating proliferation and differentiation of host stem cells [49]. In MSC-based tissue engineering approaches, MSCs are incorporated in scaffolds that facilitate the local delivery of MSCs into the bone defects. Scaffold colonization can occur either by cell culture prior to scaffold creation, or by simultaneous deposition of cells and biomaterials [74].

Transplanted MSCs have been shown to proliferate and differentiate into an osteogenic phenotype [75]. However, their short lifespan after implantation becomes a major limitation, mainly due to poor adherence to the matrix, ischemia, and low glucose levels. Cells colonize the defect, proliferate, and differentiate into mature osteoblasts, promoting the formation of new bone tissue. However, the lack of a vascular network upon implantation impedes cells survival in the site of implantation. In this framework, different strategies can be followed to promote cell and rapid vascularization in the defect area [49]. For instance, the association of oxygen carriers with BTE scaffolds has been shown to improve survival and the bone regeneration capacity of the cells [49]. Moreover, several studies have sought to mimic the initial stages of endochondral ossification by chondrogenic priming of MSCs, which can significantly increase osteogenic differentiation and mineralization, even to a higher extent than culturing cells in osteogenic growth factors alone [76].

Thus far, bone healing has been shown to be improved when utilizing MSCs with metals, ceramics, and polymeric and composite materials [74]. The scaffolds should provide the proper microenvironment for cells to survive, proliferate, and differentiate in vitro and in vivo. For instance, a system comprising PLGA membranes incorporating BMP-2-loaded microspheres and rat mesenchymal stem cells (rMSC) with their Smad ubiquitin regulatory factor-1 (Smurf1) expression knocked down was evaluated in a rat calvaria, a critical size defect by Rodríguez-Évora et al. [77], showing a defect repair of 85% after 8 weeks.

The interdependence between macrophages and osteoblasts is also essential for the resolution of the inflammatory process, since it has been demonstrated that some macrophages are involved in particle clean up and the up-regulation of osteolytic and pro-inflammatory cytokines, including IL-6 and tumoral necrosis factor (TNF-α) [42]. Further research has shown that the use of macrophage-recruiting agents combined with platelet-rich plasma in a hydrogel induced bone formation [78].

Still, bone tissue biology depends on the action of growth factors (GFs), which control cell behavior through specific receptors on the target cell membrane. In a bone regeneration context, these factors diffuse signals at the defect site through the ECM, facilitating the migration of progenitors and inflammatory cells to initiate the healing process [79].

Therefore, incorporation of GFs into the scaffold biomaterial is thought to improve osteogenesis and angiogenesis, limiting excessive bone formation and accelerating the healing process [47,79]. Thus, bone tissue engineering strategies pursue the combination of cells and engineering materials with growth factors. The main factors involved in bone healing have been mentioned in previous sections and can be grouped into several families: osteogenic (BMPs, activins, among others), angiogenic (such as platelet-derived growth factor (PDGF) and vascular endothelial growth factor (VEGF)), inflammation control (e.g., TNF-α, interleukins, interferon-γ), and systemic factors (vitamin D, growth hormone, calcitonin, PTH) [47,80].

Among them, the use of BMP-2 and BMP-7 has been incorporated in FDA-approved devices for bone regeneration, showing a clinical performance comparable to autografts in certain BTE applications [79]. Still, large doses of recombinant BMP-2 are required to promote bone formation, sometimes leading to adverse effects (e.g., heterotopic ossification and osteolysis). In this context, BMP-9 has emerged as a potential alternative, described as the most potent BMP in osteogenic differentiation. Indeed, it has been shown to completely close rat critical-sized calvaria defects when loaded into a microparticle (MPs)–hydrogel scaffold [81]. Furthermore, BMP-2 treatment has been shown to fail to regenerate articular cartilage structures such as joints, where BMP-9 has been proven to stimulate regeneration. For this reason, the sequential administration of BMP-2 and BMP-9 has resulted in regeneration of both bone and joints, providing the adequate environment for bone regeneration [82].

In addition, molecules such as N-acetyl cysteine have been exploited to promote runt-related transcription factor 2 (RUNX2) expression, which is involved in osteogenic differentiation of MSCs [80]. A product based on β-tricalcium phosphate carrying rhPDGF (Augment® Bone Graft, BioMimetic Therapeutics, (Franklin, TN, USA)) is also commercially available to treat foot, ankle, and distal radius fractures in the USA [80]. Moreover, local delivery of angiogenic growth factors such as VEGF and basic fibroblast growth factor (bFGF) has been shown to accelerate vascularization through recruitment of endothelial progenitor cells (EPCs) [40].

Despite the success of numerous bone-promoting growth factor-based products, several complications have been reported related to their clinical utilization. Specifically, inflammation, pleiotropic effects, hypotension, and teratogenic effects constitute some of the main concerns. In this regard, carriers with reliable release kinetics could help in the adoption of this therapeutical strategy [80]. Additionally, proper dosage of GFs has been shown to affect the quality of the vessels. For this reason, the addition of growth factors that stimulate the recruitment of smooth muscle cells or pericytes has been considered to help vessels stabilize and mature [40].

Likewise, scaffolds loaded with soluble molecules such as antibiotics and chemotherapeutic agents that can be delivered in the environment have also been exploited. An extensive review on the clinical application of bone-targeted drug delivery for bone malignancies is presented by Ferracini [83], showing a promising route to treat osteomyelitis, bone metastasis, OS, osteoarthritis, osteonecrosis, and delayed/non-unions, among other bone disorders.

5. Cell–Biomaterial Interactions beyond Microenvironment

Despite the recent advances in BTE, utilization of biomaterials has barely translated to human clinical trials, mainly due to a lack of studies about the interaction between biomaterials and host cells. Particularly, cell–material interactions occur at micro- and nanoscales, where cells physically contact the ECM, altering their response. As has been mentioned in Section 4.2, tuning 3D scaffold chemistry, topography, and stiffness can help selectively guide cell proliferation and differentiation within the bulk material. A better understanding of the effect that scaffold parameters exert on host cells might help map out the future path for BTE translation.

5.1. Cell Response to Biomaterial Chemistry

Biomaterial surface chemistry is somehow the most manageable parameter to control its effect on cell behavior. At the macroscale, coating approaches seek to increase cell adhesion or specifically select cell types for cell attachment.

There are a variety of inorganic and organic compounds, such as collagen, fibronectin, gelatin, or poly-L-Lysine, that have been used for covering substrates. Interestingly, culture surfaces have been frequently ornamented with adhesion-derived peptides, such as RGD at 1 pmol/mm^2 [84], that enhance cell attachment in 2D. To avoid degradation or detachment issues of the coated compound, normally, the substrate chemistry is modified, or ligands are added as presenting proteins. Biomaterials functionalized with RGD peptides have been shown to direct cell adhesion, migration, and differentiation in numerous tissues, including bone, neural, endothelial, liver, and cancer cells [85]. It has been found that RGD density positively regulates osteoblast mineralization [86]. RGD sequence interaction with integrins is further modulated by RGD conformation (cyclic penta- and hexapeptide), which leads to specific integrin affinity. In the case of osteogenic cells, functionalization of PMMA and PEG-PLA substrates with RGD favors osteoblast adhesion, proliferation, and bone formation through selective engagement of $\alpha_v\beta_3$ and $\alpha_v\beta_5$ integrins [87,88]. Moreover, Gly-Phe-Hyp-Gly-Glu-Arg (GFOGER)-functionalized hydrogel leads to superior osteogenic differentiation and bone formation of human mesenchymal stromal cells, compared to RGD-functionalized hydrogel both in vitro and in vivo [89].

Patterning at the microscale is a potent tool to control the cell shape, location, and density. Combining non-adhesive regions (normally treated with PEG) with adhesive regions (a variety of cell adhesion proteins (CAPs)) can generate a multitude of patterns and cell spots, which can be especially useful in printing methods [90,91].

Using fibronectin micropatterned material, McBeatch et al. [92] demonstrated that cell shape regulated human mesenchymal stem cell (hMSC) differentiation. Thus, hMSCs allowed to adhere, spread, and flatten were differentiated into osteoblasts, whereas those that did not attach formed spherical cells that resulted in adipocytes. Furthermore, modeling techniques can be used in co-culture assays where two or more types of cells are selectively adhered by controlling their cell–cell contact, spacing, and microenvironment interactions across flow-through microfluidic channels [93,94], by stamping with a stencil-based approach [95], or by seeding on surfaces that dynamically switch from cell adhesive to cell repulsive [96,97]. Advances in high-throughput chemical interaction approaches permit a large screening of cell–ECM, cell–biomaterial, or cell–cell interaction at the nanoliter scale. Recently, microarrays of biomaterials have been generated by robotic spotters that dispense and immobilize nanoliters of materials to test the interaction of stem cells with extracellular proteins [98].

5.2. Cell Response to Biomaterial Topography

Cell behavior can be regulated by topographical signals from the underlying substrate. In this regard, micro- and nanofabrication methods that reproduce in the substrate the topographical cues of the cell niche have become crucial [99].

Topography represents the different structures that exist on the surface of biomaterials. The majority of biological surfaces contain non-organized features at the macro- and microscale, being more organized at the nanoscale [100]. Cells have been shown to respond to topographical cues down to 5 nm, affecting proliferation, gene expression [101], cell adhesion [102], motility [103], alignment, differentiation [104], and matrix production [105].

At the microscale, cell spreading directly correlates to the substrate exposure to ECM proteins, being topography independent. Osteoblasts [102] and endothelial cells [106] have demonstrated a reproducible response to surface texture. Polarization or cell alignment generally rises with increasing groove depth and decreasing groove spacing [106], although the response to substrate topography is highly dependent on cell type. At the nanoscale, several reports have suggested that cells can sense and respond to features of 10–30 nm in size [107]. Indeed, the repetition of similar patterns has the greatest effect and provides the most predictable results [108,109]. Proteomic-derived studies have shown that human osteoprogenitor cells respond to nanosized pits and pores in asymmetrical patterns, favoring differentiation and matrix production [110].

Altogether, advances in domineering topography would provide an alternative to exogenous biological stimulation, diminishing fabrication costs and avoiding its adverse effects. For instance, intra-articular injections of TGF-β result in osteophyte formation in the murine joint [111].

5.3. Cell Response to Biomaterial Elasticity

Cells are also affected by physical and mechanical properties (stiffness or rigidity) of the substrate. Stiffness constitutes the resistance of a solid material to deformation, being defined by elastic modulus (E) and reported in "Pascals" (Pa). Bones usually range from 10–20×10^9 Pa, even though most of the tissues have elastic moduli in the range of 10^1–10^6 Pa, lower than most culture surfaces, such as TCP (3–3.5×10^9 Pa).

The rigidity of a material hence regulates cell adhesion, spreading, and migration. In particular, the mechanotaxis phenomenon induces cells to migrate preferentially towards stiff surfaces in 2D cultures [112]. Moreover, elasticity has also been proven to trigger the differentiation of MSCs. For instance, Engler et al. [113] demonstrated that MSCs cultured on collagen-coated material with stiffness variability can differentiate into neuronal, myogenic, and osteogenic lineages.

5.4. Cell Response to Mechanical Deformation

Elongation or compression of a material (2D) or matrix (3D) can lead to cell alignment in the direction of the applied load, resulting in elongated morphology in both 2D and 3D cultures [114,115]. In vitro, cyclic strain in both tensile and compressive loading enhances osteoblast mineralization [116]. In this context, bioreactors capable of applying physiologic loads have been fabricated to selectively produce and align extracellular matrix in a number of tissues, including bone [117], cartilage [118], and tendon [119].

5.5. Organ-on-a-Chip 3D Culture

Organ-on-a-chip models have arisen as a powerful means to mimic the 3D in vivo environment, since 2D culture lacks many native tissue aspects (such as microfluidic flow) [120]. An organ-on-a-chip is composed of a 3D culture system with dynamic flow through microchannels, achieved by integration of knowledge on microfluidics, microfabrication, and bioreactors. Cells can be exposed to flow pressure, topographical signals, and stimulation by embedded biomolecules and microelectrodes. The result can then be registered using microsensors [121] which will detect and control changes on a continuous basis, allowing real-time monitoring [122].

5.6. Extracellular Matrix and Cell–Biomaterial Interactions

ECMs are composed of noncellular biological materials, including (1) fibrillar, structural, and adhesive proteins such as collagen, elastin, and fibronectin; (2) amorphous matrix macromolecules like proteoglycans, glycosaminoglycans, and hyaluronan; and (3) growth factors, cytokines, and hormones. Biophysical properties of the ECM include strain, viscoelasticity, topography, and permeability [123].

At the tissue level, the ECM acts as a scaffold that provides structural and biomechanical support. At the cellular level, the ECM acts as a biophysical medium in which cells can attach and function. Moreover, the ECM also constitutes a reservoir for bioactive molecules such as growth factors and cytokines [123]. Cells interact with the ECM mainly through transmembrane adhesion proteins that are primarily integrins. Integrin–ECM ligand interactions are regulated by extracellular divalent cations (Ca^{2+} and/or Mg^{2+}) and by the conformation of extracellular portion of integrins [124].

To stimulate cell–biomaterial interaction, ECM molecules and mimetic adhesive peptides can be introduced into scaffolds to reproduce biophysical and biochemical tissue properties, hence allowing the targeting of specific integrins and/or other receptors. In bone, fibronectin-specific $\alpha_5\beta_1$ and collagen-specific $\alpha_2\beta_1$ integrins are critical in bone marrow MSCs for osteoblastic differentiation [125,126].

5.7. Effect of Mechanical Forces on Cells and Tissues

Julius Wolff detailed in 1892 how structural bone remodeling was influenced by mechanical forces [127]. The evidence that mechanical forces rule tissue remodeling was one of the first insights into mechanosensing in biological systems and later became known as Wolff's law. Broadly, cellular mechanosensing can be classified into: (1) focal adhesion and mechanosensing at the ECM, (2) cytoskeletal mechanotransduction, and (3) nuclear mechanotransduction (Figure 3).

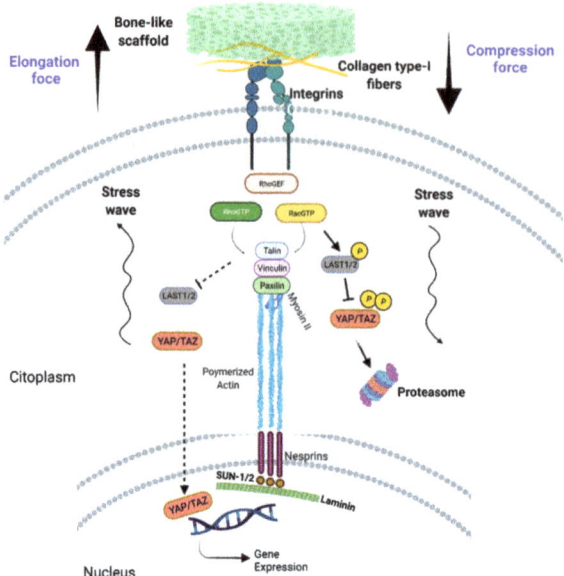

Figure 3. Canonical signaling pathway during cell–ECM interaction with a bone-like scaffold. Mechanical deformation induced by elongation and compression forces triggers recruitment of focal adhesion proteins (vinculin, talin, and paxillin). Focal adhesion kinase (FAK) proteins induce polymerization of actin from the cell cytoskeleton, transmitting the deformation cue to the nucleus cytoskeleton. In parallel, YAP/TAZ molecules are translocated to the nucleus in a mechanical-dependent manner, controlling the expression of genes implicated in proliferation and migration.

Focal adhesion consists of multiprotein frameworks composed of integrins that create a mechanical link between the cell's cytoskeleton and the local microenvironment [128,129]. The canonical model of cell adhesion is based on integrin activation, which leads to Rho and Rac protein activation [130] and subsequent recruitment of focal adhesion-associated proteins (e.g., vinculin, talin, and paxillin) [131]. These associated proteins sense mechanical tension across the focal adhesions [132]. In this sense, TGF-α mechanosignaling has been shown to be involved in the connection between endothelial cells and cancer [133].

Cytoskeleton mechanotransduction is based on focal adhesion complex activation, which triggers actin filaments and non-muscle myosine II to polymerize and rearrange into stress fibers [134]. Forces applied at focal adhesions can be passed on to the nucleus either through signal molecules or direct mechanical forces (Figure 3) [135]. Nuclear envelope spectrin repeat proteins (nesprins) are located on the outside of the nuclear envelope, allowing attachment of actin filaments and microtubules to the nucleus [136]. The generated structures are also known as "linker of nucleoskeleton and cytoskeleton" (LINC), and allow direct transmission of mechanical forces to the chromatin [137]. Major mediators of mechanosignaling are the transcriptional regulators YAP and TAZ (YAP/TAZ), which are crucial in the Hippo signaling pathway [138]. The tension on LINC proteins causes nuclear deformation, which favors YAP/TAZ nuclear entry and subsequent transcription of genes related to proliferation and migration [139,140].

5.8. Mechanical Forces in the Bone

Osteocytes are considered mechanosensors, since they respond to mechanical forces (principally to shear stress [141]), releasing prostaglandins and transmitting signals to other bone cells and the matrix through channels or cell–cell gap junctions, mainly formed by connexin43 [142]. Bone loss caused by a sedentary lifestyle, limb paralysis, or microgravity during space flight has proven the positive effects of physiological loading on skeletal tissues [143].

The compact bone matrix withstands compressive forces that range from 0.04–0.3%, limiting the transfer of force to the cells. Indeed, in vitro studies have concluded that strains must be 1–10% to induce cellular responses. Unmineralized bone matrix around osteocytes is more permeable than mineralized bone, creating lacuna–canalicular porosities for interstitial fluid flow that is mainly sensed by the osteoclasts [143]. Exercise-stimulated bone remodeling may be the response of osteoblasts to interstitial fluid flow [144].

In this sense, a recent elegant work showed that running exercise, in a murine model, control osteolectin$^+$ cell content. Osteolectin-positive cells include osteoblasts, a subset of stromal cell leptin receptor-positive cells (LeptinR$^+$), osteocytes, and hypertrophic chondrocytes in the bone marrow. Consequently, an increase in osteolectin levels activates osteogenesis. Osteolectin binds to $\alpha 11\beta 1$ integrin, triggering Wnt pathway activation, which is necessary for the osteogenic response, revealing a new mechanism for maintenance of adult bone mass [145,146].

6. Computational Modeling
6.1. Bone Mechanobiology

Computational modeling has emerged as an excellent means to improve, predict, and optimize the clinical potential in terms of tissue-level phenomena, such as cell proliferation and differentiation, tissue growth, adaptation, and maintenance [12]. Cell incorporation into artificially engineered matrices has been commonly used in tissue engineering. As has been mentioned, most of the dynamic cell processes, such as growth, differentiation, or migration, are somehow controlled by mechanotransduction [147].

Although it is possible to mechanically stimulate bone and quantify changes at tissue levels in experimental techniques, it is extremely difficult to simultaneously describe and predict cellular and molecular mechanisms that underlie those changes. For this reason, computational mechanobiology has focused on elucidating the cell stimulation and on modeling individual bone cells to predict tissue differentiation. To do so, mechanoregulation algorithms and cell models for predicting mechanobiological changes have been developed [148].

Among mechanoregulation algorithms, two different approaches can be distinguished. First, algorithms based on the fact that tissue differentiation can be regulated by mechanical stimulation. For instance, Lacroix et al. proposed a poroelastic model based on the finite element (FE) method that was able to simulate direct periosteal bone formation, endochondral ossification in the external callus, stabilization during bridging, and resorption. The model successfully predicted tissue differentiation in a rabbit bone chamber and during osteochondral defect healing [148].

The second approach considers that musculoskeletal tissues also adapt to mechanical loading through changes in mass and shape. Studies based on tissue growth were initiated by Heegaard et al. [149], who reported a model to describe how the stresses generated by joint motion may affect the growth, leading to a congruent articular surface. Particularly, they developed a planar biomechanical model of the proximal interphalangeal joint and FE analysis to simulate joint kinematics and stress distribution resulting from muscle contraction [148].

Continuum methods such as FE simulations allow for examining mechanical experiments on cells and in vivo mechanical environments. These models include single cell–biomaterial interaction models; cell population–biomaterial interaction models; and indirect mechanistic models in tissue engineering [147]. Among them, Byrne et al. [150] and Sanz-Herrera et al. [151] simulated how scaffold design parameters such as porosity, Young's modulus, and dissolution rate influence tissue growth.

6.2. Cell Adhesion

Numerous models for the analysis of adhesion have been developed to date. Among them, molecular models take place at the protein level, focusing on the ligand linkage between a cell and the ECM. In these models, steered molecular dynamics (SMD) allow computational modeling of molecular structure unbinding by applying an external force. Thus far, SMD has provided some insights on fibronectin-integrin binding and also on biotin–streptavidin, both of them crucial in ECM–substrate contact [147]. However, molecular models do not consider essential proteins such as cytoskeleton structures, which are relevant for achieving a proper modeling of adhesion.

On the other hand, information regarding adhesion surface modeling is primarily based on kinetics and chemomechanical models. This type of models interrelate the kinetic rates or binding affinities and the mechanical variables, combining two concepts: the mechanics of adhesive tape peeling and the thermodynamics of L-R binding, which relate to kinetic energy of the adhesive bonds [147].

6.3. Optimization of Scaffold Design

Computer-aided simulation can be of use in designing scaffold architectures for a wide range of situations, since it is possible to simulate different strain fields and mechanical properties [152].

Broadly, multi-scale modeling utilizes the rigid body model at the system level to estimate the body loading and boundary conditions. Then, an FE analysis of the organ level can estimate the tissue stress [153]. The combination of a system-level model and organ-level model prevents many models from being successful, as they lead to misinterpretation of simulation outcomes. Dao et al. have presented a fully integrated multiscale modeling workflow to account for the interscale synergies, applying the model to a case study on the bone remodeling process of the human jaw [154].

6.4. Machine Learning for 3D Printing

The design of scaffolds for tissue engineering can be optimized through three-dimensional printing technologies, which offer unparalleled control over the design of constructs with complex architecture. In particular, extrusion-based 3D printing constitutes a widespread manufacturing technique for scaffold fabrication, due to its low cost and compatibility for processing of a wide range of biomaterials. Optimization of processing parameters, such as speed, pressure, and temperature of the printing process [155], often involves time- and labor-intensive experiments.

In this framework, artificial intelligence (AI) techniques based on machine learning (ML) have arisen to improve 3D printing of materials by analyzing underlying behaviors within a given dataset. The three ML approaches that have been used in these studies are to (1) predict and optimize printing parameters to maximize the structure's properties, (2) optimize printability of the material, and (3) assess the quality of the prints [156]. For instance, a convolutional neural network trained with a database of hundreds of thousands of geometries from FE analysis was used to design and 3D print composite constructs with superior mechanical properties. In this work, the ML model could identify the geometrical configurations of soft and stiff materials that resulted in the highest toughness and strength when 3D printed as composite structures [157].

6.5. Computerized Multiscale Diagnostic System

Bone structure analysis in a patient-specific fashion is often limited to models that incorporate only macro and micro levels. Thus, achieving specific models below the microscale level might lead to significant advances in medical treatment of bone disorders. A conceptual representation of a comprehensive computerized diagnostic system has been proposed by Podshivalov et al. for patient-specific treatment of metabolic bone diseases, fractures, and bone cancer. The diagnostic system is thought to include the following: (a) high-resolution images of human bone at different scales; (b) image processing;

(c) 3D reconstruction and multiscale modeling of bone at different structural levels to obtain highly accurate and complete 3D bone models; (d) analysis of bone architecture by applying 3D bone microstructural and topological parameters; (e) multiscale FE analysis of bone structure; and (f) patient-specific scaffolds and/or implants for damaged bone tissue replacement. The system could be also utilized for follow-up and treatment assessment after medication and local therapy procedures [63].

7. Current Challenges and Future Directions

To date, numerous biomaterials have been proven to contribute to the development of BTE. However, clinical implementation of these biomaterials is still at its first stages, mainly due to a lack of knowledge about the mechanisms that underlie cell–biomaterial interactions [57]. Particular limitations of current approaches include cell death due to poor nutrient transport in biomaterial scaffolds, inadequate integration of regenerated tissue with the host tissue, and poor mechanical rigidity to provide load-bearing functions [42].

In this context, emerging technologies applied to BTE together with a better understanding of bone biology allow the combination of scaffolds, cells, and growth factors for successful bone repair and regeneration. In order to optimize their implementation, more effective cell isolation, seeding, and culturing methods need to be developed [6]. Moreover, the scaffold properties, discussed in this review, need to mimic those of the native tissue in order to stimulate cell adhesion, migration, proliferation, and differentiation [42].

Overall, the complex scenario present in bone regeneration is extremely dependent on the local microenvironment, including factors such as patient age, injury type, early inflammatory response, ECM composition, physiological adaptation, and angiogenic capacity [61]. One of the concerns that should be addressed is related to adverse effects caused by the presence of biomaterial degradation products for a long period of time. This causes inflammation processes and macrophage polarization from M1 to M2, affecting cytokines such as TNF α and IL 6, which play a crucial role at the initial stage of the healing process. Thus, further fundamental research should be carried out to describe the mechanisms that control cell–biomaterial interactions [57].

Cell incorporation in BTE scaffolds has been predominantly focused on MSCs. However, induced pluripotent stem cells and embryonic stem cells could be appropriate alternatives to be used for specific disease states [49].

Animal models constitute a major limitation in the preclinical research of effective BTE strategies. Particularly, works on small animals (i.e., mice) have not resulted in relevant results due to major differences in graft size and healing properties. For this reason, it is thought that load-bearing large animal models should be used to assess graft functionality [40]. In this regard, long-bone segmental defects have been modeled in dogs, pigs, goats, and most commonly in sheep, due to their similar body weight to adult humans, well-known mechanical loading, and analogous metabolic and bone remodeling rates [158]. Still, Zeiter et al. [159] performed in 2020 an evaluation of preclinical models in BTE, reporting a lack of standardized and accepted models, and showing the need for optimizing translational aspects (i.e., adaptation to the targeted patient population and justification of the animal model in scientific publications).

Computational approaches might be a useful strategy to optimize and predict substrate performance on bone tissue. However, the translation of computational models from bench to bedside is limited by several issues. First, the determination of patient-specific parameter values becomes difficult when information is limited or of insufficient quality. In addition, current computational models are only validated in animal models, whereas a thorough assessment of the in silico predictive models is critical to encourage health care providers [160]. Furthermore, computational modeling can help improve both scaffold design and the use of high-resolution bioprinting technologies, allowing the design at the cell-specific level at the micro- and nanoscale [42].

Altogether, the future of BTE should integrate fundamental knowledge in bone microenvironment, scaffold design, and simulation and prediction of bone tissue phenomena.

Therefore, a multidisciplinary perspective becomes essential for upcoming treatments in bone disorders.

Author Contributions: Conceptualization, J.S.-L.; investigation, S.G.P. and J.S.-L.; resources, P.L.-S.; writing—original draft preparation, S.G.P. and J.S.-L.; writing—review and editing, S.G.P., J.S.-L. and P.L.-S.; supervision, P.L.-S.; project administration, P.L.-S.; funding acquisition, P.L.-S. All authors have read and agreed to the published version of the manuscript.

Funding: The project that gave rise to these results received the support of a fellowship from "la Caixa" Foundation (ID 100010434). The fellowship code is LCF/BQ/DR20/11790025. National grant received from Ministerio de Ciencia e Innovacción, project PID2020/117091RB-I00.

Institutional Review Board Statement: Not applicable.

Informed Consent Statement: Not applicable.

Data Availability Statement: Not applicable.

Acknowledgments: We would like to thank the Smart Biomaterials laboratory from Universidad Complutense de Madrid (UCM, Spain) for their support and advice. The figures in this article were created with Biorender.

Conflicts of Interest: The authors declare no conflict of interest.

Abbreviations

bFGF	Basic Fibroblast Growth Factor
BMD	Bone Mineral Density
BMP	Bone Morphogenic Protein
BMU	Basic Multicellular Unit
BRC	Bone Remodeling Compartment
BTE	Bone Tissue Engineering
CAP	Cell Adhesion Protein
CPC	Calcium Phosphate Ceramic
CS	Chitosan
CSF-1	Colony-stimulating Factor 1
ECM	Extracellular Matrix
ESC	Embryonic Stem Cell
EPC	Endothelial Progenitor Cell
FAK	Focal Adhesion Kinase
FDA	Food and Drug Administration
GF	Growth Factor
GFOGER	Gly-Phe-Hyp-Gly-Glu-Arg
HA	Hydroxyapatite
hMSC	Human Mesenchymal Stem Cell
IL	Interleukin
iPSC	Induced Pluripotent Stem Cell
LINC	Linker of Nucleoskeleton and Cytoskeleton
MLaHA/CS	Magnetic Lanthanum (La)-doped HA Nanoparticles/Chitosan Scaffolds
MMP	Matrix Metalloproteinase
MP	Microparticle
MSC	Mesenchymal Stem Cell
MSN	Mesoporous Silica Nanoparticle
MWCNT	Multi-walled Carbon Nanotube
NP	Nanoparticle
OPG	Osteoprotegerin
OS	Osteosarcoma
PEEK	Polyether Ether Ketone

PCL	Poly(caprolactone)
PDGF	Platelet-derived Growth Factor
PEG	Polyethylene Glycol
PGA	Poly(glycolic acid)
PLA	Poly(lactic acid)
PLGA	Poly Lactic-co-Glycolic Acid
PMMA	Poly (methyl metacrylate)
PPF	Polypropylene Fumarate
PTH	Parathyroid Hormone
PTHrP	Parathyroid Hormone-related Peptide
RANKL	Receptor Activator of NF-κB Ligand
RGD	Arg-Gly-Asp
rMSC	Rat Mesenchymal Stem Cell
RUNX2	Runt-related Transcription Factor 2
SF	Silk Fibroin
Smurf1	Smad Ubiquitin Regulatory Factor-1
TCP	Tricalcium Phosphate
TNF	Tumoral Necrosis Factor
TGF-β	Transcription Growth Factor β
VEGF	Vascular Endothelial Growth Factor

References

1. Florencio-Silva, R.; da Silva Sasso, G.R.; Sasso-Cerri, E.; Simões, M.J.; Cerri, P.S. Biology of Bone Tissue: Structure, Function, and Factors That Influence Bone Cells. *BioMed Res. Int.* **2015**, *2015*, 421746. [CrossRef]
2. Li, J.J.; Ebied, M.; Xu, J.; Zreiqat, H. Current Approaches to Bone Tissue Engineering: The Interface between Biology and Engineering. *Adv. Healthc. Mater.* **2018**, *7*, 1701061. [CrossRef] [PubMed]
3. Raggatt, L.J.; Partridge, N.C. Cellular and Molecular Mechanisms of Bone Remodeling. *J. Biol. Chem.* **2010**, *285*, 25103–25108. [CrossRef] [PubMed]
4. Dimitriou, R.; Jones, E.; McGonagle, D.; Giannoudis, P.V. Bone Regeneration: Current Concepts and Future Directions. *BMC Med.* **2011**, *9*, 66. [CrossRef] [PubMed]
5. Qasim, M.; Chae, D.S.; Lee, N.Y. Advancements and Frontiers in Nano-Based 3D and 4D Scaffolds for Bone and Cartilage Tissue Engineering. *IJN* **2019**, *14*, 4333–4351. [CrossRef]
6. Roseti, L.; Parisi, V.; Petretta, M.; Cavallo, C.; Desando, G.; Bartolotti, I.; Grigolo, B. Scaffolds for Bone Tissue Engineering: State of the Art and New Perspectives. *Mater. Sci. Eng. C* **2017**, *78*, 1246–1262. [CrossRef]
7. Ng, P.Y.; Ong, A.J.; Gale, L.S.; Dass, C.R. Treatment of Bone Disorders with Parathyroid Hormone: Success and Pitfalls. *Pharmazie* **2016**, *71*, 427–433.
8. Wubneh, A.; Tsekoura, E.K.; Ayranci, C.; Uludağ, H. Current State of Fabrication Technologies and Materials for Bone Tissue Engineering. *Acta Biomater.* **2018**, *80*, 1–30. [CrossRef]
9. Vieira, S.; Vial, S.; Reis, R.L.; Oliveira, J.M. Nanoparticles for Bone Tissue Engineering. *Biotechnol. Prog.* **2017**, *33*, 590–611. [CrossRef]
10. Ansari, M. Bone Tissue Regeneration: Biology, Strategies and Interface Studies. *Prog. Biomater.* **2019**, *8*, 223–237. [CrossRef]
11. Roddy, E.; DeBaun, M.R.; Daoud-Gray, A.; Yang, Y.P.; Gardner, M.J. Treatment of Critical-Sized Bone Defects: Clinical and Tissue Engineering Perspectives. *Eur. J. Orthop. Surg. Traumatol.* **2018**, *28*, 351–362. [CrossRef]
12. Carlier, A.; Lammens, J.; Van Oosterwyck, H.; Geris, L. Computational Modeling of Bone Fracture Non-Unions: Four Clinically Relevant Case Studies. *Silico. Cell Tissue Sci.* **2015**, *2*, 1. [CrossRef]
13. Buck, D.W.; Dumanian, G.A. Bone Biology and Physiology: Part I. The Fundamentals. *Plast. Reconstr. Surg.* **2012**, *129*, 7. [CrossRef]
14. Sommerfeldt, D.W.; Rubin, C.T. Biology of Bone and How It Orchestrates the Form and Function of the Skeleton. *Eur. Spine J.* **2001**, *10*, S86–S95. [CrossRef]
15. Katsimbri, P. The Biology of Normal Bone Remodelling. *Eur. J. Cancer Care* **2017**, *26*, e12740. [CrossRef]
16. Xiao, W.; Wang, Y.; Pacios, S.; Li, S.; Graves, D.T. Cellular and Molecular Aspects of Bone Remodeling. In *Frontiers of Oral Biology*; Kantarci, A., Will, L., Yen, S., Eds.; S. Karger AG: Basel, Switzerland, 2015; Volume 18, pp. 9–16, ISBN 978-3-318-05479-8.
17. Langdahl, B.; Ferrari, S.; Dempster, D.W. Bone Modeling and Remodeling: Potential as Therapeutic Targets for the Treatment of Osteoporosis. *Ther. Adv. Musculoskelet. Dis.* **2016**, *8*, 225–235. [CrossRef]
18. Bernhardt, A.; Wolf, S.; Weiser, E.; Vater, C.; Gelinsky, M. An Improved Method to Isolate Primary Human Osteocytes from Bone. *Biomed. Eng. Biomed. Tech.* **2020**, *65*, 107–111. [CrossRef]
19. Datta, H.K.; Ng, W.F.; Walker, J.A.; Tuck, S.P.; Varanasi, S.S. The Cell Biology of Bone Metabolism. *J. Clin. Pathol.* **2008**, *61*, 577–587. [CrossRef]

20. Brown, J.L.; Kumbar, S.G.; Laurencin, C.T. Bone Tissue Engineering. In *Biomaterials Science*; Elsevier: Amsterdam, The Netherlands, 2013; pp. 1194–1214, ISBN 978-0-12-374626-9.
21. Perić Kačarević, Ž.; Rider, P.; Alkildani, S.; Retnasingh, S.; Pejakić, M.; Schnettler, R.; Gosau, M.; Smeets, R.; Jung, O.; Barbeck, M. An Introduction to Bone Tissue Engineering. *Int. J. Artif. Organs* **2020**, *43*, 69–86. [CrossRef]
22. Matsumoto, M.A.; Biguetti, C.C.; Fonseca, A.C.; Saraiva, P.P. Bone Tissue Healing Dynamics: From Damage to Reconstruction. *J. Mol. Signal. Updates* **2016**, *1*, 33–40.
23. Kenkre, J.S.; Bassett, J. The Bone Remodelling Cycle. *Ann. Clin. Biochem.* **2018**, *55*, 308–327. [CrossRef]
24. Fuchs, R.K.; Warden, S.J.; Turner, C.H. Bone anatomy, physiology and adaptation to mechanical loading. In *Bone Repair Biomaterials*; Elsevier: Amsterdam, The Netherlands, 2009; pp. 25–68. ISBN 978-1-84569-385-5.
25. Clarke, B. Normal Bone Anatomy and Physiology. *CJASN* **2008**, *3*, S131–S139. [CrossRef] [PubMed]
26. Hadjidakis, D.J.; Androulakis, I.I. Bone Remodeling. *Ann. N. Y. Acad. Sci.* **2006**, *1092*, 385–396. [CrossRef] [PubMed]
27. Zang, J.; Lu, L.; Yaszemski, M.J. Bone Disorders. In *Materials for Bone Disorders*; Elsevier: Amsterdam, The Netherlands, 2017; pp. 83–118, ISBN 978-0-12-802792-9.
28. Jimi, E.; Hirata, S.; Osawa, K.; Terashita, M.; Kitamura, C.; Fukushima, H. The Current and Future Therapies of Bone Regeneration to Repair Bone Defects. *Int. J. Dent.* **2012**, *2012*, 148261. [CrossRef] [PubMed]
29. Frohlich, M.; Grayson, W.; Wan, L.; Marolt, D.; Drobnic, M.; Vunjak- Novakovic, G. Tissue Engineered Bone Grafts: Biological Requirements, Tissue Culture and Clinical Relevance. *CSCR* **2008**, *3*, 254–264. [CrossRef]
30. Cawthray, J.; Wasan, E.; Wasan, K. Bone-Seeking Agents for the Treatment of Bone Disorders. *Drug Deliv. Transl. Res.* **2017**, *7*, 466–481. [CrossRef] [PubMed]
31. Feng, X.; McDonald, J.M. Disorders of Bone Remodeling. *Annu. Rev. Pathol. Mech. Dis.* **2011**, *6*, 121–145. [CrossRef]
32. Griz, L.; Fontan, D.; Mesquita, P.; Lazaretti-Castro, M.; Borba, V.Z.C.; Borges, J.L.C.; Fontenele, T.; Maia, J.; Bandeira, F. Diagnosis and Management of Paget?S Disease of Bone. *Arq. Bras. Endocrinol. Metab.* **2014**, *58*, 587–599. [CrossRef]
33. Michael, J.W.-P.; Schlüter-Brust, K.U.; Eysel, P. The Epidemiology, Etiology, Diagnosis, and Treatment of Osteoarthritis of the Knee. *Dtsch. Aerzteblatt. Online* **2010**, *107*, 152. [CrossRef]
34. Morbach, H.; Hedrich, C.M.; Beer, M.; Girschick, H.J. Autoinflammatory Bone Disorders. *Clin. Immunol.* **2013**, *147*, 185–196. [CrossRef]
35. Stern, S.M.; Ferguson, P.J. Autoinflammatory Bone Diseases. *Rheum. Dis. Clin. North. Am.* **2013**, *39*, 735–749. [CrossRef]
36. Macedo, F.; Ladeira, K.; Pinho, F.; Saraiva, N.; Bonito, N.; Pinto, L.; Gonçalves, F. Bone Metastases: An Overview. *Oncol. Rev.* **2017**, *11*, 321.
37. Sun, W.; Ge, K.; Jin, Y.; Han, Y.; Zhang, H.; Zhou, G.; Yang, X.; Liu, D.; Liu, H.; Liang, X.-J.; et al. Bone-Targeted Nanoplatform Combining Zoledronate and Photothermal Therapy To Treat Breast Cancer Bone Metastasis. *ACS Nano* **2019**, *13*, 7556–7567. [CrossRef]
38. Nguyen, D.T.; Burg, K.J.L. Bone Tissue Engineering and Regenerative Medicine: Targeting Pathological Fractures: Bone Tissue Engineering and Regenerative Medicine. *J. Biomed. Mater. Res.* **2015**, *103*, 420–429. [CrossRef]
39. O'Keefe, R.J.; Mao, J. Bone Tissue Engineering and Regeneration: From Discovery to the Clinic—An Overview. *Tissue Eng. Part. B: Rev.* **2011**, *17*, 389–392. [CrossRef]
40. Amini, A.R.; Laurencin, C.T.; Nukavarapu, S.P. Bone Tissue Engineering: Recent Advances and Challenges. *Crit. Rev. Biomed. Eng.* **2012**, *40*, 363–408. [CrossRef]
41. Nguyen, L.H.; Annabi, N.; Nikkhah, M.; Bae, H.; Binan, L.; Park, S.; Kang, Y.; Yang, Y.; Khademhosseini, A. Vascularized Bone Tissue Engineering: Approaches for Potential Improvement. *Tissue Eng. Part. B: Rev.* **2012**, *18*, 363–382. [CrossRef]
42. Fernandez-Yague, M.A.; Abbah, S.A.; McNamara, L.; Zeugolis, D.I.; Pandit, A.; Biggs, M.J. Biomimetic Approaches in Bone Tissue Engineering: Integrating Biological and Physicomechanical Strategies. *Adv. Drug Deliv. Rev.* **2015**, *84*, 1–29. [CrossRef]
43. Kalsi, S.; Singh, J.; Sehgal, S.S.; Sharma, N.K. Biomaterials for Tissue Engineered Bone Scaffolds: A Review. *Mater. Today: Proc.* **2021**, in press.
44. Henkel, J.; Woodruff, M.A.; Epari, D.R.; Steck, R.; Glatt, V.; Dickinson, I.C.; Choong, P.F.M.; Schuetz, M.A.; Hutmacher, D.W. Bone Regeneration Based on Tissue Engineering Conceptions — A 21st Century Perspective. *Bone Res.* **2013**, *1*, 216–248. [CrossRef]
45. Qu, H.; Fu, H.; Han, Z.; Sun, Y. Biomaterials for Bone Tissue Engineering Scaffolds: A Review. *RSC Adv.* **2019**, *9*, 26252–26262. [CrossRef]
46. Koons, G.L.; Diba, M.; Mikos, A.G. Materials Design for Bone-Tissue Engineering. *Nat. Rev. Mater.* **2020**, *5*, 584–603. [CrossRef]
47. Ghassemi, T.; Shahroodi, A.; Ebrahimzadeh, M.H.; Mousavian, A.; Movaffagh, J.; Moradi, A. Current Concepts in Scaffolding for Bone Tissue Engineering. *Arch. Bone Jt. Surg.* **2018**, *6*, 90–99. [PubMed]
48. Donnaloja, F.; Jacchetti, E.; Soncini, M.; Raimondi, M.T. Natural and Synthetic Polymers for Bone Scaffolds Optimization. *Polymers* **2020**, *12*, 905. [CrossRef] [PubMed]
49. Maisani, M.; Pezzoli, D.; Chassande, O.; Mantovani, D. Cellularizing Hydrogel-Based Scaffolds to Repair Bone Tissue: How to Create a Physiologically Relevant Micro-Environment? *J. Tissue Eng.* **2017**, *8*, 204173141771207. [CrossRef]
50. Griffin, K.S.; Davis, K.M.; McKinley, T.O.; Anglen, J.O.; Chu, T.-M.G.; Boerckel, J.D.; Kacena, M.A. Evolution of Bone Grafting: Bone Grafts and Tissue Engineering Strategies for Vascularized Bone Regeneration. *Clin. Rev. Bone Min. Metab.* **2015**, *13*, 232–244. [CrossRef]

51. Lamers, E.; te Riet, J.; Domanski, M.; Luttge, R.; Figdor, C.; Gardeniers, J.; Walboomers, X.; Jansen, J. Dynamic Cell Adhesion and Migration on Nanoscale Grooved Substrates. *eCM* **2012**, *23*, 182–194. [CrossRef]
52. Stevens, M.M. Biomaterials for Bone Tissue Engineering. *Mater. Today* **2008**, *11*, 18–25. [CrossRef]
53. Yan, L.-P.; Silva-Correia, J.; Correia, C.; Caridade, S.G.; Fernandes, E.M.; Sousa, R.A.; Mano, J.F.; Oliveira, J.M.; Oliveira, A.L.; Reis, R.L. Bioactive Macro/Micro Porous Silk Fibroin/Nano-Sized Calcium Phosphate Scaffolds with Potential for Bone-Tissue-Engineering Applications. *Nanomedicine* **2013**, *8*, 359–378. [CrossRef]
54. Collins, M.N.; Ren, G.; Young, K.; Pina, S.; Reis, R.L.; Oliveira, J.M. Scaffold Fabrication Technologies and Structure/Function Properties in Bone Tissue Engineering. *Adv. Funct. Mater.* **2021**, *31*, 2010609. [CrossRef]
55. Cheng, Q.; Rutledge, K.; Jabbarzadeh, E. Carbon Nanotube–Poly(Lactide-Co-Glycolide) Composite Scaffolds for Bone Tissue Engineering Applications. *Ann. Biomed. Eng* **2013**, *41*, 904–916. [CrossRef]
56. Cha, W.; Fan, R.; Miao, Y.; Zhou, Y.; Qin, C.; Shan, X.; Wan, X.; Li, J. Mesoporous Silica Nanoparticles as Carriers for Intracellular Delivery of Nucleic Acids and Subsequent Therapeutic Applications. *Molecules* **2017**, *22*, 782. [CrossRef]
57. Lee, J.; Byun, H.; Perikamana, S.K.M.; Lee, S.; Shin, H. Current Advances in Immunomodulatory Biomaterials for Bone Regeneration. *Adv. Healthc. Mater.* **2019**, *8*, 1801106. [CrossRef]
58. Woodard, J.R.; Hilldore, A.J.; Lan, S.K.; Park, C.J.; Morgan, A.W.; Eurell, J.A.C.; Clark, S.G.; Wheeler, M.B.; Jamison, R.D.; Wagoner Johnson, A.J. The Mechanical Properties and Osteoconductivity of Hydroxyapatite Bone Scaffolds with Multi-Scale Porosity. *Biomaterials* **2007**, *28*, 45–54. [CrossRef]
59. Ghayor, C.; Weber, F.E. Osteoconductive Microarchitecture of Bone Substitutes for Bone Regeneration Revisited. *Front. Physiol.* **2018**, *9*, 960. [CrossRef]
60. Zhang, J.; Wehrle, E.; Rubert, M.; Müller, R. 3D Bioprinting of Human Tissues: Biofabrication, Bioinks, and Bioreactors. *IJMS* **2021**, *22*, 3971. [CrossRef]
61. Ho-Shui-Ling, A.; Bolander, J.; Rustom, L.E.; Johnson, A.W.; Luyten, F.P.; Picart, C. Bone Regeneration Strategies: Engineered Scaffolds, Bioactive Molecules and Stem Cells Current Stage and Future Perspectives. *Biomaterials* **2018**, *180*, 143–162. [CrossRef]
62. Turnbull, G.; Clarke, J.; Picard, F.; Riches, P.; Jia, L.; Han, F.; Li, B.; Shu, W. 3D Bioactive Composite Scaffolds for Bone Tissue Engineering. *Bioact. Mater.* **2018**, *3*, 278–314. [CrossRef]
63. Podshivalov, L.; Fischer, A.; Bar-Yoseph, P.Z. On the Road to Personalized Medicine: Multiscale Computational Modeling of Bone Tissue. *Arch. Comput. Methods Eng* **2014**, *21*, 399–479. [CrossRef]
64. Kim, H.D.; Amirthalingam, S.; Kim, S.L.; Lee, S.S.; Rangasamy, J.; Hwang, N.S. Biomimetic Materials and Fabrication Approaches for Bone Tissue Engineering. *Adv. Healthc. Mater.* **2017**, *6*, 1700612. [CrossRef]
65. Bisht, B.; Hope, A.; Mukherjee, A.; Paul, M.K. Advances in the Fabrication of Scaffold and 3D Printing of Biomimetic Bone Graft. *Ann. Biomed. Eng* **2021**, *49*, 1128–1150. [CrossRef] [PubMed]
66. Asadi-Eydivand, M.; Solati-Hashjin, M.; Fathi, A.; Padashi, M.; Abu Osman, N.A. Optimal Design of a 3D-Printed Scaffold Using Intelligent Evolutionary Algorithms. *Appl. Soft Comput.* **2016**, *39*, 36–47. [CrossRef]
67. Ni, P.; Ding, Q.; Fan, M.; Liao, J.; Qian, Z.; Luo, J.; Li, X.; Luo, F.; Yang, Z.; Wei, Y. Injectable Thermosensitive PEG–PCL–PEG Hydrogel/Acellular Bone Matrix Composite for Bone Regeneration in Cranial Defects. *Biomaterials* **2014**, *35*, 236–248. [CrossRef] [PubMed]
68. Lin, Z.; Cao, S.; Chen, X.; Wu, W.; Li, J. Thermoresponsive Hydrogels from Phosphorylated ABA Triblock Copolymers: A Potential Scaffold for Bone Tissue Engineering. *Biomacromolecules* **2013**, *14*, 2206–2214. [CrossRef]
69. Watson, B.M.; Kasper, F.K.; Engel, P.S.; Mikos, A.G. Synthesis and Characterization of Injectable, Biodegradable, Phosphate-Containing, Chemically Cross-Linkable, Thermoresponsive Macromers for Bone Tissue Engineering. *Biomacromolecules* **2014**, *15*, 1788–1796. [CrossRef]
70. Marolt, D.; Campos, I.M.; Bhumiratana, S.; Koren, A.; Petridis, P.; Zhang, G.; Spitalnik, P.F.; Grayson, W.L.; Vunjak-Novakovic, G. Engineering Bone Tissue from Human Embryonic Stem Cells. *Proc. Natl. Acad. Sci. USA* **2012**, *109*, 8705–8709. [CrossRef]
71. Tang, M.; Chen, W.; Weir, M.D.; Thein-Han, W.; Xu, H.H.K. Human Embryonic Stem Cell Encapsulation in Alginate Microbeads in Macroporous Calcium Phosphate Cement for Bone Tissue Engineering. *Acta Biomater.* **2012**, *8*, 3436–3445. [CrossRef]
72. Bastami, F.; Nazeman, P.; Moslemi, H.; Rezai Rad, M.; Sharifi, K.; Khojasteh, A. Induced Pluripotent Stem Cells as a New Getaway for Bone Tissue Engineering: A Systematic Review. *Cell Prolif.* **2017**, *50*, e12321. [CrossRef]
73. Ardeshirylajimi, A. Applied Induced Pluripotent Stem Cells in Combination With Biomaterials in Bone Tissue Engineering. *J. Cell. Biochem.* **2017**, *118*, 3034–3042. [CrossRef]
74. Battafarano, G.; Rossi, M.; De Martino, V.; Marampon, F.; Borro, L.; Secinaro, A.; Del Fattore, A. Strategies for Bone Regeneration: From Graft to Tissue Engineering. *IJMS* **2021**, *22*, 1128. [CrossRef]

75. Prosecká, E.; Rampichová, M.; Litvinec, A.; Tonar, Z.; Králíčková, M.; Vojtová, L.; Kochová, P.; Plencner, M.; Buzgo, M.; Míčková, A.; et al. Collagen/Hydroxyapatite Scaffold Enriched with Polycaprolactone Nanofibers, Thrombocyte-Rich Solution and Mesenchymal Stem Cells Promotes Regeneration in Large Bone Defect in Vivo: Coll/HA SCAFFOLD ENRICHED WITH PCL, MSCs AND TRS IN VIVO. *J. Biomed. Mater. Res.* **2015**, *103*, 671–682. [CrossRef]
76. Checa, S.; Prendergast, P.J. Effect of Cell Seeding and Mechanical Loading on Vascularization and Tissue Formation inside a Scaffold: A Mechano-Biological Model Using a Lattice Approach to Simulate Cell Activity. *J. Biomech.* **2010**, *43*, 961–968. [CrossRef]
77. Rodríguez-Évora, M.; García-Pizarro, E.; del Rosario, C.; Pérez-López, J.; Reyes, R.; Delgado, A.; Rodríguez-Rey, J.C.; Évora, C. Smurf1 Knocked-Down, Mesenchymal Stem Cells and BMP-2 in an Electrospun System for Bone Regeneration. *Biomacromolecules* **2014**, *15*, 1311–1322. [CrossRef]
78. Kim, Y.-H.; Furuya, H.; Tabata, Y. Enhancement of Bone Regeneration by Dual Release of a Macrophage Recruitment Agent and Platelet-Rich Plasma from Gelatin Hydrogels. *Biomaterials* **2014**, *35*, 214–224. [CrossRef]
79. De Witte, T.-M.; Fratila-Apachitei, L.E.; Zadpoor, A.A.; Peppas, N.A. Bone Tissue Engineering via Growth Factor Delivery: From Scaffolds to Complex Matrices. *Regen. Biomater.* **2018**, *5*, 197–211. [CrossRef]
80. Mishra, R.; Bishop, T.; Valerio, I.L.; Fisher, J.P.; Dean, D. The Potential Impact of Bone Tissue Engineering in the Clinic. *Regen. Med.* **2016**, *11*, 571–587. [CrossRef]
81. Gaihre, B.; Bharadwaz, A.; Unagolla, J.M.; Jayasuriya, A.C. Evaluation of the Optimal Dosage of BMP-9 through the Comparison of Bone Regeneration Induced by BMP-9 versus BMP-2 Using an Injectable Microparticle Embedded Thermosensitive Polymeric Carrier in a Rat Cranial Defect Model. *Mater. Sci. Eng. C* **2021**, *127*, 112252. [CrossRef]
82. Yu, L.; Dawson, L.A.; Yan, M.; Zimmel, K.; Lin, Y.-L.; Dolan, C.P.; Han, M.; Muneoka, K. BMP9 Stimulates Joint Regeneration at Digit Amputation Wounds in Mice. *Nat. Commun.* **2019**, *10*, 424. [CrossRef]
83. Ferracini, R.; Martínez Herreros, I.; Russo, A.; Casalini, T.; Rossi, F.; Perale, G. Scaffolds as Structural Tools for Bone-Targeted Drug Delivery. *Pharmaceutics* **2018**, *10*, 122. [CrossRef]
84. Chollet, C.; Chanseau, C.; Remy, M.; Guignandon, A.; Bareille, R.; Labrugère, C.; Bordenave, L.; Durrieu, M.-C. The Effect of RGD Density on Osteoblast and Endothelial Cell Behavior on RGD-Grafted Polyethylene Terephthalate Surfaces. *Biomaterials* **2009**, *30*, 711–720. [CrossRef]
85. Hersel, U.; Dahmen, C.; Kessler, H. RGD Modified Polymers: Biomaterials for Stimulated Cell Adhesion and Beyond. *Biomaterials* **2003**, *24*, 4385–4415. [CrossRef]
86. Harbers, G.M.; Healy, K.E. The Effect of Ligand Type and Density on Osteoblast Adhesion, Proliferation, and Matrix Mineralization. *J. Biomed. Mater. Res.* **2005**, *75*, 855–869. [CrossRef]
87. Kantlehner, M.; Schaffner, P.; Finsinger, D.; Meyer, J.; Jonczyk, A.; Diefenbach, B.; Nies, B.; Hölzemann, G.; Goodman, S.L.; Kessler, H. Surface Coating with Cyclic RGD Peptides Stimulates Osteoblast Adhesion and Proliferation as Well as Bone Formation. *Chembiochem* **2000**, *1*, 107–114. [CrossRef]
88. Lieb, E.; Hacker, M.; Tessmar, J.; Kunz-Schughart, L.A.; Fiedler, J.; Dahmen, C.; Hersel, U.; Kessler, H.; Schulz, M.B.; Göpferich, A. Mediating Specific Cell Adhesion to Low-Adhesive Diblock Copolymers by Instant Modification with Cyclic RGD Peptides. *Biomaterials* **2005**, *26*, 2333–2341. [CrossRef] [PubMed]
89. Shekaran, A.; García, J.R.; Clark, A.Y.; Kavanaugh, T.E.; Lin, A.S.; Guldberg, R.E.; García, A.J. Bone Regeneration Using an Alpha 2 Beta 1 Integrin-Specific Hydrogel as a BMP-2 Delivery Vehicle. *Biomaterials* **2014**, *35*, 5453–5461. [CrossRef]
90. Khademhosseini, A.; Langer, R.; Borenstein, J.; Vacanti, J.P. Microscale Technologies for Tissue Engineering and Biology. *Proc. Natl. Acad. Sci. USA* **2006**, *103*, 2480–2487. [CrossRef] [PubMed]
91. Khademhosseini, A.; Jon, S.; Suh, K.Y.; Tran, T.-N.T.; Eng, G.; Yeh, J.; Seong, J.; Langer, R. Direct Patterning of Protein- and Cell-Resistant Polymeric Monolayers and Microstructures. *Adv. Mater.* **2003**, *15*, 1995–2000. [CrossRef]
92. McBeath, R.; Pirone, D.M.; Nelson, C.M.; Bhadriraju, K.; Chen, C.S. Cell Shape, Cytoskeletal Tension, and RhoA Regulate Stem Cell Lineage Commitment. *Dev. Cell* **2004**, *6*, 483–495. [CrossRef]
93. Chiu, D.T.; Jeon, N.L.; Huang, S.; Kane, R.S.; Wargo, C.J.; Choi, I.S.; Ingber, D.E.; Whitesides, G.M. Patterned Deposition of Cells and Proteins onto Surfaces by Using Three-Dimensional Microfluidic Systems. *Proc. Natl. Acad. Sci. USA* **2000**, *97*, 2408–2413. [CrossRef]
94. Takayama, S.; Ostuni, E.; LeDuc, P.; Naruse, K.; Ingber, D.E.; Whitesides, G.M. Subcellular Positioning of Small Molecules. *Nature* **2001**, *411*, 1016. [CrossRef]
95. Chen, C.S.; Mrksich, M.; Huang, S.; Whitesides, G.M.; Ingber, D.E. Micropatterned Surfaces for Control of Cell Shape, Position, and Function. *Biotechnol. Prog.* **1998**, *14*, 356–363. [CrossRef]
96. Edahiro, J.; Sumaru, K.; Tada, Y.; Ohi, K.; Takagi, T.; Kameda, M.; Shinbo, T.; Kanamori, T.; Yoshimi, Y. In Situ Control of Cell Adhesion Using Photoresponsive Culture Surface. *Biomacromolecules* **2005**, *6*, 970–974. [CrossRef]
97. Kikuchi, K.; Sumaru, K.; Edahiro, J.-I.; Ooshima, Y.; Sugiura, S.; Takagi, T.; Kanamori, T. Stepwise Assembly of Micropatterned Co-Cultures Using Photoresponsive Culture Surfaces and Its Application to Hepatic Tissue Arrays. *Biotechnol. Bioeng.* **2009**, *103*, 552–561. [CrossRef]
98. Anderson, D.G.; Levenberg, S.; Langer, R. Nanoliter-Scale Synthesis of Arrayed Biomaterials and Application to Human Embryonic Stem Cells. *Nat. Biotechnol.* **2004**, *22*, 863–866. [CrossRef]

99. Metavarayuth, K.; Sitasuwan, P.; Zhao, X.; Lin, Y.; Wang, Q. Influence of Surface Topographical Cues on the Differentiation of Mesenchymal Stem Cells in Vitro. *ACS Biomater. Sci. Eng.* **2016**, *2*, 142–151. [CrossRef]
100. Fratzl, P. When the Cracks Begin to Show. *Nat. Mater.* **2008**, *7*, 610–612. [CrossRef]
101. Carinci, F.; Pezzetti, F.; Volinia, S.; Francioso, F.; Arcelli, D.; Marchesini, J.; Scapoli, L.; Piattelli, A. Analysis of Osteoblast-Like MG63 Cells' Response to A Rough Implant Surface by means of DNA Microarray. *J. Oral Implantol.* **2003**, *29*, 215–220. [CrossRef]
102. Hamilton, D.W.; Brunette, D.M. The Effect of Substratum Topography on Osteoblast Adhesion Mediated Signal Transduction and Phosphorylation. *Biomaterials* **2007**, *28*, 1806–1819. [CrossRef]
103. Clark, P.; Connolly, P.; Curtis, A.S.G.; Dow, J.A.T.; Wilkinson, C.D.W. Topographical Control of Cell Behaviour. *Development* **1990**, *108*, 635–644. [CrossRef]
104. Martínez, E.; Lagunas, A.; Mills, C.; Rodríguez-Seguí, S.; Estévez, M.; Oberhansl, S.; Comelles, J.; Samitier, J. Stem Cell Differentiation by Functionalized Micro- and Nanostructured Surfaces. *Nanomedicine* **2009**, *4*, 65–82. [CrossRef]
105. Hacking, S.A.; Harvey, E.; Roughley, P.; Tanzer, M.; Bobyn, J. The Response of Mineralizing Culture Systems to Microtextured and Polished Titanium Surfaces. *J. Orthop. Res.* **2008**, *26*, 1347–1354. [CrossRef]
106. Bettinger, C.J.; Orrick, B.; Misra, A.; Langer, R.; Borenstein, J.T. Microfabrication of Poly (Glycerol–Sebacate) for Contact Guidance Applications. *Biomaterials* **2006**, *27*, 2558–2565. [CrossRef]
107. Dalby, M.J.; Riehle, M.O.; Johnstone, H.; Affrossman, S.; Curtis, A.S.G. In Vitro Reaction of Endothelial Cells to Polymer Demixed Nanotopography. *Biomaterials* **2002**, *23*, 2945–2954. [CrossRef]
108. Ball, M.D.; Prendergast, U.; O'Connell, C.; Sherlock, R. Comparison of Cell Interactions with Laser Machined Micron- and Nanoscale Features in Polymer. *Exp. Mol. Pathol.* **2007**, *82*, 130–134. [CrossRef]
109. Curtis, A.S.G.; Gadegaard, N.; Dalby, M.J.; Riehle, M.O.; Wilkinson, C.D.W.; Aitchison, G. Cells React to Nanoscale Order and Symmetry in Their Surroundings. *IEEE Trans. Nanobioscience* **2004**, *3*, 61–65. [CrossRef]
110. Kantawong, F.; Burchmore, R.; Gadegaard, N.; Oreffo, R.O.C.; Dalby, M.J. Proteomic Analysis of Human Osteoprogenitor Response to Disordered Nanotopography. *J. R. Soc. Interface.* **2009**, *6*, 1075–1086. [CrossRef]
111. van Beuningen, H.M.; Glansbeek, H.L.; van der Kraan, P.M.; van den Berg, W.B. Osteoarthritis-like Changes in the Murine Knee Joint Resulting from Intra-Articular Transforming Growth Factor-β Injections. *Osteoarthr. Cartil.* **2000**, *8*, 25–33. [CrossRef]
112. Lo, C.-M.; Wang, H.-B.; Dembo, M.; Wang, Y. Cell Movement Is Guided by the Rigidity of the Substrate. *Biophys. J.* **2000**, *79*, 144–152. [CrossRef]
113. Engler, A.J.; Sen, S.; Sweeney, H.L.; Discher, D.E. Matrix Elasticity Directs Stem Cell Lineage Specification. *Cell* **2006**, *126*, 677–689. [CrossRef] [PubMed]
114. Haghighipour, N.; Tafazzoli-Shadpour, M.; Shokrgozar, M.A.; Amini, S.; Amanzadeh, A.; Taghi Khorasani, M. Topological Remodeling of Cultured Endothelial Cells by Characterized Cyclic Strains. *Mol. Cell Biochem.* **2007**, *4*, 189–199.
115. Henshaw, D.R.; Attia, E.; Bhargava, M.; Hannafin, J.A. Canine ACL Fibroblast Integrin Expression and Cell Alignment in Response to Cyclic Tensile Strain in Three-Dimensional Collagen Gels. *J. Orthop. Res.* **2006**, *24*, 481–490. [CrossRef] [PubMed]
116. Ravichandran, A.; Lim, J.; Chong, M.S.K.; Wen, F.; Liu, Y.; Pillay, Y.T.; Chan, J.K.Y.; Teoh, S.-H. In Vitro Cyclic Compressive Loads Potentiate Early Osteogenic Events in Engineered Bone Tissue: Compressive Stimulation for Bone Tissue Engineering. *J. Biomed. Mater. Res.* **2017**, *105*, 2366–2375. [CrossRef] [PubMed]
117. Griensven, M.; Diederichs, S.; Roeker, S.; Boehm, S.; Peterbauer, A.; Wolbank, S.; Riechers, D.; Stahl, F.; Kasper, C. Mechanical Strain Using 2D and 3D Bioreactors Induces Osteogenesis: Implications for Bone Tissue Engineering. In *Advances in Biochemical Engineering/Biotechnology*; Springer: Berlin/Heidelberg, Germany, 2008.
118. Preiss-Bloom, O.; Mizrahi, J.; Elisseeff, J.; Seliktar, D. Real-Time Monitoring of Force Response Measured in Mechanically Stimulated Tissue-Engineered Cartilage. *Artif. Organs* **2009**, *33*, 318–327. [CrossRef]
119. Riboh, J.; Chong, A.K.S.; Pham, H.; Longaker, M.; Jacobs, C.; Chang, J. Optimization of Flexor Tendon Tissue Engineering With a Cyclic Strain Bioreactor. *J. Hand Surg.* **2008**, *33*, 1388–1396. [CrossRef]
120. Zheng, F.; Fu, F.; Cheng, Y.; Wang, C.; Zhao, Y.; Gu, Z. Organ-on-a-Chip Systems: Microengineering to Biomimic Living Systems. *Small* **2016**, *12*, 2253–2282. [CrossRef]
121. Shin, S.R.; Kilic, T.; Zhang, Y.S.; Avci, H.; Hu, N.; Kim, D.; Branco, C.; Aleman, J.; Massa, S.; Silvestri, A.; et al. Label-Free and Regenerative Electrochemical Microfluidic Biosensors for Continual Monitoring of Cell Secretomes. *Adv. Sci.* **2017**, *4*, 1600522. [CrossRef]
122. Ashammakhi, N.; Elkhammas, E.; Hasan, A. Translating Advances in Organ-on-a-chip Technology for Supporting Organs. *B Appl. Biomater.* **2019**, *107*, 2006–2018. [CrossRef]
123. Frantz, C.; Stewart, K.M.; Weaver, V.M. The Extracellular Matrix at a Glance. *J. Cell Sci.* **2010**, *123*, 4195–4200. [CrossRef]
124. Zhang, K.; Chen, J. The Regulation of Integrin Function by Divalent Cations. *Cell Adhes. Migr.* **2012**, *6*, 20–29. [CrossRef]
125. Moursi, A.; Globus, R.; Damsky, C. Interactions between Integrin Receptors and Fibronectin Are Required for Calvarial Osteoblast Differentiation in Vitro. *J. Cell Sci.* **1997**, *110*, 2187–2196. [CrossRef]
126. Mizuno, M.; Fujisawa, R.; Kuboki, Y. Type I Collagen-Induced Osteoblastic Differentiation of Bone-Marrow Cells Mediated by Collagen-α2β1 Integrin Interaction. *J. Cell. Physiol.* **2000**, *184*, 207–213. [CrossRef]
127. Wolff, J. *The Law of Bone Remodelling*; Springer: Berlin/Heidelberg, Germany, 1986; ISBN 978-3-642-71033-9.
128. Harburger, D.S.; Calderwood, D.A. Integrin Signalling at a Glance. *J. Cell Sci.* **2009**, *122*, 1472. [CrossRef]

129. Geiger, B.; Yamada, K.M. Molecular Architecture and Function of Matrix Adhesions. *Cold Spring Harb. Perspect. Biol.* **2011**, *3*, a005033. [CrossRef]
130. Buchsbaum, R.J. Rho Activation at a Glance. *J. Cell Sci.* **2007**, *120*, 1149–1152. [CrossRef]
131. Parsons, J.T.; Horwitz, A.R.; Schwartz, M.A. Cell Adhesion: Integrating Cytoskeletal Dynamics and Cellular Tension. *Nat. Rev. Mol. Cell Biol* **2010**, *11*, 633–643. [CrossRef]
132. Grashoff, C.; Hoffman, B.D.; Brenner, M.D.; Zhou, R.; Parsons, M.; Yang, M.T.; McLean, M.A.; Sligar, S.G.; Chen, C.S.; Ha, T.; et al. Measuring Mechanical Tension across Vinculin Reveals Regulation of Focal Adhesion Dynamics. *Nature* **2010**, *466*, 263–266. [CrossRef]
133. Wei, S.C.; Fattet, L.; Tsai, J.H.; Guo, Y.; Pai, V.H.; Majeski, H.E.; Chen, A.C.; Sah, R.L.; Taylor, S.S.; Engler, A.J.; et al. Matrix Stiffness Drives Epithelial–Mesenchymal Transition and Tumour Metastasis through a TWIST1–G3BP2 Mechanotransduction Pathway. *Nat. Cell Biol.* **2015**, *17*, 678–688. [CrossRef] [PubMed]
134. Vicente-Manzanares, M.; Ma, X.; Adelstein, R.S.; Horwitz, A.R. Non-Muscle Myosin II Takes Centre Stage in Cell Adhesion and Migration. *Nat. Rev. Mol. Cell Biol.* **2009**, *10*, 778–790. [CrossRef]
135. Wang, N.; Tytell, J.D.; Ingber, D.E. Mechanotransduction at a Distance: Mechanically Coupling the Extracellular Matrix with the Nucleus. *Nat. Rev. Mol. Cell Biol.* **2009**, *10*, 75–82. [CrossRef]
136. Haque, F.; Lloyd, D.J.; Smallwood, D.T.; Dent, C.L.; Shanahan, C.M.; Fry, A.M.; Trembath, R.C.; Shackleton, S. SUN1 Interacts with Nuclear Lamin A and Cytoplasmic Nesprins To Provide a Physical Connection between the Nuclear Lamina and the Cytoskeleton. *Mol. Cell Biol.* **2006**, *26*, 3738–3751. [CrossRef]
137. Sosa, B.A.; Rothballer, A.; Kutay, U.; Schwartz, T.U. LINC Complexes Form by Binding of Three KASH Peptides to Domain Interfaces of Trimeric SUN Proteins. *Cell* **2012**, *149*, 1035–1047. [CrossRef]
138. Dupont, S. Role of YAP/TAZ in Cell-Matrix Adhesion-Mediated Signalling and Mechanotransduction. *Exp. Cell Res.* **2016**, *343*, 42–53. [CrossRef] [PubMed]
139. Totaro, A.; Panciera, T.; Piccolo, S. YAP/TAZ Upstream Signals and Downstream Responses. *Nat. Cell Biol* **2018**, *20*, 888–899. [CrossRef] [PubMed]
140. Elosegui-Artola, A.; Andreu, I.; Beedle, A.E.M.; Lezamiz, A.; Uroz, M.; Kosmalska, A.J.; Oria, R.; Kechagia, J.Z.; Rico-Lastres, P.; Le Roux, A.-L.; et al. Force Triggers YAP Nuclear Entry by Regulating Transport across Nuclear Pores. *Cell* **2017**, *171*, 1397–1410.e14. [CrossRef]
141. Jiang, J.X. Roles of Gap Junctions and Hemichannels in Bone Cell Functions and in Signal Transmission of Mechanical Stress. *Front. Biosci.* **2007**, *12*, 1450. [CrossRef]
142. Zhao, D.; Liu, R.; Li, G.; Chen, M.; Shang, P.; Yang, H.; Jiang, J.X.; Xu, H. Connexin 43 Channels in Osteocytes Regulate Bone Responses to Mechanical Unloading. *Front. Physiol.* **2020**, *11*, 299. [CrossRef]
143. Orr, A.W.; Helmke, B.P.; Blackman, B.R.; Schwartz, M.A. Mechanisms of Mechanotransduction. *Dev. Cell* **2006**, *10*, 11–20. [CrossRef]
144. Reich, K.M.; Gay, C.V.; Frangos, J.A. Fluid Shear Stress as a Mediator of Osteoblast Cyclic Adenosine Monophosphate Production. *J. Cell. Physiol.* **1990**, *143*, 100–104. [CrossRef]
145. Yue, R.; Shen, B.; Morrison, S.J. Clec11a/Osteolectin Is an Osteogenic Growth Factor That Promotes the Maintenance of the Adult Skeleton. *eLife* **2016**, *5*, e18782. [CrossRef]
146. Shen, B.; Vardy, K.; Hughes, P.; Tasdogan, A.; Zhao, Z.; Yue, R.; Crane, G.M.; Morrison, S.J. Integrin Alpha11 Is an Osteolectin Receptor and Is Required for the Maintenance of Adult Skeletal Bone Mass. *eLife* **2019**, *8*, e42274. [CrossRef]
147. Sanz-Herrera, J.A.; Reina-Romo, E. Cell-Biomaterial Mechanical Interaction in the Framework of Tissue Engineering: Insights, Computational Modeling and Perspectives. *IJMS* **2011**, *12*, 8217–8244. [CrossRef] [PubMed]
148. Giorgi, M.; Verbruggen, S.W.; Lacroix, D. In Silico Bone Mechanobiology: Modeling a Multifaceted Biological System: *In Silico* Bone Mechanobiology. *WIREs Syst. Biol. Med.* **2016**, *8*, 485–505. [CrossRef] [PubMed]
149. Carter, D.R.; Wong, M. Modelling Cartilage Mechanobiology. *Phil. Trans. R. Soc. Lond. B* **2003**, *358*, 1461–1471. [CrossRef]
150. Byrne, D.P.; Lacroix, D.; Planell, J.A.; Kelly, D.J.; Prendergast, P.J. Simulation of Tissue Differentiation in a Scaffold as a Function of Porosity, Young's Modulus and Dissolution Rate: Application of Mechanobiological Models in Tissue Engineering. *Biomaterials* **2007**, *28*, 5544–5554. [CrossRef]
151. Sanzherrera, J.; Garciaaznar, J.; Doblare, M. On Scaffold Designing for Bone Regeneration: A Computational Multiscale Approach. *Acta Biomater.* **2009**, *5*, 219–229. [CrossRef]
152. Dias, M.R.; Guedes, J.M.; Flanagan, C.L.; Hollister, S.J.; Fernandes, P.R. Optimization of Scaffold Design for Bone Tissue Engineering: A Computational and Experimental Study. *Med. Eng. Phys.* **2014**, *36*, 448–457. [CrossRef]
153. Halloran, J.P.; Sibole, S.; van Donkelaar, C.C.; van Turnhout, M.C.; Oomens, C.W.J.; Weiss, J.A.; Guilak, F.; Erdemir, A. Multiscale Mechanics of Articular Cartilage: Potentials and Challenges of Coupling Musculoskeletal, Joint, and Microscale Computational Models. *Ann. Biomed. Eng.* **2012**, *40*, 2456–2474. [CrossRef]
154. Dao, T.T. Advanced Computational Workflow for the Multi-Scale Modeling of the Bone Metabolic Processes. *Med. Biol Eng Comput.* **2017**, *55*, 923–933. [CrossRef]
155. Roopavath, U.K.; Malferrari, S.; Van Haver, A.; Verstreken, F.; Rath, S.N.; Kalaskar, D.M. Optimization of Extrusion Based Ceramic 3D Printing Process for Complex Bony Designs. *Mater. Des.* **2019**, *162*, 263–270. [CrossRef]

156. Conev, A.; Litsa, E.E.; Perez, M.R.; Diba, M.; Mikos, A.G.; Kavraki, L.E. Machine Learning-Guided Three-Dimensional Printing of Tissue Engineering Scaffolds. *Tissue Eng. Part. A* **2020**, *26*, 1359–1368. [CrossRef]
157. Dellinger, J.G.; Wojtowicz, A.M.; Jamison, R.D. Effects of Degradation and Porosity on the Load Bearing Properties of Model Hydroxyapatite Bone Scaffolds. *J. Biomed. Mater. Res.* **2006**, *77*, 563–571. [CrossRef]
158. McGovern, J.A.; Griffin, M.; Hutmacher, D.W. Animal Models for Bone Tissue Engineering and Modelling Disease. *Dis. Models Mech.* **2018**, *11*, dmm033084. [CrossRef]
159. Zeiter, S.; Koschitzki, K.; Alini, M.; Jakob, F.; Rudert, M.; Herrmann, M. Evaluation of Preclinical Models for the Testing of Bone Tissue-Engineered Constructs. *Tissue Eng. Part. C: Methods* **2020**, *26*, 107–117. [CrossRef]
160. Carlier, A.; Geris, L.; Lammens, J.; Van Oosterwyck, H. Bringing Computational Models of Bone Regeneration to the Clinic: Bringing Computational Models of Bone Regeneration to the Clinic. *WIREs Syst. Biol. Med.* **2015**, *7*, 183–194. [CrossRef]

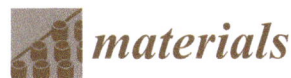

Article

Utilizing Osteocyte Derived Factors to Enhance Cell Viability and Osteogenic Matrix Deposition within IPN Hydrogels

Laurens Parmentier [1,2,3], Mathieu Riffault [1,2,4] and David A. Hoey [1,2,4,*]

1. Trinity Centre for Biomedical Engineering, Trinity Biomedical Sciences Institute, Trinity College Dublin, Dublin 2 D02 R590, Ireland
2. Department of Mechanical and Manufacturing Engineering, School of Engineering, Trinity College Dublin, Dublin 2 D02 DK07, Ireland
3. Polymer Chemistry and Biomaterials Group, Centre of Macromolecular Chemistry (CMaC), Department of Organic and Macromolecular Chemistry, Ghent University, 9000 Ghent, Belgium
4. Advanced Materials and Bioengineering Research Centre, Trinity College Dublin & RCSI, Dublin 2 D02 VN51, Ireland
* Correspondence: dahoey@tcd.ie; Tel.: +353-18961359

Received: 23 February 2020; Accepted: 1 April 2020; Published: 4 April 2020

Abstract: Many bone defects arising due to traumatic injury, disease, or surgery are unable to regenerate, requiring intervention. More than four million graft procedures are performed each year to treat these defects making bone the second most commonly transplanted tissue worldwide. However, these types of graft suffer from a limited supply, a second surgical site, donor site morbidity, and pain. Due to the unmet clinical need for new materials to promote skeletal repair, this study aimed to produce novel biomimetic materials to enhance stem/stromal cell osteogenesis and bone repair by recapitulating aspects of the biophysical and biochemical cues found within the bone microenvironment. Utilizing a collagen type I–alginate interpenetrating polymer network we fabricated a material which mirrors the mechanical and structural properties of unmineralized bone, consisting of a porous fibrous matrix with a young's modulus of 64 kPa, both of which have been shown to enhance mesenchymal stromal/stem cell (MSC) osteogenesis. Moreover, by combining this material with biochemical paracrine factors released by statically cultured and mechanically stimulated osteocytes, we further mirrored the biochemical environment of the bone niche, enhancing stromal/stem cell viability, differentiation, and matrix deposition. Therefore, this biomimetic material represents a novel approach to promote skeletal repair.

Keywords: bone; collagen type I; alginate; conditioned medium; viability; MSC; osteogenesis

---

1. Introduction

Bone defects arise due to traumatic injury, disease, or orthopedic surgeries and many of these are unable to regenerate requiring intervention [1]. More than four million graft procedures are performed each year to treat these defects making bone the second most commonly transplanted tissue worldwide [2]. The prevalence of bone defects, their associated morbidity, and socio-economic cost necessitates the need for new materials to promote skeletal repair through regeneration [3]. It is intuitive that a material which mimics the native tissue may be optimal to promote repair and it is autografts that are currently used as the clinical gold standard. However, these types of grafts suffer from a limited supply, a second surgical site, donor site morbidity, and pain [4]. Allografts on the other hand carry the risk of transmission of infections or an enhanced immune response [5,6]. Therefore, bone substitute materials are gaining much interest as an alternative to grafts. These materials should be designed in such a way so that they provide both biochemical and biophysical cues similar to that found in the native extracellular matrix (ECM) inductive of bone and the marrow cavity, that can promote cell attachment, migration, proliferation, and osteogenesis [7].

There are numerous biochemical and biophysical cues present within the bone niche which promote progenitor cell osteogenesis. For example, physical cues derived from the substrate can dramatically influence cell behavior. Substrate stiffness in the range of 25–40 kPa has been shown to be osteogenic mimicking the non-mineralized osteoid tissue deposited by osteoblasts during bone formation [8]. The surface topography presented to a cell is also a mediator for stem cell fate since it influences the extent a cell can spread over the surface. A higher degree of spreading commits the mesenchymal stromal/stem cell (MSC) to the osteogenic lineage [9–12]. Furthermore, a more disordered surface topography results in a higher osteogenic stimulus [13]. In addition, an average roughness on the micrometer range has been found to be the most favorable for the osteogenic differentiation of MSCs [14]. The biochemical makeup of the material can also greatly influence cell behavior. The native composition of bone tissue is mainly comprised of collagen type I, interspersed with mineral crystals [15]. Collagen type I, the major protein present in the tissue, comprises a number of adhesive ligands which influences the degree of cell attachment, spreading and hence the osteogenic differentiation of resident cells [9,10]. Therefore, there is a need for a synthetic alternative to autograft which aspires to recapitulate the various structural and physical properties of bone ECM in a 3D environment [16].

In addition to biophysical cues derived from the cell substrate, biochemical cues within the bone niche arise predominately from resident cells via paracrine signaling. Bone is exquisitely mechanosensitive and can structurally adapt to its mechanical environment to maintain function [17]. Macroscopic loading resulting in tissue deformation leads to fluid flow at the cellular level in the lacuno-canalicular system [18]. The fluid flow translates in various stimuli at the cell level but it has been shown that stimulation through a fluid-flow induced shear stress has the greatest capacity for mechanical activation and prevention of apoptosis [19–21]. Osteocytes are the most abundant cell type within bone and are largely believed to be the master orchestrator of bone physiology [22]. Factors secreted by mature bone cells, such as osteocytes, have been shown to drive mesenchymal stem cell recruitment, proliferation, and osteogenic differentiation, with medium collected from mechanically stimulated osteocytes demonstrating a greater capacity for osteogenesis [23–26]. This therefore demonstrates that factors secreted by resident bone cells may represent novel anabolic agents to functionalize materials to enhance bone repair.

Taken together, this study aims to produce novel biomimetic materials to enhance stem/stromal cell osteogenesis and bone repair by recapitulating aspects of the biophysical (ECM structure/stiffness) and biochemical cues (osteocyte secretome) found within the bone microenvironment.

2. Materials and Methods

2.1. Interpenetrating Polymer Network (IPN) Synthesis

Interpenetrating polymer network hydrogels were made with a final rat tail collagen type I (COL-I) (Corning, Bedford, MA, USA) concentration of 1.5 mg/mL mixed in a 1:1 ratio with either a final concentration of 5 (interpenetrating polymer network (IPN) 5), 10 (IPN 10), or 15 (IPN 15) mg/mL of ultrapure, low-viscosity, and high glucuronic acid (LVG) alginate (ALG) (Novamatrix, Sandvika, Norway) in phosphate buffered saline (PBS) (Thermo Fisher Scientific, Carlsbad, CA, USA). According to the manufacturer's instructions, collagen was brought to alkalinity to assist in the gelling procedure. The alginate stock solution was first centrifuged at 650 g for 5 min, diluted to 10, 20, and 30 mg/mL, mixed with the collagen solution and added to custom-made molds. These molds were then placed in petri dishes for collagen gelation at 37 °C for 30 min. In the meantime, 20 mM calcium chloride (Sigma, Arklow, Ireland) in ultrapure water was prepared and brought up to a pH of 7.2 using 1 N NaOH. The calcium chloride was used to ionically crosslink the alginate present in the IPN hydrogels for an additional 3 h at 37 °C. Control sample hydrogels were made that completely consisted of 1.5 mg/mL collagen type I by following the same gelation procedure as outlined above. The samples for compressive testing were stored in ultrapure water whereas the samples for histology and scanning electron microscopy (SEM) were washed with PBS, fixed with 4% paraformaldehyde (PFA) for 4 h, subjected to 30 min of 30% ethanol (EtOH) and stored in 50% EtOH.

2.2. Compressive Testing

Unconfined compressive testing was performed on hydrogels submersed in PBS up to 30% strain at a strain rate of 1 mm/min (Zwick Roell Z005, Herefordshire, UK, 5 N load cell). A 0.005 N pre-load was applied so that the impermeable compressive plates touch the sample on both sides. The compressive modulus was then calculated as the slope in the linear region of the stress-strain curve between 0% and 30% strain.

2.3. Scanning Electron Microscopy

The fixed IPN samples that were stored in 50% EtOH were further dehydrated in concentrated EtOH baths (70% EtOH, 90% EtOH, and absolute ethanol) before being transferred to a critical point dryer (Quorum Technologies, Lewes, UK) for further dehydration. The samples were then adhered to sample stubs using carbon tape, sputter coated with 5 mm of platinum-palladium (Cressington sputter coater, Cressington Scientific Instruments Ltd., Watford, UK) and imaged with a scanning electron microscope (Zeiss Ultra Plus, Cambourne, UK).

2.4. Cell Culture

The MLO-Y4 cell line (Kerafast, Boston, MA, USA) [27] is a murine derived osteocyte cell line that was cultured, as previously described [28], on 0.15 mg/mL rat tail collagen type I (Sigma)-coated culture flasks with α-modification of Eagle's minimal essential medium (α-MEM) (Labtech, Heathfield, UK) supplemented with 5% fetal bovine serum (FBS) (Labtech), 5% calf serum (CS) (Sigma), 1% penicillin/streptomycin (Pen/Strep) (Sigma), and 1% L-glutamine (Sigma). Human mesenchymal stromal/stem cells (hMSCs) (Lonza, Huddersfield, UK) were cultured with low glucose Dulbecco's modified Eagle's medium (DMEM) (Sigma) supplemented with 10% FBS and 1% Pen/Strep. Standard incubator culture conditions (37 °C, 5% CO_2) were used for all cell types. MLO-Y4 cells were used between passage numbers 33 and 36 and HMSCs between passage numbers 3 and 4.

2.5. Conditioned Medium Production

MLO-Y4 cells were seeded on 0.15 mg/mL rat tail collagen type I-coated 6-well plates at a density of 11,600 cells/cm^2 in 2 mL of α-MEM supplemented with 2.5% FBS, 2.5% CS, 1% Pen/Strep, and 1% L-glutamine per well. After 48 h of culture, these cells were either subjected to mechanical stimulation or left in culture for an extra 2 h. For mechanical stimulation, 6-well plates were placed on an orbital shaker (Carl Roth, Karlsruhe, Germany) for 2 h at a rotational speed of 100 rpm in an incubator. Both the statically cultured as well as the mechanically activated osteocytes were then washed with 2 mL of PBS and 833 μL of serum free media was applied onto the cells. After 24 h of culture, both the static (S-CM) as well as the mechanically activated (MA-CM) conditioned medium was collected, centrifuged at 3000 g for 10 min at 4 °C to remove debris after which the supernatant was used or stored at −20 °C.

2.6. Conditioned Medium Osteogenesis Study

hMSCs were seeded at a density of 5000 cells/cm^2 in 6-well plates in either 2 mL of growth medium (α-MEM + 1% Pen/Strep + 1% L-glutamine) with the addition of 10% FBS as a negative control (GM), static osteocyte conditioned medium supplemented with 10% FBS and osteogenic factors (100 nM dexamethasone (Sigma), 10 mM β-glycerol phosphate (Sigma) and 0.28 mM ascorbic acid (Sigma)) (S-CM^{ost}), mechanically activated osteocyte conditioned medium with the addition of 10% FBS and osteogenic factors (MA-CM^{ost}) or growth medium supplemented with 10% FBS and osteogenic factors as a positive control (GM^{ost}). These four different media groups were cultured for 21 days with a medium change twice a week.

2.6.1. DNA Analysis

After 21 days of culture, the hMSC monolayer was washed with cold PBS where after 100 µL of lysis buffer (DNAse free water (Thermo Fisher Scientific) with 0.2% Triton X100 (Sigma), 10 mM Tris pH8 (Thermo Fisher Scientific), and 0.5% phenylmethylsulfonyl fluoride (PMSF) (Sigma)) was added per well. Cells were then detached with a cell scraper, transferred to a microtube, vortexed, sonicated, frozen at −80 °C, thawed and homogenized with a needle. A quant-it picogreen dsDNA assay kit (Invitrogen, Carlsbad, CA, USA) was used to quantify the amount of DNA present in the cell lysate samples with reference to set standards. The samples and standards were excited at 480 nm and their emission was captured at 520 nm.

2.6.2. Collagen Production

Collagen was stained and quantified through a protocol previously described [29,30]. The hMSC monolayer was fixed with 10% formalin (Sigma) for 15 min with PBS washing steps both before and after the fixation procedure. After 1 mL of picrosirius red was added per well, gentle shaking was applied for 1 h at room temperature. The cell monolayer was then washed twice with 0.5% acetic acid (Sigma) and once with ultrapure water. To quantify the amount of collagen deposited by the HMSCs, 1 mL of PBS was added per well and a cell scraper was used to remove the monolayer of cells and subsequently transferred to a microtube. After centrifugation at 14,000 g for 10 min at room temperature, the pellet was resuspended in 0.5 M NaOH and vortexed until the stain was dissolved. The samples were then compared against a collagen standard (Corning) that was centrifuged and resuspended in 0.5 M NaOH. The absorbance of both standards and samples was read at 550 nm.

2.6.3. Mineral Production

Mineral deposits were stained and quantified through a protocol previously described [29,30]. The hMSC monolayer was fixed with 10% formalin for 15 min with PBS washing steps both before and after the fixation procedure. The fixed monolayers were incubated with 2 mL of alizarin red S (ARS) solution (Sigma) at a pH of 4.1 for 20 min at room temperature with gentle shaking. Afterwards, the cells were washed with excess ultrapure water until the background staining was maximally cleared. To quantify the amount of mineral that was produced by the differentiating hMSCs, 1.6 mL of 10% acetic acid was added to each well. The plates were then incubated for 30 min at room temperature while shaking at 150 rpm on an orbital shaker. The monolayer of cells were detached using a cell scraper, transferred to a microtube, vortexed, and heated to 85 °C for 10 min after which these tubes were transferred to ice for 5 min. Once the tubes were fully cooled, they were centrifuged at 20,000 g for 15 min. After adding 200 µL of 10% ammonium hydroxide to 500 µL of the supernatant, the samples were quantified against serial dilutions of ARS solution by reading their absorbance at 405 nm.

2.7. IPN + Conditioned Medium Osteogenesis Study

Both static as well as mechanically activated osteocyte conditioned medium were concentrated up to 10 mg/mL of protein content using a Speedvac concentrator (Savant, Carlsbad, CA, USA). The S-CM was then diluted to 0.5 mg/mL (S-CM$_{0.5}$) whereas the MA-CM was both diluted to 5 (MA-CM$_5$) and 0.5 (MA-CM$_{0.5}$) mg/mL. All the conditioned media was then sterile filtered and 10% FBS was added to the media.

Human mesenchymal stromal/stem cells were resuspended into either growth medium with the addition of 10% FBS (GM) or the different conditioned media solutions that were prepared as described before with an appropriate cell density to obtain 500,000 hMSCs per IPN construct. The hydrogels were then cultured for either 1 (GM D1) or 21 days (GM D21, S-CM$_{0.5}$, MA-CM$_{0.5}$, and MA-CM$_5$) in osteogenic medium (growth medium with the addition of 10% FBS and osteogenic factors) with a medium change twice a week. The complete experimental planning for this study is shown in Figure 1.

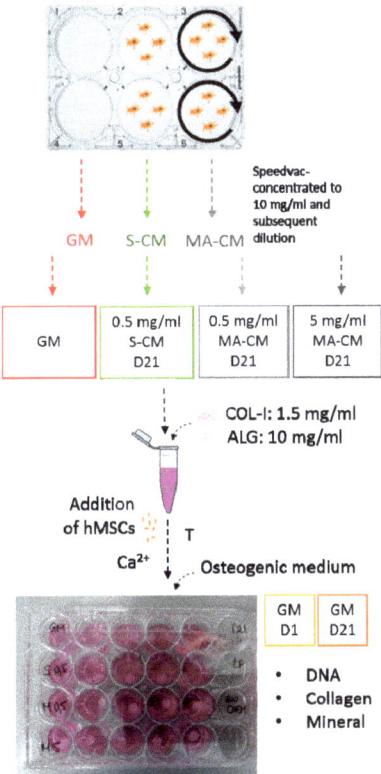

Figure 1. Experimental outline investigating the effect of osteocyte secreted factors on human mesenchymal stromal/stem cells (hMSC) osteogenesis within interpenetrating polymer network (IPN) hydrogels comprising collagen type I (COL-I) and alginate (ALG). Five different groups are investigated: GM = growth medium (α-modification of Eagle's minimal essential medium (α-MEM) supplemented with 10% fetal bovine serum (FBS), 1% Pen/Strep, and 1% L-glutamine), 0.5 mg/mL statically cultured osteocyte conditioned media (S-CM) supplemented with 10% FBS, 0.5 mg/mL mechanically activated osteocyte conditioned media (MA-CM), and 5 mg/mL MA-CM supplemented with 10% FBS. hMSCs were resuspended into these media groups and incorporated into the COL-I/ALG hydrogel subsequently exposed to thermal gelation (T), ionic crosslinking (Ca^{2+}), and cultured for 21 days in osteogenic medium. DNA content, collagen, and mineral deposition was quantified at D1 and D21, n = 5.

Either after 1 or 21 days, the osteogenic media was removed and the IPN was washed with PBS. The materials for biochemical assessment were cut in two and put into 1.5 mL microtubes for either papain or hydrochloric acid digestion. These microtubes were then stored overnight at −80 °C. The histology samples were fixed with 4% PFA for 4 h, dehydrated in 30% EtOH, and stored in 50% EtOH.

2.7.1. DNA Analysis

A papain buffer extract (PBE) was made by adding 0.7098 g of dibasic anhydrous sodium phosphate (Sigma), 0.5998 g monobasic sodium phosphate (Sigma), and 1 mL of 500 mM EDTA to 90 mL of ultrapure water. The pH was brought to 6.5 by adding 38% HCl (Sigma). Ultrapure water was then added up to 100 mL and the solution was sterile filtered to remove dust particles. The papain digestion buffer was activated by adding 63 mg of L-cysteine hydrochloride hydrate (Sigma) together with 3.88 units/mL of papain enzyme to 40 mL of PBE. Samples were removed from the freezer and 472.5 µL of the activated papain buffer extract was added to each microtube before being put on a rocker for 18 h at 60 °C. Then, 27.5 µL of a 1 M sodium citrate solution was subsequently added to fully digest the IPN sample. The samples were then vortexed and centrifuged at 15,000 g for 10 min at 4 °C and the amount of DNA within these samples was obtained with a quant-it picogreen dsDNA assay kit (Invitrogen) by referring to set standards. The emission of both samples and standards was captured at 520 nm after excitation at 480 nm.

2.7.2. Collagen Production

A hydroxyproline assay was performed to quantify the amount of collagen present in the samples as previously described [31]. Briefly, the papain digested sample was combined with PBE and 38% hydrochloric acid. The samples were then incubated at 110 °C for 18 h, cooled, centrifuged, allowed to dry in a fume hood and dissolved in ultrapure water. Hydroxyproline standards were made by serial dilution of the hydroxyproline stock solution. Both standards and samples were subsequently added to a 96-well plate in triplicate. A citrate stock buffer was made as the basis of the assay buffer and the chloramine T reagent which were added to both standards and samples in the 96-well plate. After the oxidation of hydroxyproline, (dimethylamino)benzaldehyde (DMBA) reagent was added and the absorbance of the plate was read at 570 nm. Qualification of the collagen content in the IPN samples was obtained through picrosirius red staining. The histology samples stored in 50% EtOH were further dehydrated in more concentrated EtOH and xylene baths before being embedded in paraffin wax. A microtome was used to slice the samples where after these were put in a water bath and mounted on a glass slide. After drying overnight, picrosirius red staining was applied and a bright-field microscope was used to image with a 2× and 10× objective.

2.7.3. Mineral Production

A calcium assay kit (Sentinel Diagnostics, Milan, Italy) was used to quantify the amount of calcium present in the samples compared to standards which were made as serial dilutions of a 20 µg/mL and 100 µg/mL stock solution based on calcium chloride and hydrochloric acid solutions. Mineral depositions were also visualized through alizarin red staining of the sliced IPN samples. These were then subsequently imaged with a bright-field microscope using a 2× and 10× objective.

2.8. Statistical Analysis

The data obtained in this study was subjected to a statistical analysis with GraphPad Prism v8.2.0 (GraphPad Software, La Jolla, CA, USA) presented as mean ± standard deviation. The different experimental groups were compared using an ordinary one-way ANOVA with Tukey's multiple comparison test. A p-value less than 0.05 was accepted as a significant difference between groups.

3. Results

3.1. Fabrication of an IPN Material with Mechanical Properties Mirroring the Bone Marrow/Osteoid Niche

Figure 2a gives an overview of the IPN hydrogel synthesis where the constant collagen concentration is mixed with different concentrations of alginate. Unconfined compressive testing was performed to quantify the compressive modulus of the developed polymer networks (Figure 2b). Addition of alginate results in a significant considerable increase in the modulus of the material. Whereas the modulus of collagen type I (COL-1) lies around 0.3 kPa, it is increased to around 25 kPa with the addition of 5 mg/mL of alginate (IPN 5). Further addition of alginate results in significantly increased moduli of around 60 kPa (IPN 10) and 85 kPa (IPN 15). To determine the influence of alginate addition to the microstructure of the materials, each IPN was observed under SEM (Figure 2c).

The collagen type I network on its own possesses a fibrillar structure with small pore spaces between the fibers. Addition of 5 mg/mL of alginate reduces these pore spaces and tends to break up the fibrillar structure. When 10 mg/mL of alginate is added to the collagen type I network, the fibrillar microstructure is restored with enlarged pore spaces between the fibers making the structure more open. The pore spaces are further enlarged by the addition of 15 mg/mL of alginate. As the IPN 10 hydrogel possesses both a compressive modulus and a fibrillar porous architecture similar to that previously shown to enhance osteogenesis, this material was utilized for all further experimentation.

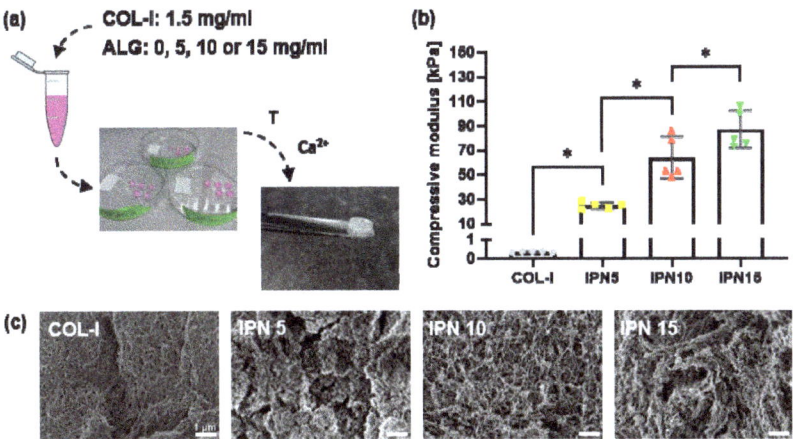

Figure 2. Fabrication of an IPN material mirroring the bone marrow/osteoid niche (**a**) Overview of the IPN synthesis with a 1.5 mg/mL collagen type I (COL-I) concentration and a varying alginate (ALG) concentration of 0, 5, 10, and 15 mg/mL subjected to a collagen type I gelation phase at 37 °C (T) for 30 min next to an ionic crosslinking (Ca^{2+}) phase of alginate at 37 °C for 3 h; (**b**) unconfined compressive modulus compared for four different materials: a collagen type I hydrogel (COL-I), a COL-I/ALG IPN hydrogel with 5 mg/mL alginate (IPN 5), a COL-I/ALG IPN hydrogel with 10 mg/mL alginate (IPN 10), and a COL-I/ALG IPN hydrogel with 15 mg/mL alginate (IPN 15) (n = 5); (**c**) SEM images of COL-I, IPN 5, IPN 10, and IPN 15 (scale bar: 1 µm).

3.2. Paracrine Factors Released by Osteocytes Can Enhance Osteogenic Matrix Deposition by hMSCs in Monolayer Culture

In Figure 3a, an overview of the different media groups is given that will be used in subsequent experiments, i.e., growth media (GM), statically cultured osteocyte conditioned media (S-CM), and mechanically activated osteocyte conditioned media (MA-CM). The proliferation of hMSCs over 21 days was quantified through a picogreen dsDNA assay (Figure 3b). The addition of osteogenic supplements resulted in a significant 2.4-fold increase in proliferation of hMSCs when compared to standard growth medium ($p < 0.05$, n = 5). While an increase in hMSC proliferation was also seen following treatment with S-CM (1.6-fold) and MA-CM (1.7-fold) when compared to GM, this was not significant. This is likely due to the depletion of nutrients in the media during the conditioning procedure. There was also no difference in hMSC proliferation when comparing S-CM to MA-CM.

To determine the effect of osteocyte secreted factors on hMSC matrix deposition, we next analyzed collagen and matrix deposition after 21 days. As expected, the addition of osteogenic supplements resulted in a significant 4-fold ($p < 0.05$, n = 5) increase in collagen deposition (Figure 3c). An increase in collagen deposition following treatment with S-CM (2-fold) and MA-CM (2-fold) was also identified when compared to GM, but this was significantly less than that seen with GM^{ost}. This trend mirrors that seen in the DNA analysis. Interestingly, mineral deposition was significantly altered by factors secreted by osteocytes (Figure 3d). Both the S-CM and MA-CM groups significantly enhanced mineral deposition over both GM and GM^{ost} ($p < 0.05$, n = 5). However, there was no difference in mineralization when comparing S-CM to MA-CM.

Taken together, this data demonstrates that paracrine factors released by osteocytes can enhance osteogenic matrix deposition by hMSCs in monolayer culture, and thus represent potential factors to enhance bone regeneration.

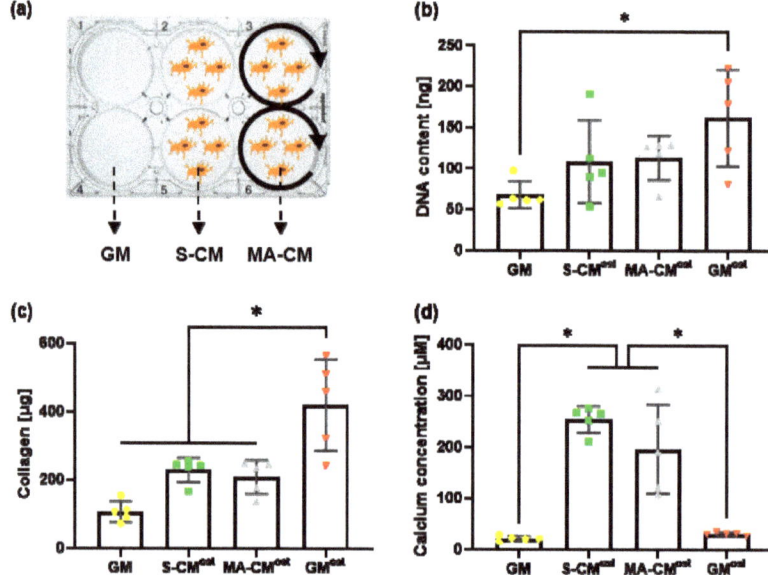

Figure 3. Effect of paracrine factors released by osteocytes on hMSC behavior in 2D cell culture. (a) Overview of the different media groups including growth medium (GM), conditioned medium collected from statically cultured osteocytes (S-CM) and conditioned medium collected from mechanically activated osteocytes (MA-CM); (b) quantification of the DNA content through a picogreen dsDNA kit for hMSCs treated with GM, S-CM^{ost}, MA-CM^{ost}, and the growth medium group supplemented with osteogenic factors (GM^{ost}) (n = 5); (c) quantification of collagen deposition through the amount of bound picrosirius red staining for each medium group (n = 5); (d) quantification of mineral deposition through the amount of bound alizarin red staining for every medium group (n = 5).

3.3. Osteocyte Derived Paracrine Factors Maintain hMSC Viability in Biomimetic IPN Hydrogels

We next looked to combine the paracrine factors released by osteocytes with the IPN materials to achieve a scaffold that recapitulates some of the biochemical and biophysical cues similar to that seen in the bone niche. Figure 4a schematically displays how both the hMSCs and the conditioned medium were incorporated into the IPN 10 material. A picogreen dsDNA assay was used to quantify the viability and proliferation of hMSCs within the IPN hydrogel over 21 days (Figure 4b). All groups show a significant decrease in DNA content compared to the day 1 group, demonstrating that these materials can have adverse effects on viability over long term culture. However, the addition of osteocyte secreted biochemical factors significantly improved cell viability approximately 2-fold ($p < 0.05$, n = 5) when compared to GM alone at day 21. As seen in 2D culture, no difference was seen between S-CM and MA-CM, nor was it influenced by CM concentration.

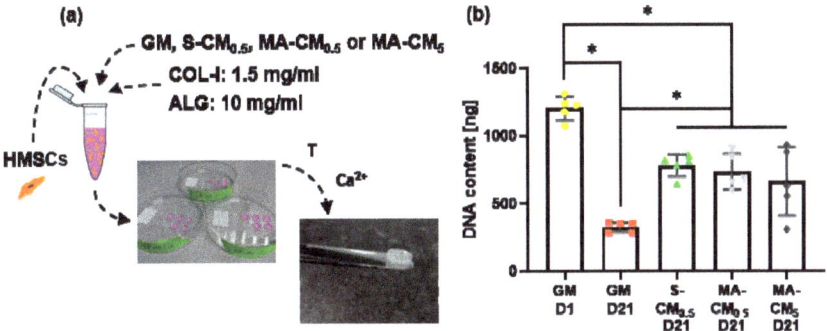

Figure 4. Effect of osteocyte derived paracrine factors on cell viability in IPN 10 hydrogels. (**a**) Schematic overview of the different media groups supplemented with 10% FBS and osteogenic factors including growth medium quantified at both day 1 and day 21 after incorporating the hMSCs into the IPN hydrogel (GM D1 and GM D21), Speedvac-concentrated static osteocyte conditioned medium diluted to a protein content of 0.5 mg/mL quantified at day 21 after hMSC incorporation (S-CM$_{0.5}$ D21), Speedvac-concentrated mechanically activated osteocyte conditioned medium diluted to a protein content of 0.5 mg/mL quantified at day 21 after hMSC incorporation (MA-CM$_{0.5}$ D21), and Speedvac-concentrated mechanically activated osteocyte conditioned medium diluted to a protein content of 5 mg/mL quantified at day 21 after hMSC incorporation (MA-CM$_5$ D21); (**b**) quantification of the DNA content through a picogreen dsDNA kit for the different media groups (n = 5).

3.4. IPN Hydrogels Functionalised with Osteocyte Derived Biochemical Factors Enhance hMSC Osteogenic Matrix Deposition

We next examined whether the osteocyte derived biochemical factors could enhance osteogenic matrix deposition within biomimetic IPN 10 hydrogels. The picrosirius red collagen staining is evident across both the complete IPN hydrogel (Figure 5a, inset) and at a higher magnification (Figure 5a). Furthermore, at high magnification, punctate collagen staining is seen surround entrapped cells demonstrating collagen production by encapsulated cells. Interestingly there is no increase in collagen deposition over 21 days in the GM group but an increasing trend in deposition is seen following the addition of osteocyte secreted factors. The mechanically activated osteocyte conditioned media groups have an overall higher amount of staining across the hydrogels when analyzing the magnified images which is also confirmed in the quantification shown in Figure 5b. This increase in collagen deposition reaches significance in the higher concentration MA-CM compared to the growth media groups ($p < 0.05$, n = 5). The dose-dependent effect can also be observed when comparing both MA-CM groups. This data demonstrates the osteocyte derived factors can enhance hMSC collagen deposition in IPN hydrogels, although high concentrations are required.

Mineralization, as measured by Alizarin red staining, is evident across all groups by day 21 shown in Figure 5c. Interestingly, the GM IPN demonstrated poor mineralization within the center of the material while each of the osteocyte CM IPNs demonstrated good mineralization throughout, with high intensity staining observed surrounding encapsulated cells. Quantifying the mineral deposited, there is significant ~10-fold increase in calcium content after 21 days culture (Figure 5d). The osteocyte CM groups did not significantly influence the total concentration of mineral deposited when compared to GM at day 21 except for the MA-CM at 0.5 mg/mL which demonstrated a reduced total mineral. However, this was corrected when MA-CM concentration was increased to 5 mg/mL. Therefore, osteocyte derived factors do not increase overall quantity of mineral in IPN hydrogels but improves the distribution of mineral throughout the material.

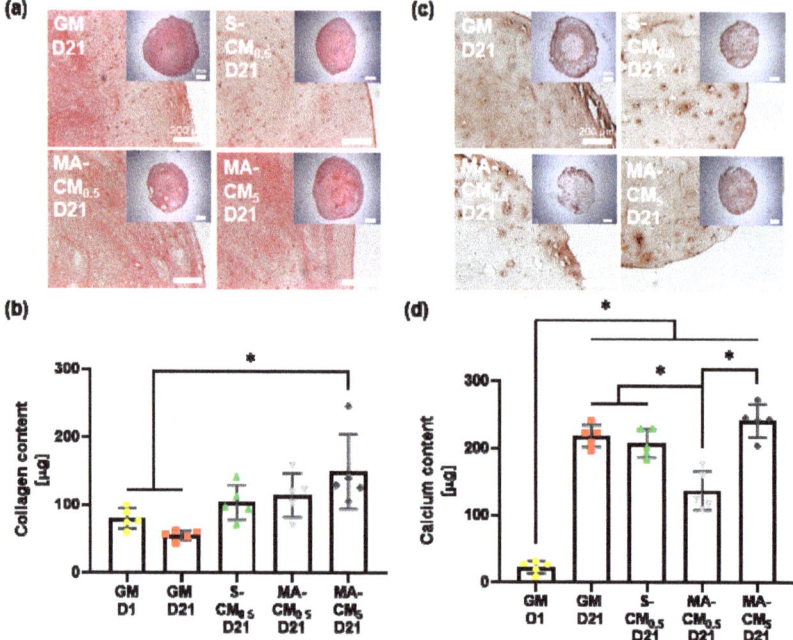

Figure 5. IPN hydrogels functionalized with osteocyte derived biochemical factors enhance hMSC osteogenic matrix deposition. (**a**) Collagen production qualified through picrosirius red staining for the different media groups supplemented with 10% FBS and osteogenic factors including growth media GM D1 and GM D21, osteocyte conditioned medium at 0.5 mg/mL quantified at day 21 after hMSC incorporation (S-$CM_{0.5}$ D21), mechanically activated osteocyte conditioned medium at 0.5 mg/mL and 5 mg/mL quantified at day 21 after hMSC incorporation (MA-$CM_{0.5}$ D21 and MA-CM_5 D21) (scale bar: 200 µm, scale bar inset: 1 mm); (**b**) collagen content quantified with a hydroxyproline assay for every medium group (n = 5); (**c**) mineral production qualified through alizarin red staining for the different media groups (scale bar: 200 µm, scale bar inset: 1 mm); (**d**) mineral content quantified with a calcium assay for every medium group (n = 5).

4. Discussion

Due to the unmet clinical need for new materials to promote skeletal repair, this study aimed to produce novel biomimetic materials to enhance stem/stromal cell osteogenesis and bone repair by recapitulating aspects of the biophysical and biochemical cues found within the bone microenvironment. Utilizing a collagen type I–alginate interpenetrating polymer network we fabricated a material which mirrors the mechanical and structural properties of unmineralized bone, consisting of a porous fibrous matrix with a young's modulus of 64 kPa, both of which have been shown to enhance MSC osteogenesis. Moreover, by combining this material with biochemical paracrine factors released by statically cultured and mechanically stimulated osteocytes, we furthered mirrored the biochemical environment of the bone niche, enhancing stromal/stem cell viability, differentiation and matrix deposition. Therefore, this biomimetic material represents a novel approach to promote skeletal repair.

Various cues have been shown to affect the lineage commitment of bone marrow stromal/stem cells. Collagen type I was selected for this study as this structural protein is the most abundant protein found in bone and exhibits a fibrillar architecture that facilitates cell adherence which has been shown to favor osteogenic differentiation [9,10]. However, collagen alone displays poor mechanical properties. By adding alginate to collagen type I, forming an interpenetrating polymer network, we were able to significantly improve the mechanical properties of the material in terms of compressive modulus.

The IPNs containing 5 and 10 mg/mL alginate possess compressive moduli that lie within the range predicted to be optimal for osteogenesis [8]. The reported electrostatic complexation with alginate further adds to the roughness of the material on the microstructural level which has also been shown to be favorable and hence further adds to the stimulating environment for osteogenic differentiation [14]. Increasing the alginate content of the IPN also resulted in a more open network structure. This can be explained by a reduced number of available nucleation sites for collagen fibrillogenesis due to the choice for a low concentration of collagen type I present in the IPN material as well as the formation of an electrostatic complex with alginate leading to the inhibition of the branching lateral addition of collagen molecules [32]. It was hypothesized that this more open structure would facilitate cell migration and the diffusion of nutrients. Ultimately, the IPN with 10 mg/mL alginate was chosen since it has the highest ability to incorporate both biophysical and biochemical cues present in the bone marrow stromal cell niche.

In vivo, mechanical loading leads to bone formation by recruiting or activating osteoprogenitor cells from the marrow stroma and along the bone surface which subsequently differentiate into bone forming osteoblasts [33,34]. Osteocytes have been shown to play a key role in this bone mechanoadaptation [26,35]. To decipher the potential regenerative properties of biochemical factors released by osteocytes, we collected the secretome of statically cultured and mechanically stimulated osteocytes and utilized this to treat human MSCs and evaluate cell viability/proliferation and osteogenic matrix deposition in 2D culture. Conditioned media, either static or mechanically activated, was found to have a minimal effect on stem cell proliferation, which is consistent with previous findings by Birmingham et al. [23]. This is partially in contrast to Brady et al. who identified a significant increase in murine MSC proliferation following treatment in mechanically activated osteocyte conditioned medium. [25]. However, this discrepancy in proliferative effect may be due to the different species, the different mechanical stimulus that was applied (a rocking platform versus an orbital shaker), the difference in duration of mechanical activation (24 h instead of the 2 h time frame used in this experiment), and finally due to the use of a shorter time point at which proliferation was quantified (day 3 versus day 21). This minimal effect of the osteocyte secretome was also seen in terms of collagen deposition. However, this is in contrast to the mineral production of the conditioned media groups which was significantly increased compared to controls. This is consistent with data obtained by Heino et al. for static osteocyte conditioned medium [24]. Brady et al. found that the normalized calcium concentration of both the mechanically activated osteocyte conditioned medium and the positive control was significantly upregulated compared to static osteocyte conditioned medium and the negative control group [25]. This discrepancy arises possibly because no osteogenic factors were added in their conditioned media groups or, as discussed earlier, due to either a different mechanical activation or the use of another cell type. In conclusion, the main effect of adding osteocyte conditioned medium in terms of matrix deposition can be found in the production of mineral deposits. However, the orbital shaker mechanically activated osteocyte conditioned medium shows the same mineral production as the one observed with static osteocyte conditioned medium, suggesting that a more robust mechanical stimulation regimen is required to harness the benefits of physical loading previously identified.

To elucidate the combined effect of the cues presented in the paracrine signaling of osteocytes and the cues incorporated into the biomaterial, an osteogenic differentiation study was conducted that evaluated both cell viability as well as matrix deposition in 3D cell culture. It was hypothesized that the experimental biomaterial groups that incorporated the conditioned medium would have a more favorable effect on the osteogenic differentiation. Moreover, it was speculated that the concentrated mechanically activated conditioned media group would lead to an enhanced osteogenic differentiation. The number of cells present after 21 days quantified through the amount of DNA content is significantly decreased compared to the negative control at day 1. This could be attributed to a lack of nutrients especially in the center of the hydrogel which can be seen in the histology images of both the collagen production and more pronounced in the mineral production for the growth medium group quantified at day 21. The conditioned media groups still show a significant decrease compared to day 1 although significantly less pronounced than the one identified with the negative control at day 21. This shows that the addition of conditioned medium to the hydrogel positively influences cell survival but is not able to completely turn the issue of cell death in the core of the hydrogel around.

Combining the biophysical cues within collagen based IPN hydrogels with biochemical cues derived from osteocytes, we developed a material that recapitulates aspects of the bone microenvironment, enhanced cell viability and osteogenic matrix deposition. While the IPN material presents a mimetic architecture, it was evident that cell death occurred particularly within the center of this construct over a 21-day period which is indicative of poor nutrient transport. Interestingly, the addition of biochemical factors released by osteocytes significantly improved cell viability. This positive influence of osteocyte derived factors is further evident when examining matrix deposition. Collagen deposition is significantly enhanced by concentrated mechanically activated osteocyte derived factors. Moreover, a uniform distribution of mineralization was clear throughout the material while mineralization is absent in the core of materials lacking osteocyte derived factors. While the increase in mineralization relative to GM controls seen in 2D culture was not found in the IPN materials, this is likely due the inherent osteogenic capacity of the collagen based IPN hydrogel. Taken together this data demonstrates that mimicking aspects of the bone microenvironment can be utilized as a strategy to enhance MSC osteogenesis and bone repair.

There are a number of limitations in this study. For example, the orbital shaker used here was not able to optimally activate osteocytes since the effect of the mechanically activated conditioned medium, despite some minor non-significant trends, did not differ significantly from its static counterpart, as has been previously shown using alternative bioreactors. Although shear stress values reported with the orbital shaker vary between 0.02 and 1.3 Pa, the delivered shear stress distribution might be too low and irregular to achieve a sufficient mechanical activation [36]. Future work should look at a new type of bioreactor that is able to have a higher control over the delivered shear stress distribution, whilst also enabling the generation of large volumes of media. Concentrating the conditioned media should also be explored further as a mechanism to stimulate osteogenesis next to an optimal mechanical activation.

5. Conclusions

In this study we recapitulated aspects of the biophysical and biochemical cues found within the bone microenvironment in a material as a strategy to address the clinical need for novel materials to enhance bone repair. Utilizing a collagen based interpenetrating polymer network we fabricated a material which mirrors the mechanical and structural properties of unmineralized bone, consisting of a porous fibrous matrix with a young's modulus of 64 kPa, both of which have been shown to enhance MSC osteogenesis. Moreover, by combining this material with biochemical paracrine factors released by osteocytes, we furthered mirrored the biochemical environment of the bone niche, enhancing stromal/stem cell viability, differentiation and matrix deposition. Therefore, this biomimetic material represents a novel approach to promote skeletal repair.

Author Contributions: Conceptualization, L.P., M.R. and D.A.H.; methodology, L.P. and M.R.; software, L.P.; validation, L.P.; formal analysis, L.P.; investigation, L.P. and M.R.; resources, D.A.H.; data curation, L.P.; writing—original draft preparation, L.P.; writing—review and editing, D.A.H.; visualization, L.P.; supervision, D.A.H.; project administration, D.A.H.; funding acquisition, D.A.H. All authors have read and agreed to the published version of the manuscript.

Funding: The authors would like to acknowledge funding from European Research Council (ERC) Starting and Proof of Concept Grant (336882 & 825905), Science Foundation Ireland (SFI) Support Grant SFI 13/ERC/L2864 and Interreg 2Seas 3DMed.

Acknowledgments: The authors would like to acknowledge Ian Whelan for his support in the fabrication of the interpenetrating polymer networks.

Conflicts of Interest: The authors declare no conflict of interest. The funders had no role in the design of the study; in the collection, analyses, or interpretation of data; in the writing of the manuscript, or in the decision to publish the results.

References

1. Porter, J.R.; Ruckh, T.T.; Popat, K.C. Bone tissue engineering: A review in bone biomimetics and drug delivery strategies. *Biotechnol. Prog.* **2009**, *25*, 1539–1560. [CrossRef] [PubMed]
2. Turnbull, G.; Clarke, J.; Picard, F.; Riches, P.; Jia, L.; Han, F.; Li, B.; Shu, W. 3d bioactive composite scaffolds for bone tissue engineering. *Bioact. Mater.* **2018**, *3*, 278–314. [CrossRef] [PubMed]
3. Black, C.R.; Goriainov, V.; Gibbs, D.; Kanczler, J.; Tare, R.S.; Oreffo, R.O. Bone tissue engineering. *Curr. Mol. Biol. Rep.* **2015**, *1*, 132–140. [CrossRef] [PubMed]
4. Henkel, J.; Woodruff, M.A.; Epari, D.R.; Steck, R.; Glatt, V.; Dickinson, I.C.; Choong, P.F.; Schuetz, M.A.; Hutmacher, D.W. Bone regeneration based on tissue engineering conceptions—A 21st century perspective. *Bone. Res.* **2013**, *1*, 216–248. [CrossRef] [PubMed]
5. Fishman, J.A.; Greenwald, M.A.; Grossi, P.A. Transmission of infection with human allografts: Essential considerations in donor screening. *Clin. Infect. Dis.* **2012**, *55*, 720–727. [CrossRef] [PubMed]
6. VandeVord, P.J.; Nasser, S.; Wooley, P.H. Immunological responses to bone soluble proteins in recipients of bone allografts. *J. Orthop. Res.* **2005**, *23*, 1059–1064. [CrossRef]
7. Kharkar, P.M.; Kiick, K.L.; Kloxin, A.M. Designing degradable hydrogels for orthogonal control of cell microenvironments. *Chem. Soc. Rev.* **2013**, *42*, 7335–7372. [CrossRef]
8. Engler, A.J.; Sen, S.; Sweeney, H.L.; Discher, D.E. Matrix elasticity directs stem cell lineage specification. *Cell* **2006**, *126*, 677–689. [CrossRef]
9. McBeath, R.; Pirone, D.M.; Nelson, C.M.; Bhadriraju, K.; Chen, C.S. Cell shape, cytoskeletal tension, and rhoa regulate stem cell lineage commitment. *Development. Cell.* **2004**, *6*, 483–495. [CrossRef]
10. Oh, S.; Brammer, K.S.; Li, Y.S.J.; Teng, D.; Engler, A.J.; Chien, S.; Jin, S. Stem cell fate dictated solely by altered nanotube dimension. *Proc. Natl. Acad. Sci. USA* **2009**, *106*, 2130–2135. [CrossRef]
11. Brennan, C.M.; Eichholz, K.F.; Hoey, D.A. The effect of pore size within fibrous scaffolds fabricated using melt electrowriting on human bone marrow stem cell osteogenesis. *Biomed. Mater.* **2019**, *14*, 065016. [CrossRef] [PubMed]
12. Eichholz, K.F.; Hoey, D.A. Mediating human stem cell behaviour via defined fibrous architectures by melt electrospinning writing. *Acta Biomater.* **2018**, *75*, 140–151. [CrossRef] [PubMed]
13. Dalby, M.J.; Gadegaard, N.; Tare, R.; Andar, A.; Riehle, M.O.; Herzyk, P.; Wilkinson, C.D.; Oreffo, R.O. The control of human mesenchymal cell differentiation using nanoscale symmetry and disorder. *Nat. Mater.* **2007**, *6*, 997–1003. [CrossRef] [PubMed]
14. Faia-Torres, A.B.; Guimond-Lischer, S.; Rottmar, M.; Charnley, M.; Goren, T.; Maniura-Weber, K.; Spencer, N.D.; Reis, R.L.; Textor, M.; Neves, N.M. Differential regulation of osteogenic differentiation of stem cells on surface roughness gradients. *Biomaterials* **2014**, *35*, 9023–9032. [CrossRef] [PubMed]
15. Reznikov, N.; Shahar, R.; Weiner, S. Bone hierarchical structure in three dimensions. *Acta. Biomater.* **2014**, *10*, 3815–3826. [CrossRef] [PubMed]
16. Werner, M.; Kurniawan, N.A.; Bouten, C.V. Cellular geometry sensing at different length scales and its implications for scaffold design. *Materials* **2020**, *13*, 963. [CrossRef] [PubMed]
17. Wolff, J. Das gesetz der transformation der knochen. *Dtsch. Med. Wochenschr.* **1892**, *47*, 1222–1224. [CrossRef]
18. Bonewald, L.F.; Johnson, M.L. Osteocytes, mechanosensing and wnt signaling. *Bone* **2008**, *42*, 606–615. [CrossRef]
19. Bakker, A.; Klein-Nulend, J.; Burger, E. Shear stress inhibits while disuse promotes osteocyte apoptosis. *Biochem. Biophys. Res. Commun.* **2004**, *320*, 1163–1168. [CrossRef]
20. Bakker, A.D.; Soejima, K.; Klein-Nulend, J.; Burger, E.H. The production of nitric oxide and prostaglandin e(2) by primary bone cells is shear stress dependent. *J. Biomech.* **2001**, *34*, 671–677. [CrossRef]
21. Burger, E.H.; Klein-Nulend, J. Mechanotransduction in bone - Role of the lacuno-canalicalur network. *Fed. Am. Soc. Exp. Biol.* **1999**, *13*, 101–112.
22. Schaffler, M.B.; Kennedy, O.D. Osteocyte signaling in bone. *Curr. Osteoporos. Rep.* **2012**, *10*, 118–125. [CrossRef] [PubMed]
23. Birmingham, E.; Niebur, G.L.; McHugh, P.E.; Shaw, G.; Barry, F.P.; McNamara, L.M. Osteogenic differentiation of mesenchymal stem cells is regulated by osteocyte and osteoblast cells in a simplified bone niche. *Eur. Cells Mater.* **2012**, *23*, 13–27. [CrossRef] [PubMed]

24. Heino, T.J.; Hentunen, T.A.; Vaananen, H.K. Conditioned medium from osteocytes stimulates the proliferation of bone marrow mesenchymal stem cells and their differentiation into osteoblasts. *Exp. Cell. Res.* **2004**, *294*, 458–468. [CrossRef] [PubMed]
25. Brady, R.T.; O'Brien, F.J.; Hoey, D.A. Mechanically stimulated bone cells secrete paracrine factors that regulate osteoprogenitor recruitment, proliferation, and differentiation. *Biochem. Biophys. Res. Commun.* **2015**, *459*, 118–123. [CrossRef]
26. Hoey, D.A.; Kelly, D.J.; Jacobs, C.R. A role for the primary cilium in paracrine signaling between mechanically stimulated osteocytes and mesenchymal stem cells. *Biochem. Biophys. Res. Commun.* **2011**, *412*, 182–187. [CrossRef] [PubMed]
27. Kato, Y.; Windle, J.J.; Koop, B.A.; Mundy, G.R.; Bonewald, L.F. Establishment of an osteocyte-like cell line, mlo-y4. *J. Bone Miner. Res.* **1997**, *12*, 2014–2023. [CrossRef]
28. Rosser, J.; Bonewald, L.F. Studying osteocyte function using the cell lines mlo-y4 and mlo-a5. In *Bone Research Protocols*; Springer Humana Press: Totowa, NJ, USA, 2012; pp. 67–81.
29. Stavenschi, E.; Corrigan, M.A.; Johnson, G.P.; Riffault, M.; Hoey, D.A. Physiological cyclic hydrostatic pressure induces osteogenic lineage commitment of human bone marrow stem cells: A systematic study. *Stem. Cell. Res. Ther.* **2018**, *9*, 276. [CrossRef]
30. Corrigan, M.A.; Coyle, S.; Eichholz, K.F.; Riffault, M.; Lenehan, B.; Hoey, D.A. Aged osteoporotic bone marrow stromal cells demonstrate defective recruitment, mechanosensitivity, and matrix deposition. *Cells Tissues. Organs.* **2019**, *207*, 83–96. [CrossRef]
31. Kafienah, W.; Sims, T.J. Biochemical methods for the analysis of tissue-engineered cartilage. In *Biopolymer Methods in Tissue Engineering*; Hollander, A.P., Hatton, P.V., Eds.; Humana Press: Totowa, NJ, USA, 2004; pp. 217–229.
32. Sang, L.; Wang, X.; Chen, Z.; Lu, J.; Gu, Z.; Li, X. Assembly of collagen fibrillar networks in the presence of alginate. *Carbohydr. Polym.* **2010**, *82*, 1264–1270. [CrossRef]
33. Liu, C.; Cabahug-Zuckerman, P.; Stubbs, C.; Pendola, M.; Cai, C.; Mann, K.A.; Castillo, A.B. Mechanical loading promotes the expansion of primitive osteoprogenitors and organizes matrix and vascular morphology in long bone defects. *J. Bone. Miner. Res.* **2019**, *34*, 896–910. [CrossRef] [PubMed]
34. Turner, C.H.; Owan, I.; Alvey, T.; Hulman, J.; Hock, J.M. Recruitment and proliferative responses of osteoblasts after mechanical loading in vivo determined using sustained-release bromodeoxyuridine. *Bone* **1998**, *22*, 463–469. [CrossRef]
35. Klein-Nulend, J.; van der Plas, A.; Semeins, C.M.; Ajubi, N.E.; Frangos, J.A.; Nijweide, P.J.; Burger, E.H. Sensitivity of osteocytes to biomechanical stress in vitro. *FASEB J.* **1995**, *9*, 441–445. [CrossRef] [PubMed]
36. Salek, M.M.; Sattari, P.; Martinuzzi, R.J. Analysis of fluid flow and wall shear stress patterns inside partially filled agitated culture well plates. *Ann. Biomed. Eng.* **2012**, *40*, 707–728. [CrossRef]

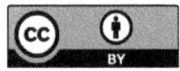

© 2020 by the authors. Licensee MDPI, Basel, Switzerland. This article is an open access article distributed under the terms and conditions of the Creative Commons Attribution (CC BY) license (http://creativecommons.org/licenses/by/4.0/).

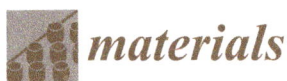

Article

Human Olfactory Mucosa Stem Cells Delivery Using a Collagen Hydrogel: As a Potential Candidate for Bone Tissue Engineering

Sara Simorgh [1,2], Peiman Brouki Milan [1,2,*], Maryam Saadatmand [3], Zohreh Bagher [2,4], Mazaher Gholipourmalekabadi [1,2], Rafieh Alizadeh [4], Ahmad Hivechi [1], Zohreh Arabpour [5,6], Masoud Hamidi [7] and Cédric Delattre [8,9,*]

1 Cellular and Molecular Research Centre, Iran University of Medical Sciences, Tehran 1591639675, Iran; srsimorgh@gmail.com (S.S.); mazaher.gholipour@gmail.com (M.G.); ahmadhivechi2020@gmail.com (A.H.)
2 Department of Tissue Engineering and Regenerative Medicine, Faculty of Advanced Technologies in Medicine, Iran University of Medical Sciences, Tehran 1591639675, Iran; Baharebagher@gmail.com
3 Department of Chemical and Petroleum Engineering, Sharif University of Technology, Tehran 111559465, Iran; m.saadatmand@sharif.edu
4 ENT and Head and Neck Research Center and Department, Hazrat Rasoul Akram Hospital, The Five Senses Health Institute, Iran University of Medical Sciences, Tehran 1445613111, Iran; nafiseh.alizadeh@gmail.com
5 Department of Tissue Engineering and Applied Cell Sciences, School of Advanced Technologies in Medicine, Tehran University of Medical Sciences, Tehran 1417613151, Iran; arabpourzohreh@gmail.com
6 Iranian Tissue Bank & Research Center, Tehran University of Medical Sciences, Teheran 1419733141, Iran
7 Department of Medical Biotechnology, Faculty of Paramedicine, Guilan University of Medical Sciences, Rasht 4477166595, Iran; Masoud.Hamidi@ulb.be
8 Université Clermont Auvergne, Clermont Auvergne INP, CNRS, Institut Pascal, F-63000 Clermont-Ferrand, France
9 Institut Universitaire de France (IUF), 1 Rue Descartes, 75005 Paris, France
* Correspondence: brouki.p@iums.ac.ir (P.B.M.); cedric.delattre@uca.fr (C.D.)

Abstract: For bone tissue engineering, stem cell-based therapy has become a promising option. Recently, cell transplantation supported by polymeric carriers has been increasingly evaluated. Herein, we encapsulated human olfactory ectomesenchymal stem cells (OE-MSC) in the collagen hydrogel system, and their osteogenic potential was assessed in vitro and in vivo conditions. Collagen type I was composed of four different concentrations of (4 mg/mL, 5 mg/mL, 6 mg/mL, 7 mg/mL). SDS-Page, FTIR, rheologic test, resazurin assay, live/dead assay, and SEM were used to characterize collagen hydrogels. OE-MSCs encapsulated in the optimum concentration of collagen hydrogel and transplanted in rat calvarial defects. The tissue samples were harvested after 4- and 8-weeks post-transplantation and assessed by optical imaging, micro CT, and H&E staining methods. The highest porosity and biocompatibility were confirmed in all scaffolds. The collagen hydrogel with 7 mg/mL concentration was presented as optimal mechanical properties close to the naïve bone. Furthermore, the same concentration illustrated high osteogenic differentiation confirmed by real-time PCR and alizarin red S methods. Bone healing has significantly occurred in defects treated with OE-MSCs encapsulated hydrogels in vivo. As a result, OE-MSCs with suitable carriers could be used as an appropriate cell source to address clinical bone complications.

Keywords: tissue engineering; collagen hydrogel; cell delivery; bone regeneration; olfactory ectomesenchyme stem cells

1. Introduction

Bone defects represent a primary concern of disability worldwide [1]. Although there have been enormous advances in developing new drugs, surgical methods and treatment modalities, clinical outcomes remain fundamentally undesirable in many patients. Autologous bone grafting has been popularized as a therapeutic tool, accelerating the overgrowth of cells that can regenerate new bone tissue [2]. Restricted access to bone tissue has been widely challenged in the clinic [3]. Hence, developing new strategies for bone regeneration is highly required. As a new area with a clinical prospect, tissue engineering has emerged as powerful platforms for tissue reconstruction [4].

Biomaterials as a main component of tissue engineering have emerged as effective cell delivery systems to accelerate their survival and proliferation rate and differentiation capacity [5]. Up to now, many types of polymeric materials and bone substitutes have been studied and developed to regenerate bone defects. Among them, hydrogels contain hydrophilic cross-linked networks with water-swelling capacity have a great potential to increase cell adhesion and migration with biodegradation property [6]. Therefore, these bioactive three-dimensional scaffolds provide appropriate conditions for cell proliferation and differentiation. Living cells can be encapsulated in hydrogels as a cell delivery system and can be easily transferred to the target region for tissue regeneration [7].

Collagen is one of the most important structural proteins in the extracellular matrix (ECM). A large and growing body of literature has emphasized the application of collagen in medicine owing to its supreme biocompatibility and low immunogenicity [8]. Since bone ECM is composed of hydroxyapatite mineral deposits in collagen type I substrate, collagen hydrogel can be a suitable candidate for stem cell encapsulation with flexibility analogous to natural tissue features for bone regeneration [9]. Additionally, the different type of stem cell has been examined in the tissue engineering field and can be isolated from adult and embryonic tissues [10]. Immunomodulatory effects, releasing paracrine molecules, and remarkable angiogenic capacity are known as the leading mechanisms for tissue regeneration [11]. Various mesenchymal stem cells (MSC) sources, such as dental pulp MSCs, human amniotic MSCs, placental-derived MSCs, and mesenchymal cell derived from bone marrow and adipose tissue, have been identified for bone regeneration [12]. Clinical trials of autologous adult stem cells transplantation for bone repair exhibited long term safety and efficacy [13]. Researchers have shown a growing trend towards using olfactory-derived ectomesenchymal stem cells (OE-MSC) as an appropriate available stem cell source for therapeutic strategies [14–16]. Human olfactory mucosa consists of two layers, lamina propria, and the epithelial layer. The globose and basal cells lay quiescent in the epidermal layer of olfactory mucosa, involving epithelial regeneration. The olfactory mucosa also contains multipotent cells in the lamina propria with neuronal and mesenchymal properties. These stem cells have been considered as a new family of MSCs due to their easy accessibility and autologous grafting ability [17,18] to solve immune system rejection and ethical issues in clinical trials [19].

There has been exciting research that recognized the critical immunomodulatory role played by olfactory-derived stem cells via releasing TGF-B and IL10 [20]. Moreover, it has been shown that OE-MSCs have a higher differentiation capacity into osteocyte than progenitor cells found in the umbilical cord [15,21]. OE-MSCs have been successfully used for nerve regeneration [22,23]. Due to its capacity to osteocyte [17], It can be appropriate sources for in vivo study of bone regeneration. However, no comprehensive research has been performed on OE-MSCs and their application in vivo condition for bone tissue engineering.

The main questions have been raised about the behavior of human OE-MSCs in an osteogenic microenvironment. Accordingly, in this research, we encapsulated human OE-MSCs in a collagen hydrogel system, and their osteogenic potential was evaluated in vitro conditions. After optimization of collagen concentration, we transplanted this system to assess in vivo bone condition in a rat calvaria defection.

2. Materials and Methods

2.1. Materials

Ethylenediaminetetraacetic acid (EDTA) was purchased from Gibco, Canada Inc. Ethanol, methanol, and acetic acid (100%) were obtained from Merck, Germany. Polyacrylamide, Alizarin Red, Dil, The fetal bovine serum was given by Gibco (FBS). Primers and cDNA synthesis kit were obtained from Sinaclon, IRAN. B-glycerophosphate and dexamethasone were prepared from SANTA CRUZ biotechnology. The SYBR-Green PCR Master Mix was given by ThermoFisher Scientific in the United Kingdom.

2.2. Ethics

This investigation was confirmed by IUMS Ethical Committee (NO; IR.IUMS.REC. 1399.020). All procedure performed according to the University guidelines.

2.3. Experimental Studies

2.3.1. Isolation and Characterization of Cells

Olfactory mucosa samples were harvested from human sources and processed, as previously defined [1]. Shortly, the tissue pieces were minced and transferred to a sterile dish, and OE-MSCs isolation was carried out as previously reported [2]. The isolated cells were cultured in DMEM/F12 nutrient mixture and proliferated. After that, cells were characterized by flow cytometry assessment for specific proteins like CD90, CD29, CD105, CD31, and CD34. The adipogenic and osteogenic capacity of stem cells were assessed on day 21. Moreover, to detect mesenchymal cells markers, immunocytochemistry was done, and the expression of nestin and vimentin were assessed.

2.3.2. Collagen Extraction, Hydrogel Preparation, and Characterization

Rat Tail Collagen Type I Extraction

First of all, we harvested tendons from the rat tails [3]. Tissue samples transferred to a petri dish containing 70% ethanol. The tendons then were separated from the sheath attached to the vertebrae. The extracted tendons were transferred in 0.02% acetic acid under moderate vibration at 4 °C. After that, the solution was centrifuged for 1 h at $12,000 \times g$ and deposited at -80 °C. The frozen solution was transferred to a freeze dryer machine to obtain dried collagen.

Fourier Transform Infrared Spectroscopy (FTIR)

The detection of amide bands was done using Fourier transform infrared spectroscopy (FTIR) [4]. The spectra were collected in a Nicolet 6700 spectrometer (Mundelein, IL, USA) and documented with a resolution of 4 cm in 1 over 64 scans.

Gel Electrophoresis

Gel electrophoresis sodium dodecyl sulfate-polyacrylamide (SDS-PAGE) was carried out to detect collagen type I according to previous studies [5]. Gel electrophoresis was prepared by a combination of running and stacking gels. After electrophoresis, the gels were set and dyed in Coomassie Blue R-250 (0.1%) for four hours at 60 °C in a 25% solution; then several rinses in a decolorizer solution containing methanol, acetic acid, and water (2:3:35, V/V) dissolved the residual stain.

Hydrogel Preparation and OE-MSCs Encapsulation

Collagen type I extracted from rat tail was dissolved in 1 mL acetic acid 2 N. This solution was mixed with phosphate buffer saline (10 × PBS) and NaOH (1N) at pH 7.4 while kept on ice [6] and was prepared in four final separate concentrations including 4 mg/mL, 5 mg/mL, 6 mg/mL, and 7 mg/mL. The human OE-MSCs pellet was resuspended in cell culture medium and 1×10^4 cells/mL mixed into the non-gelated collagen mixture, followed by immediate gelation in 37 °C incubation, and the cell culture medium was added on top of the gelated hydrogels [7].

Field Emission Scanning Electron Microscopy

The morphology and elemental composition of the specimens were determined using digital field emission scanning electron microscopy [8]. OE-MSCs had been cultured separately on four concentrations of hydrogels (4 mg/mL, 5 mg/mL, 6 mg/mL, and 7 mg/mL)

for 48 h; until drying with a critical point dryer, the encapsulated OE-MSCs in four concentrations of collagen hydrogels is dehydrated in a graded sequence of ethanol concentrations. Gold was sputtered on the dried specimens. The spectrum was mapped and analyzed using energy dispersive spectroscopy (TESCAN CLARA, Brno-Kohoutovice, Czechia).

Porosity Assessment

To determine porosity of scaffolds, the liquid displacement method was done [9]. Ethanol was applied for liquid displacement because it did not cause shrinking or swelling of the scaffold. The scaffolds were weighed, soaked in ethanol for 30 min, and then the weight of the scaffolds in ethanol [10] was determined. The filter paper was used to extract the ethanol from the scaffold base, and the weight of the wet scaffold (ww) was also calculated ($n = 3$). The scaffold porosity was estimated by Equation:

$$\text{Porosity (\%)} = (ww - wd)/(ww - wl) \times 100$$

Rheological Analysis

The effect of concentration on the storage (G') and loss modulus (G'') of collagen hydrogels was evaluated by rheometric mechanical spectroscopy (RMS) tests using an MCR300 rheometer (Anton Paar, Graz, Austria) equipped with a cone-plate geometry [11]. For sample preparation, the hydrogels were poured into a mold and then placed on the plate of the rheometer; and before beginning the procedure, surface water was carefully removed with tissue paper. Frequency sweeps were performed at frequencies ranging from 0.01 to 100 Hz. At a stable temperature of 37 °C, both tests were carried out.

OE-MSCs Viability and Proliferation Assessment

The viability of human OE-MSCs was quantified using a live/dead viability package (ThermoFisher, Berlin, Germany), following the manufacturer's staining protocol [11]. Briefly, after stem cell encapsulation in collagen hydrogels on days 1, 7, and 14, the samples were dyed for 10 min after the culture medium was extracted. The cells were then washed with PBS and observed under the fluorescence microscope. By staining the hydrogels with fluorescent diacetate (FDA) and propidium iodide (PI), the existence of encapsulated OE-MSCs was determined. FDA indicates living cells with green fluorescence, while PI indicates dead cells with red fluorescence. Furthermore, for proliferation quantitative evaluation, resazurin kit (Kiazist, Tehran, Iran) was used at various time points (1st, 7th, and 14th days after stem cell encapsulation). Following the removal of the media, 10 mL of resazurin reagent containing 180 mL of serum-free medium was applied to each well of a 96-well plate and incubated for 4 h at 37 °C. Using a microplate reader, the absorbance values of each well were calculated at 570 nm.

Osteogenic Differentiation

Encapsulated OE-MSCs were included in collagen hydrogels containing 10% minimum essential medication eagle alpha modification (Alpha MEM) supplemented with fetal bovine serum, 1% PS, 50 g/mL L-ascorbic acid, 100 nM dexamethasone, and 10 mM b-glycerophosphate in the osteogenic separation media [12]. For two to three weeks, the culture medium was updated twice a week.

ECM Mineralization

Alizarin Red S staining as a quantitative and qualitative evaluation was done to extracellular matrix mineralization study on day 21. The samples were set in 10% formalin at room temperature before being stained with Alizarin Red (catalogue N 5533-25G, Sigma–Aldrich) for 30 min at a pH of 4.1 to 4.5. The samples were then washed three times with purified water and photographed under a microscope in each well. The 10% acetic acid was applied to samples and incubated for 30 min at room temperature to determine calcium content. After being heated for 10 min at 85 °C, the sample was put on ice for 5 min before being centrifuged at 20,000 g for 15 min. A total of 200 µL of supernatant is combined with 75 µL of 10% ammonium hydroxide. Alizarin red staining was assessed using a plate reader (BioTek, Oxfordshire, UK) set to 405 nm and light microscopic images [13].

Gene Expression of Bone Markers

On days 14 and 21, gene expression for the osteogenic markers runt-related transcription factor 2 (Runx2), collagen type I (Col 1), osteopontin (OPN), osteocalcin [14], and alkaline phosphatase was determined using real-time PCR. According to manufacturer protocol [15], max RNA was collected from the samples of five classes using an RNX-plus solution (PRIMA Scientific Co, Favorgen, Thai). Then, using oligo [16] primers and a cDNA synthesis package (QIAGEN-BIOTECH, Hilden, Germany), complete RNA was transformed to cDNA, and real-time RT-PCR analysis was performed using PCR master mix green-high RoxA325402, and the operation was built using the ABI step one unit (Applied Biosystems, Sequences Detection Systems, Foster City, CA, USA) for 40 cycles.

2.4. In Vivo Study

2.4.1. Calvarial Defect Model

Parietal calvarial defects were made in two-month-old male rats with an average weight of 200 to 250 g. The animals were anaesthetized by intramuscular injection of ketamine hydrochloride (35 mg/kg) and xylazine (2 mg/kg). To expose the parietal bone, a break was made just outside the sagittal midline. To avoid dora perforation, the pericranium was cut, and a 7 mm defect on the calvaria was produced with a trifoliate drill [17]. The surgical site was cleaned with a saline solution. The rats were randomly divided into three groups ($n = 5$) as follows: group 1: calvarial defection without any treatment as a control group; group 2: calvarial defection treated by 7 mg/mL collagen hydrogel (blank scaffold); and group 3: calvarial defection treated by OE-MSCs that encapsulated in 7 mg/mL collagen hydrogel (OE MSCs).

2.4.2. OE-MSCs Labelling and Implantation

DiI dye was used as a fluorescent lipophilic cationic carbocyanine to tag OE-MSCs membranes. According to the protocol mentioned in a previous study [18,19], OE-MSCs were tagged with 4 µg/mL DiI for 30 min at 37 °C and then OE-MSCs were washed twice with PBS. Each defect in the Hydrogel+OE-MSCs group was filled with 1×10^6 OE-MSCs encapsulated in 1 mL of 7 mg/mL collagen hydrogel. The skin was sutured after implantation.

2.4.3. Optical Imaging

DiI-labelled human OE-MSCs tracing was performed to evaluate the survival of OE-MSCs after 72 h in rat calvaria defection [20]. Therefore, 72 h after transplantation, optical images were taken by Kodak FX (Connecticut 06511, USA) pro system to stem cell tracing.

2.4.4. Micro-Computed Tomography

Four and eight weeks after surgical implantation, samples were taken. At any time point, the animals were sacrificed by CO_2 asphyxiation with cervical dislocation. The calvaria of the skull was removed and retained in 10% formalin. The reconstructed cranium morphology was assessed using a micro-CT system (LOTUS-NDT, Behin Negareh Co., Tehran, Iran). The voltage and current of the X-ray tube are set to 80 kV and 85 A, respectively. In this analysis, no additional filtration was used. The scan took about 2 h, with a nominal resolution of 10 microns. The LOTUS NDT-ACQ program handled both protocol configurations. LOTUS NDT-REC was used to reconstruct the acquired 3D data using a simple Feldkamp, Davis, Kress (FDK) algorithm [21]. On the defect field, a 7 mm diameter volume of interest (VOI) was chosen. Then, because the sample had soft tissue and different parts, thresholding was used for the segmentation of VOI into other parts. Then, by calculating the number of voxels related to newly formed bone, bone volume

(BV) was obtained, and the amount of bone volume fraction in VOI was calculated with BV/TV. TV: total volume of regenerated bone, pores, and soft tissue trapped in analyzed 3D volume of interest (VOI) selected on structures (unit: mm^3). BV: volume of regenerated bone-in analyzed 3D volume of interest (VOI) selected on structures (unit: mm^3). Bone volume fraction: The fraction of BV/TV (unit: percent).

2.4.5. Hematoxylin and Eosin (H&E) Staining

In order to evaluate bone formation, H&E staining was carried out [22]. After fixing the samples in 4% paraformaldehyde, After decalcification, the tissues were dehydrated in an ascending sequence of ethanol and then placed in paraffin. Sections that were 5 m thick were prepared and stained with (H&E). The reconstructed bone tissue photograph obtained under a microscope (ZEISS Axio Scope A1, Oberkochen, Germany) was quantified using ImageJ software.

2.5. Statistical Evaluation

The statistical analysis in this article was performed using the Graph Pad PRISM 7.03 software. All findings were evaluated using Student's t-tests for two comparisons and one-way ANOVA analysis of variance followed by Tukey's test. Both statistical data are shown using the mean and standard deviation of the mean. The statistical significance level was set at $p \leq 0.05$.

3. Results

3.1. Collagen Type I Extracted from Rat Tail and Characterized Next Prepared Collagen Hydrogel

Collagen type I was lyophilized and dissolved at a concentration of 7 mg/mL in acetic acid. The self-assembly of collagen was done in pH 7.4 and 37 °C. The hydrogel was injected easily and continually via a 0.7 mm diameter syringe (Figure 1A–C).

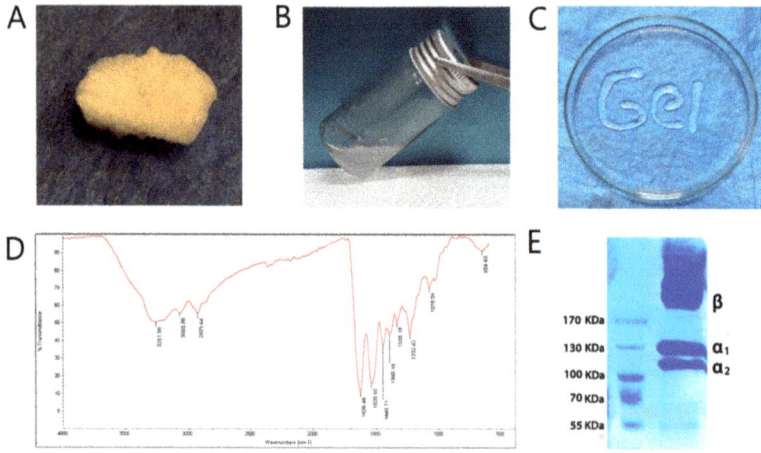

Figure 1. Characterization of collagen type I, which is extracted from rat tail. (**A**) The freeze-dried collagen; (**B**) the collagen solution at 7 mg/mL concentration; (**C**) self-assembled collagen, in pH 7.4 and 37 °C was injected via a 0.7 mm diameter syringe; (**D**) The FTIR spectrum shows the presence of specific molecular vibrations such as amide A, amide B, amide I, amide II, and amide III, which certified the attendance of type 1 collagen structure; (**E**) The inclusion of monomer α_1, α_2, and β dimers and dimers in sodium dodecyl sulfate-polyacrylamide electrophoresis data revealed collagen type I structure. In addition, the same molecular weight (MW) was found between the collagens.

The spectrum in FTIR showed the absorption peaks at 3251.95 cm^{-1} is associated with –OH. The band at 2923.64 cm^{-1} has corresponded with CH3 and CH2 symmetric stretching, respectively. At 1446.71 cm^{-1}, the C-N deformation reached its maximum. The bands at 1626.48 cm^{-1}, 1535.60 cm^{-1}, and 1232.42 cm^{-1}, respectively, reflect Amide I (C=O), Amide II (N-H stretching and C-N deformation), and Amide III (C-N deformation and N-H stretching) (Figure 1D). SDS-PAGE was carried out to certify the type of collagen extracted from the rat tail. The protein ingredients were isolated according to their electrophoresis volubility (Figure 1E). The extracted collagen showed two distinct bands that are attributed to two different types of α chain and β-chains. The molecular weight of $α_1$ collagen type I was about 125 kDa, while $α_2$ was approximately 110 kDa, and β-chains was higher than 170 kDa. Additionally, the ratio of the $α_1$ band was higher than the $α_2$ band (Figure 1E).

3.2. OE-MSCs Isolated from Human Olfactory Mucosa and Characterized

Based on the images obtained from the optical microscope, the morphology of OE-MSCs isolated from human olfactory mucosa appears to be completely homogeneous. It resembles the spindle-like mesenchymal cells (Figure 2A). Furthermore, immunocytochemistry analysis showed the significant expression of nestin and vimentin as neuronal and mesenchymal markers, respectively (Figure 2A).

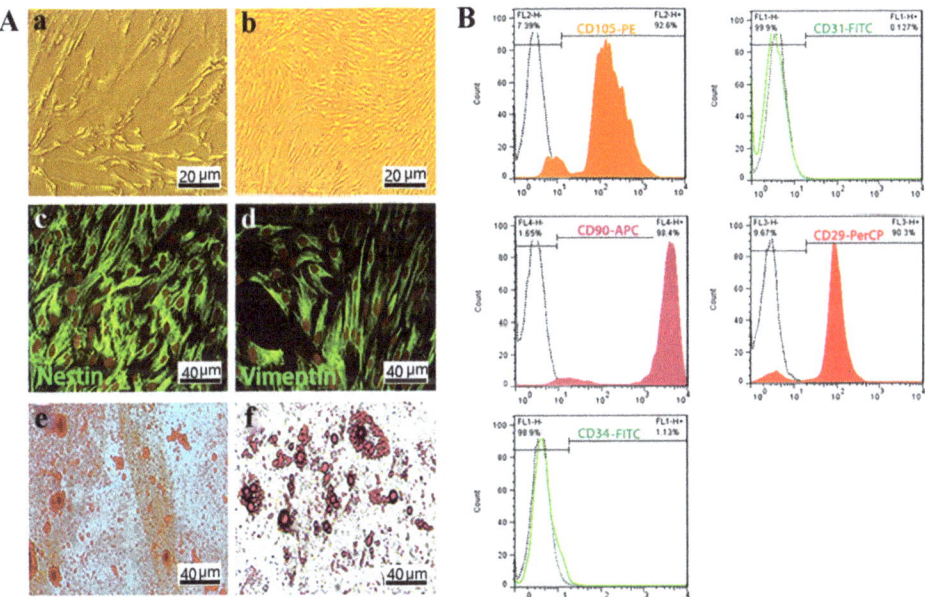

Figure 2. OE-MSCs characterization. (**A**) Morphology of OE-MSCs in passage one. Scale bar: 20 μm; (**a,b**) Morphology of OE-MSCs in passage three which was described as a spindle-like morphology. Scale bar: 10 μm; Immunocytochemistry of OE-MSCs to characterized specific neural crest and mesenchymal markers; (**c**) nestin; and (**d**) vimentin by immunofluorescence staining. Osteogenic and adipogenic differentiation of OE-MSCs, respectively; (**e,f**) Scale bar: 40 μm. (**B**) Flow cytometric assessment to characterization of OE-MSCs surface markers; including CD29 as a positive marker; CD31 as a negative marker; CD105 as a positive marker; CD90 as a positive marker; and CD34 as a negative marker.

Besides, the differentiation of human OE-MSCs into osteoblasts and adipocytes was assessed by Alizarin red S and Oil red O staining, respectively, with the results suggesting high mineralization and high adipogenic potency of OE-MSCs (Figure 2A).

The OE-MSCs is positive for CD90, CD29, and CD105 in greater than 98.4%, 90.3%, and 92.6% of the time, respectively, according to flow cytometry study as MSCs special surface markers. In addition, these cells were negative for CD31 and CD34, respectively, 0.127% and 1.13% (Figure 2B).

3.3. The Increase in the Concentration of Collagen Leads to Enhance Stem Cell Viability and Proliferation of OE-MSCs

Based on the images obtained from the live/dead assay (Figure 3A), the OE-MSCs attachment and proliferation with elongated (green) morphology in collagen hydrogel were evident in all samples. Cell proliferation was related to collagen concentration and cell culture time. On day 14, the highest cell proliferation and survival were observed in the collagen 7 mg/mL group, and cell density was higher on day 7 than on day 1. In comparison, the highest density was shown on day 14. Only a small number of dead (red) cells were visible in all samples.

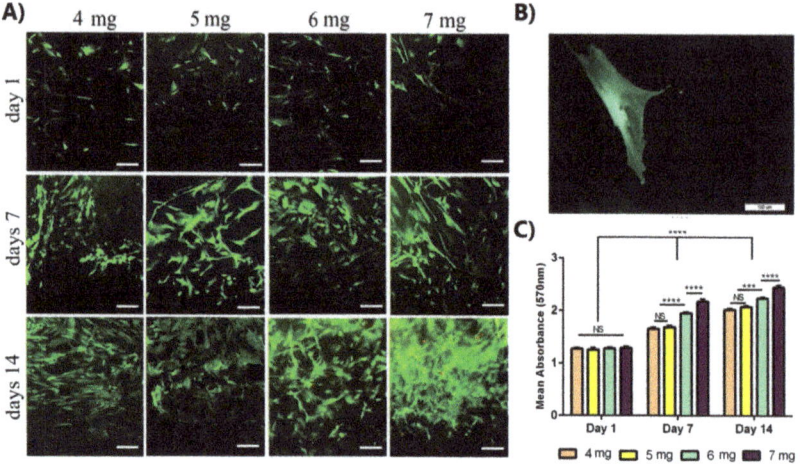

Figure 3. Evaluation of human OE-MSCs viability that encapsulated in different concentrations of collagen hydrogels for 14 days. (**A**) Live/dead fluorescence images of OE-MSCs cultured in collagen hydrogels, the green color shows the living cells, and the red color shows the dead cells (scale bar = 100 μm); (**B**) Images of OE-MSC in the bulk of collagen hydrogel (scale bar = 100 μm); (**C**) Comparison of the proliferative activity of OE-MSCs encapsulated in different concentrations of collagen hydrogels by resazurin assay (NS, no significant difference; $p < 0.05$, *** $p < 0.001$, **** $p < 0.0001$, the Scale Bars: 100 μm).

Metabolic and proliferative activity of OE-MSCs in collagen hydrogel was evaluated using the resazurin method at different time points (1, 7, and 14 days after cell culture). According to the results, as shown in Figure 3B, proliferative activity depended on collagen concentration and cell culture time for all samples. The metabolic activity was higher on day 14 than on other days. Comparing the results for different concentrations of collagen showed that the proliferative activity of human OE-MSCs was increased on days 7 and 14 with increasing collagen concentration, and on days 7 and 14, there was a significant difference between 7 mg/mL and 6 mg/mL groups. The proliferative activity of OE-MSCs encapsulated in collagen 7 mg/mL was higher than other groups at every time points.

3.4. Hydrogel Properties and Biocompatibility

FE-SEM images of acellular hydrogel (Figure 4) showed the formation of a three-dimensional high porous structure of the collagen hydrogel with uniform network connections. Evaluation of FE-SEM images after OE-MSCs encapsulated in the collagen hydrogels (Figure 4A) showed that the human OE-MSCs were alive and elongated with attached adequately to the hydrogels in all groups. Figure 4B indicates the porosity of collagen hydrogel scaffolds in different concentrations of 4 mg/mL, 5 mg/mL, 6 mg/mL, and 7 mg/mL. The results obtained in this study show that all scaffolds are very porous and above 90% porosity. As shown in Figure 4B, the percentage of porosity was associated with collagen concentration. The porosity of scaffolds containing collagen 4 mg/mL is higher than other scaffolds, and there is no significant difference between groups.

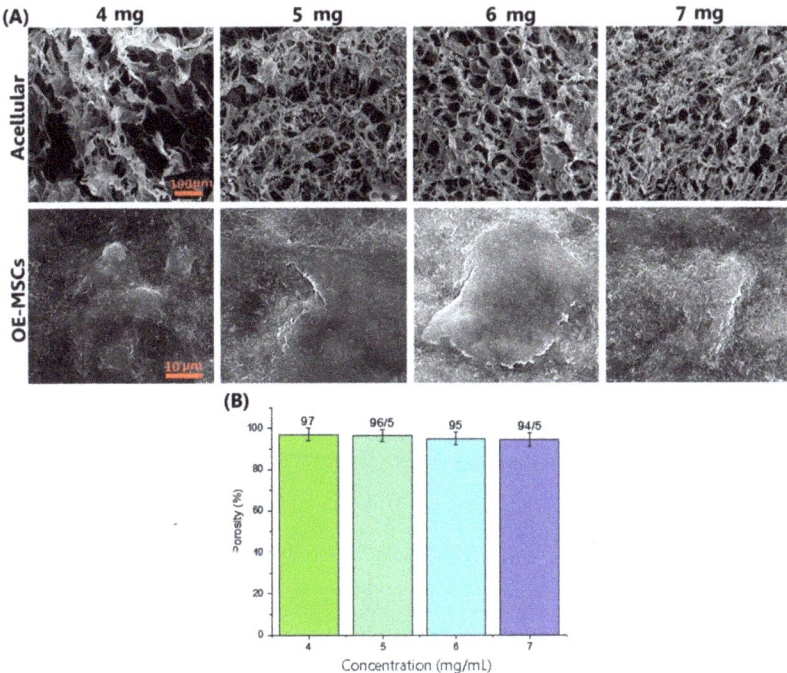

Figure 4. (A) FE-SEM images of the collagen hydrogel structures with different concentration of collagen (Scale bar: 100 μm) and OE-MSCs encapsulated in different concentration of collagen hydrogel (Scale bar: 10 μm); (B) The porosity percentage of collagen hydrogel scaffolds in different collagen concentrations, including 4 mg/mL, 5 mg/mL, 6 mg/mL, and 7 mg/mL.

3.5. Collagen Concentration of 7 mg/mL Has a Storage Modulus Comparable to the Other Concentrations

The mechanical properties include a rheological assessment characterized storage modulus (G′) and loss modulus (G″) vs. Frequency of hydrogels with different concentration of collagen (4 mg/mL, 5 mg/mL, 6 mg/mL, and 7 mg/mL) during frequency sweep analysis. G′ was better than G″, with minimal frequency dependency in all groups, according to the examined data presented in Figure 5. Rheological data analysis showed that the storage modulus was associated with collagen concentration significantly enhanced from ~875 Pa in group contained 4 mg/mL collagen to ~95,789 Pa in the group had 7 mg/mL collagen at 6 Hz.

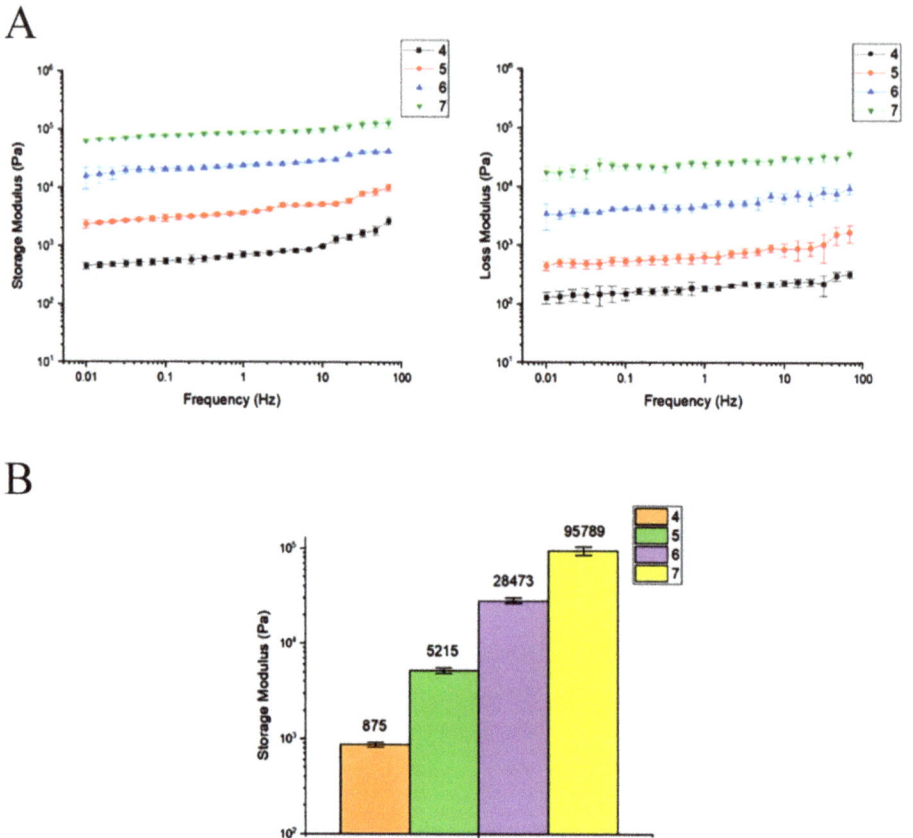

Figure 5. (**A**) Rheological evaluation of storage and loss modulus of different collagen hydrogel concentrations during frequency sweep study. (**B**) At 6 Hz, the effect of collagen concentration on hydrogel storage modulus (G′).

3.6. The Increase in the Concentration of Collagen Hydrogel Improved Osteogenic Differentiation of OE-MSCs

The ECM mineralization was evaluated on day 21 by Alizarin Red S staining. All data were assessed compared to two dimensional cultured of human OE-MSCs exposed to the osteogenic differentiation media as a control group. According to the data (Figure 6), the OE-MSCs encapsulated in all collagen concentrations showed calcium deposition. Additionally, the human OE-MSCs encapsulated in the collagen 7 mg/mL showed the highest calcium deposition than other groups. A significant difference was demonstrated between collagen 7 mg/mL absorbance and other groups (Figure 6B).

The real-time PCR was carried out to evaluate the osteogenic differentiation potency of encapsulated OE-MSCs in various concentrations to evaluate the osteogenic differentiation potency of encapsulated OE-MSCs in different concentrations of collagen hydrogel. Table 1 lists the gene primer sequences used in real-time PCR. The cycle threshold technique was used to approximate gene expression in relation to β-actin expression. The gene expression of significant osteogenic markers included Runx2, Col1, OPN, OC, and ALP, was evaluated on days 14 and 21. According to the data (Figure 6B), the up-regulation of osteogenic markers was shown in all groups during 21 days compared to the control group. These data demonstrate that the osteogenic differentiation of OE-MSCs was done in all groups, but the expression level of osteogenic markers was significantly higher on days 14. The level of gene expression was associated with collagen concentration, and the highest gene expression was obtained for encapsulated OE-MSCs in collagen 7 mg/mL in all genes. Furthermore, the significant difference between collagen 7 mg/mL and 6 mg/mL was shown in all groups.

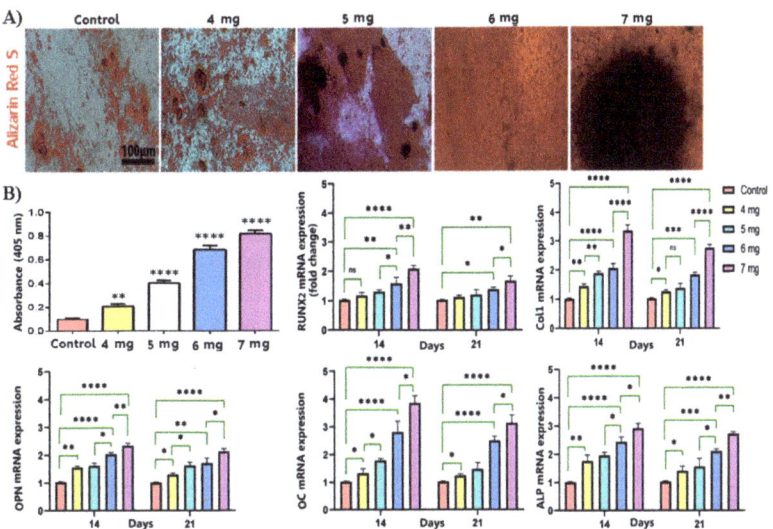

Figure 6. Osteogenic differentiation of OE-MSCs. (**A**) The extracellular matrix mineralization evaluation of encapsulated OE-MSCs in different concentration of collagen; The extracellular matrix mineralization was stained by Alizarin red S; quantifying the level of calcium production by Alizarin red S; (**B**) Osteogenic-related gene expression. Relative osteogenic marker expression of Runx2, Col1, OPN, OC, and ALP ($n = 3$, * $p < 0.05$; ** $p < 0.01$; *** $p < 0.001$; **** $p < 0.0001$), (scale bar: 100 μm).

Table 1. Primer sequences for real-time RT-PCR.

Gene Name	Primer
RUNX2	F GCCTCCAAGGTGGTAGCCC R CGTTACCCGCCATGAGAGTA
Collagen I (Col1)	F TCCGACCTCTCTCCTCTGAA R GAGTGGGGTTATGGAGGGAT
Osteopontin (OPN)	F GACCTGACATCCAGTACCC R GTTTCAGCACTCTGGTCATC
Osteocalcin (OC)	F GCAAAGGTGCAGCCTTTGTG R GGCTCCCAGCCATTGATACAG
Alkaline Phosphatase (ALP)	F GCACCTGCCTTACTAACTC R AGACACCCATCCCATCTC
B-actin	F CTTCCTTCCTGGGCATG R GTC TTTGCGGATGTCCAC

3.7. Encapsulated DiI-Labeled Human OE-MSCs in Collagen Hydrogel Were Traced in Rat Defection

For cell tracking in the defection region, 1×10^6 cells/mL of human OE-MSCs were labeled with DiI (Figure 7A). Next, these stem cells encapsulated in 7 mg/mL collagen hydrogel were implanted in the rat calvaria defection with a 7 mm critical size defect (Figure 7(B1,B2)). In vivo monitoring of alive DiI positive OE-MSCs in the lesion of calvaria was performed using optical imaging modality. Based on the data, we observed alive human OE-MSCs in the lesion area after 72 h (Figure 7D); conversely, in the blank scaffold group (OE-MSCs free), we did not recognize any trace of cell presence (Figure 7C).

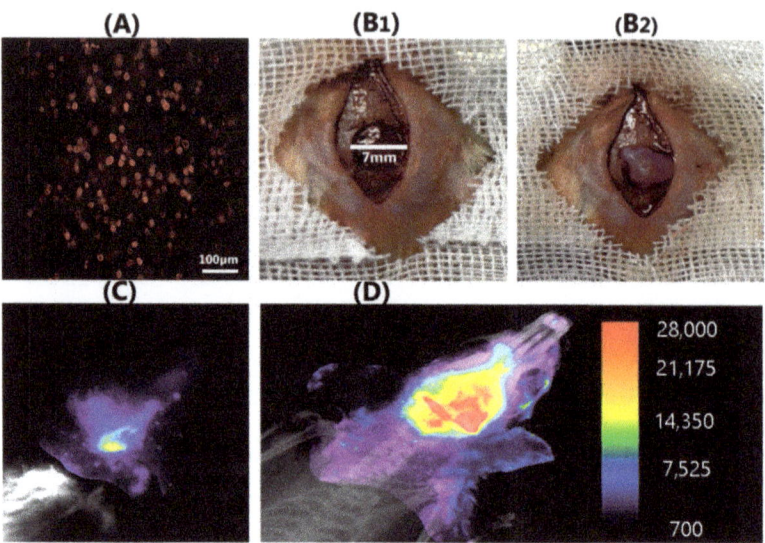

Figure 7. Human OE-MSCs labeled with DiI (**A**); and implanted with collagen hydrogel in a rat calvarial defection with critical size defect (7 mm) (**B1,B2**); Representative optical image of blank scaffold group (**C**); and covering images of X-ray and fluorescence images reveal a large number of DiI$^+$ OE-MSCs at the calvarial defective region in OE-MSCs group after 72 h (**D**) (scale bar: 100 µm).

3.8. The Highest Bone Healing Rate of Rat Calvarial Defection Observed in the OE-Mscs Group

After four weeks of implantation, H&E staining showed that the collagen hydrogel had vanished, but fibrous tissue defect had been filled (Figure 8A). Freshly formed bone tissues [15] were also evident in the OE-MSCs classes. At both 4 and 8 weeks, statistical analysis showed that the OE-MSCs group developed more NB in the calvarial defect area than the other groups. Compared to the other groups, the relative region of fresh bone tissue in the OE-MSCs population improved significantly over time in 8 weeks (Figure 8A,B). Micro-CT images also confirmed the new bone generation in the experimental groups in the rat calvarial defection (Figure 8B). The micro-CT images exhibited that the control and blank scaffold group revealed minimal bone healing (less than 5%) than OE-MSCs groups at four weeks. We also detected the highest rate of new bone formation in the OE-MSCs group than other groups after eight weeks. The region of bone growth was calculated by dividing the total defect volume by the new bone volume. In comparison, the group treated with OE-MSCs exhibited a significantly higher percentage of healing defects (about 10%) at eight weeks, associated with the osteogenic differentiation of implanted OE-MSCs that was encapsulated in collagen hydrogel (Figure 8D).

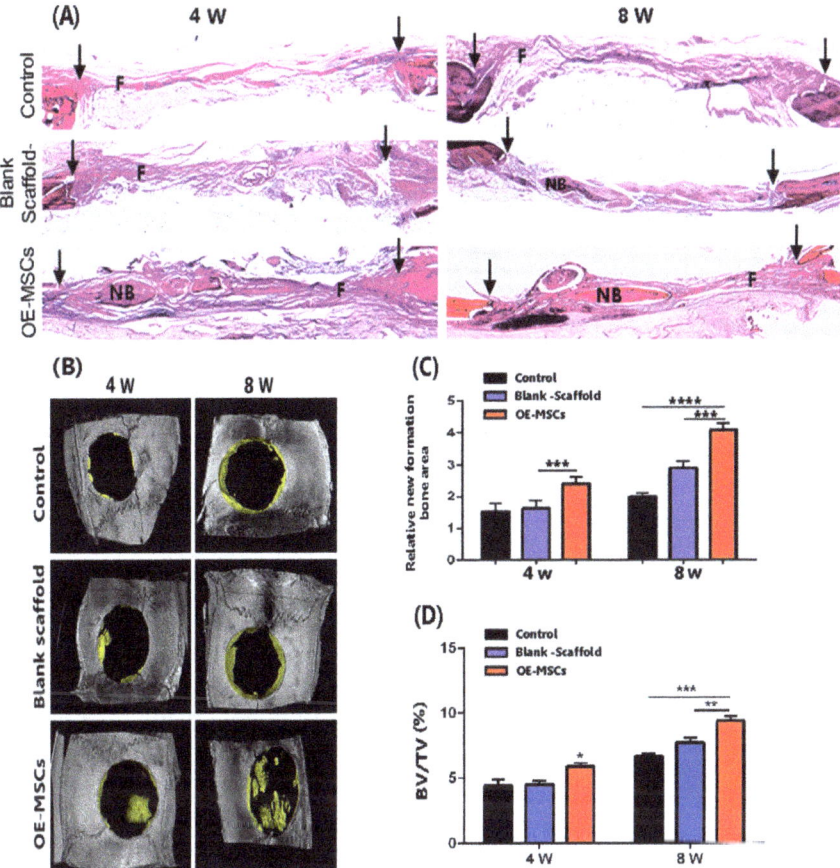

Figure 8. (**A**) After 4 and 8 weeks of implantation, H&E staining images showed new bone development in the calvarial defect area; (**B**) Representative micro-CT images of rat calvarial defects treated with or without OE-MSCs after 4 and 8 weeks; (**C**) The relative areas of fresh bone formation in three experimental groups, as determined by histological examination, (n = 5, * $p < 0.05$; ** $p < 0.01$; *** $p < 0.001$; **** $p < 0.0001$). Human OE-MSCs encapsulated in 7 mg/mL collagen hydrogel regenerate calvarial bone in vivo; (**D**) In rat calvarial defect models, summarized data showing new bone tissue volume/total defect volume (BV/TV) for newly developed bone tissue.

4. Discussion

This proof-of-concept study proposed a natural-based scaffold consisted of olfactory-derived MSCs for bone regeneration. The data from this study demonstrated that the encapsulated stem cells within collagen hydrogel cultured in osteogenic media could differentiate to osteoblasts and accelerate bone regeneration post-implantation.

Some requirements, such as biocompatibility and degradability of materials and osteoprogenitor cells, should be addressed when designing bone tissue engineering. Cell-loaded scaffolds presented an attractive option for bone formation in critical and massive defects. Additionally, there is growing interest in identifying easy available with high proliferative and osteogenic properties cell sources for bone tissue engineering. Therefore, collagen hydrogels were developed to create a supportive carrier for our study.

In 2009, Delmore et al. [14] reported a new type of undifferentiated cells with a neurogenic and osteogenic property from the olfactory mucosa defined as OE-MSCs.

Due to their easy access, higher mitotic activity, and proliferation rate than bone marrow and Wharton jelly MSCs, they have received more attention in recent years. Since these multipotent stem cells have telomere adjustment and maintain telomerase activity, they can sustain proliferative and culture ability for the long term even more than 15 weeks [2]. In other adult stem cells, the telomeres are decreased, and telomerase gradually loses its activity [23]. As expected, the morphology and characteristics of surface markers of isolated cells were like mesenchymal and ectodermal cells.

The collagen type I, which is pure and unchanged, was extracted from the rat tail. The FTIR spectrum was performed to detect the functional groups in the structure of extracted collagen. Moreover, it shows unique molecular vibrations, including amide A, amide B, amide I, amide II, and amide III. Carbonyl groups (C=O) were identified as amide I at peak 1626.48 cm^{-1}, indicating the presence of secondary structure in collagen proteins. The peak found at 1535.60 cm^{-1} indicated the tension of N-H and C-N that revealed amide II. Amide III was found at peak 1232.42 cm^{-1} and indicated the existence of C-N that confirm the presence of proline [24]. This evidence follows the data reported on similar research that has been effectively extracted collagen type I from adult tissues [25]. SDS-PAGE is a valid analysis to determine the type of collagen. Collagen type I has a striking pattern in terms of migration on an electrophoresis gel. After it runs on, the gel should be separated by α-monomer chains and β-dimer chains. The intensity and molecular weight of $α_2$ chain are lighter than $α_1$ because the collagen I triple helix is made up of two chains ($α_1$ and $α_2$). In this study, the molecular weight for $α_1$, $α_2$ was, respectively, about 125 kDa, and 110 kDa and β-chain was higher than 170 kDa, and the $α_1$ bond was heavier than the $α_2$ band. These data showed that the extracted collagen has a molecular weight similar to related published articles [26].

Collagen is a natural polymer in medical application due to high biocompatibility, suitable biodegradability, and low immunogenicity for cell encapsulation [27]. Collagen fibrils have some cell-binding sites, such as Arg-Gly-Asp (RGD) sequence, which interact and connect to cells. They significantly facilitate the attachment of cells to the hydrogel [28]. Mazzoni et al. [29], confirmed that collagen/hydroxyapatite is an ideal microenvironment for MSCs, with increased cell binding, cell augmentation, matrix synthesis, and mineralization to that shown in osteogenic condition media. The stimulation of distinct osteogenesis signaling pathways, such as extracellular signal-regulated protein kinase is mediated via collagen fibers [30].

For this reason, we investigated collagen type I hydrogel with different collagen concentrations based on some criteria, including gelation time, mechanical strength near to bone tissue and natural effect on cell attachment and proliferation.

The rheological test confirms that collagen hydrogel with 7 mg/mL concentration has optimum viscoelastic behavior. A frequency sweep was used to analyze the storage modulus (G') and loss modulus (G") of hydrogels with varying collagen concentrations. According to the obtained data, G' was higher than G" in all groups. No intersection showed the viscoelasticity and gelation rate and stability of all groups, and the storage modulus was related to collagen concentration. The viscoelasticity and gelation rate depended on collagen concentration, and the highest viscoelasticity was observed in the group containing 7 mg/mL collagen. The rheology analysis showed that collagen hydrogel storage modulus in concentrate of 7 mg/mL was close to the native bone (100 kpa) [16]. Collagen hydrogels, in particular, maintain the viability of encapsulated human OE-MSCs during in vitro tests such as live/dead and resazurin assays. The results have shown that the biocompatibility of collagen hydrogels was appropriate in all collagen concentrations. As proven in previous studies, the high concentration of collagen in the scaffold structure increases the proliferation rate of cells [31]. Therefore, this carrier provides an outstanding opportunity for cell delivery into the damaged tissue. Encapsulated human OE-MSCs maintain their morphology and live over culture time. FE-SEM images also demonstrated the cell attachment ability and the morphology of OE-MSCs on the surface of the hydrogel. As shown in Figure 4, OE-MSCs were alive and elongated with correct attachment to the hydrogels in all groups. Furthermore, the porosity of 90% is required to facilitate the flow of nutrients and metabolism and create a suitable space for the reconstruction of scaffolds [32].

In this study, collagen hydrogels' porosity containing different collagen concentrations was between 94.5–97%. The percentage of porosity was dependent on collagen concentration, and the group with 7 mg/mL collagen had lower porosity than other groups. In both classes, Alizarin red staining and real-time PCR data were used to show the osteogenic differentiation of human OE-MSCs, but gene expression was significantly better with increasing collagen concentration. The expression of RUNX2 and OPN plays a vital role in bone differentiation and formation. Additionally, Col-I and ALP genes expression are essential in the early phases of ossification and OCN in the middle and late ossification phases [33,34].

According to this study results, the 7 mg/mL collagen concentration was associated with up-regulation of ECM mineralization and the highest osteogenic gene expression of encapsulated human OE-MSCs. High regulation of osteogenic markers in 7 mg/mL collagen groups indicates this scaffold showed considerable ability to promote osteoblast proliferation and differentiation.

Optical imaging results showed that OE-MSCs labeled with DiI, which were encapsulated in collagen 7 mg/mL, could survive at the rat calvaria defection site for up to 72 h after transplantation are traceable.

Micro-CT analysis of human OE-MSCs encapsulated in 7 mg/mL collagen hydrogel in rats calvarial defects that were certified to promote bone regeneration. This group has a significant impact on bone formation after 4 and 8 weeks. Considering histological evidence and micro-CT results, bone defect in the OE-MSCs-treated rats is significantly covered by new bone compared to other groups. The most important observation from the data is that osteoblast proliferation and bone growth are induced at the defect's margins.

The previous study reports potential alternatives of bone marrow MSC-encapsulated collagen microspheres that can be differentiated into osteogenic and chondrogenic lineages in 3D collagen microspheres [35]. Collagen microspheres with committed MSCs possess osteoinductive-activities as confirmed by the ability to induce undifferentiated MSCs to commit to the osteogenic lineage [36]. We hypothesize that encapsulated human OE-MSCs in collagen hydrogel with osteoinductivity capacity have a good alternative candidate for fresh bone grafting in tissue defection.

Based on our results obtained from bone tissue regeneration, it can be declared that OE-MSCs lead to increasing osteogenesis in the defection site. This event can occur on two factors: (1) high proliferation rate and osteogenic differentiation of OE-MSCs encapsulated in collagen 7 mg/mL that was proved in vitro part; (2) OE-MSCs osteogenesis secretome can exert significant paracrine effects in the surrounding tissue defection [3]. These paracrine signals can promote osteoblast cells' survival in defection or recruit osteoblast progenitor cells from the other organs and improve bone regeneration.

5. Conclusions

A collagen-based hydrogel for human OE-MSCs delivery that allows highly efficient cell transplantation to the bone defect was fabricated and characterized. We proposed an optimum collagen concentration that meets the criteria of being a feasible carrier, biocompatible, and biodegradable. This construct provides human OE-MSCs survival and osteogenic differentiation and augmentation in vitro and shows mineralization and bone formation in vivo.

Author Contributions: P.B.M. and M.S. were in charge of conceptualization; S.S., M.G., Z.B., A.H., R.A., Z.A., M.H. and C.D. were involved in the investigation; S.S. was in charge of writing—original draft preparation; S.S. was in charge of writing—review and editing. The written edition of the manuscript has been read and approved by P.B.M. All authors have read and agreed to the published version of the manuscript.

Funding: The Iran University of Medical Sciences (IUMS) provided funding for this project under grant number 98-4-14-16643.

Institutional Review Board Statement: Not applicable.

Informed Consent Statement: Not applicable.

Data Availability Statement: Data sharing is not permitted. This analysis did not generate or review any new data. This report does not include data sharing.

Acknowledgments: Iran University of Medical Sciences provided funding for this research (IUMS). The Real time-PCR analyses and cell culture were performed by the Cellular and Molecular Research Center at IUMS, which the authors gratefully acknowledge. We'd like to thank the Behin Negareh office (BN) for their assistance with imaging.

Conflicts of Interest: There are no conflict of interest declared by the authors.

References

1. Simorgh, S.; Alizadeh, R.; Eftekharzadeh, M.; Haramshahi, S.M.A.; Milan, P.B.; Doshmanziari, M.; Ramezanpour, F.; Gholipourmalekabadi, M.; Seifi, M.; Moradi, F. Olfactory mucosa stem cells: An available candidate for the treatment of the Parkinson's disease. *J. Cell. Physiol.* **2019**, *234*, 23763–23773. [CrossRef]
2. Alizadeh, R.; Bagher, Z.; Kamrava, S.K.; Falah, M.; Hamidabadi, H.G.; Boroujeni, M.E.; Mohammadi, F.; Khodaverdi, S.; Zare-Sadeghi, A.; Olya, A. Differentiation of human mesenchymal stem cells (MSC) to dopaminergic neurons: A comparison between Wharton's Jelly and olfactory mucosa as sources of MSCs. *J. Chem. Neuroanat.* **2019**, *96*, 126–133. [CrossRef]
3. Rajan, N.; Habermehl, J.; Coté, M.-F.; Doillon, C.J.; Mantovani, D. Preparation of ready-to-use, storable and reconstituted type I collagen from rat tail tendon for tissue engineering applications. *Nat. Protoc.* **2006**, *1*, 2753. [CrossRef] [PubMed]
4. Paola, C.M.; Camila, A.M.; Ana, C.; Marlon, O.; Diego, S.; Robin, Z.; Beatriz, G.; Cristina, C. Functional textile finishing of type I collagen isolated from bovine bone for potential healthtech. *Heliyon* **2019**, *5*, e01260. [CrossRef] [PubMed]
5. Wu, J.; Li, Z.; Yuan, X.; Wang, P.; Liu, Y.; Wang, H. Extraction and isolation of type I, III and V collagens and their SDS-PAGE analyses. *Trans. Tianjin Univ.* **2011**, *17*, 111. [CrossRef]
6. Jin, G.-Z.; Kim, H.-W. Effects of type I collagen concentration in hydrogel on the growth and phenotypic expression of rat chondrocytes. *Tissue Eng. Regen. Med.* **2017**, *14*, 383–391. [CrossRef]
7. Bagheri, S.; Bagher, Z.; Hassanzadeh, S.; Simorgh, S.; Kamrava, S.K.; Nooshabadi, V.T.; Shabani, R.; Jalessi, M.; Khanmohammadi, M. Control of cellular adhesiveness in hyaluronic acid-based hydrogel through varying degrees of phenol moiety cross-linking. *J. Biomed. Mater. Res. A* **2021**, *109*, 649–658. [CrossRef]
8. Iqbal, B.; Muhammad, N.; Jamal, A.; Ahmad, P.; Khan, Z.U.H.; Rahim, A.; Khan, A.S.; Gonfa, G.; Iqbal, J.; Rehman, I.U. An application of ionic liquid for preparation of homogeneous collagen and alginate hydrogels for skin dressing. *J. Mol. Liq.* **2017**, *243*, 720–725. [CrossRef]
9. Jiankang, H.; Dichen, L.; Yaxiong, L.; Bo, Y.; Bingheng, L.; Qin, L. Fabrication and characterization of chitosan/gelatin porous scaffolds with predefined internal microstructures. *Polymer* **2007**, *48*, 4578–4588. [CrossRef]
10. Hui, T.; Cheung, K.; Cheung, W.; Chan, D.; Chan, B. In vitro chondrogenic differentiation of human mesenchymal stem cells in collagen microspheres: Influence of cell seeding density and collagen concentration. *Biomaterials* **2008**, *29*, 3201–3212. [CrossRef]
11. Karimi, S.; Bagher, Z.; Najmoddin, N.; Simorgh, S.; Pezeshki-Modaress, M. Alginate-magnetic short nanofibers 3D composite hydrogel enhances the encapsulated human olfactory mucosa stem cells bioactivity for potential nerve regeneration application. *Int. J. Biol. Macromol.* **2021**, *167*, 796–806. [CrossRef] [PubMed]
12. Apinun, J.; Honsawek, S.; Kuptniratsaikul, S.; Jamkratoke, J.; Kanokpanont, S. Osteogenic differentiation of rat bone marrow-derived mesenchymal stem cells encapsulated in Thai silk fibroin/collagen hydrogel: A pilot study in vitro. *Asian Biomed.* **2019**, *12*, 273–279. [CrossRef]
13. Souza, A.T.P.; Lopes, H.B.; Freitas, G.P.; Ferraz, E.P.; Oliveira, F.S.; Almeida, A.L.G.; Weffort, D.; Beloti, M.M.; Rosa, A.L. Role of embryonic origin on osteogenic potential and bone repair capacity of rat calvarial osteoblasts. *J. Bone Miner. Metab.* **2020**, 1–10. [CrossRef]
14. Delorme, B.; Nivet, E.; Gaillard, J.; Häupl, T.; Ringe, J.; Devèze, A.; Magnan, J.; Sohier, J.; Khrestchatisky, M.; Roman, F.S. The human nose harbors a niche of olfactory ectomesenchymal stem cells displaying neurogenic and osteogenic properties. *Stem Cells Dev.* **2010**, *19*, 853–866. [CrossRef] [PubMed]
15. Haramshahi, S.M.A.; Bonakdar, S.; Moghtadaei, M.; Kamguyan, K.; Thormann, E.; Tanbakooei, S.; Simorgh, S.; Brouki-Milan, P.; Amini, N.; Latifi, N. Tenocyte-imprinted substrate: A topography-based inducer for tenogenic differentiation in adipose tissue-derived mesenchymal stem cells. *Biomed. Mater.* **2020**, *15*, 035014. [CrossRef]
16. Liu, J.; Zheng, H.; Poh, P.S.; Machens, H.-G.; Schilling, A.F. Hydrogels for engineering of perfusable vascular networks. *Int. J. Mol. Sci.* **2015**, *16*, 15997–16016. [CrossRef] [PubMed]

17. Hamidabadi, H.G.; Shafaroudi, M.M.; Seifi, M.; Bojnordi, M.N.; Behruzi, M.; Gholipourmalekabadi, M.; Shafaroudi, A.M.; Rezaei, N. Repair of critical-sized rat calvarial defects with three-dimensional hydroxyapatite-gelatin scaffolds and bone marrow stromal stem cells. *Med. Arch.* **2018**, *72*, 88. [CrossRef]
18. Simorgh, S.; Alizadeh, R.; Shabani, R.; Karimzadeh, F.; Seidkhani, E.; Majidpoor, J.; Moradi, F.; Kasbiyan, H. Olfactory mucosa stem cells delivery via nasal route: A simple way for the treatment of Parkinson disease. *Neurotox. Res.* **2021**, *39*, 598–608. [CrossRef]
19. Ramhormozi, P.; Mohajer Ansari, J.; Simorgh, S.; Nobakht, M. Bone Marrow-Derived Mesenchymal Stem Cells Combined With Simvastatin Accelerates Burn Wound Healing by Activation of the Akt/mTOR Pathway. *J. Burn Care Res.* **2020**, *41*, 1069–1078. [CrossRef]
20. Abe, T.; Sumi, K.; Kunimatsu, R.; Oki, N.; Tsuka, Y.; Nakajima, K.; Tanimoto, K. Dynamic imaging of the effect of mesenchymal stem cells on osteoclast precursor cell chemotaxis for bone defects in the mouse skull. *J. Dent. Sci.* **2018**, *13*, 354–359. [CrossRef]
21. Feldkamp, L.A.; Davis, L.C.; Kress, J.W. Practical cone-beam algorithm. *J. Opt. Soc. Am. A* **1984**, *1*, 612–619. [CrossRef]
22. Hivechi, A.; Bahrami, S.H.; Siegel, R.A.; Siehr, A.; Sahoo, A.; Milan, P.B.; Joghataei, M.T.; Amoupour, M.; Simorgh, S. Cellulose nanocrystal effect on crystallization kinetics and biological properties of electrospun polycaprolactone. *Mater. Sci. Eng. C* **2021**, *121*, 111855. [CrossRef]
23. Banfi, A.; Bianchi, G.; Notaro, R.; Luzzatto, L.; Cancedda, R.; Quarto, R. Replicative aging and gene expression in long-term cultures of human bone marrow stromal cells. *Tissue Eng.* **2002**, *8*, 901–910. [CrossRef] [PubMed]
24. Nguyen, T.; Gobinet, C.; Feru, J.; Pasco, S.B.; Manfait, M.; Piot, O. Characterization of type I and IV collagens by Raman microspectroscopy: Identification of spectral markers of the dermo-epidermal junction. *Int. J. Spectrosc.* **2012**, *27*, 421–427. [CrossRef]
25. Carvalho, A.M.; Marques, A.P.; Silva, T.H.; Reis, R.L. Evaluation of the potential of collagen from codfish skin as a biomaterial for biomedical applications. *Mar. Drugs* **2018**, *16*, 495. [CrossRef]
26. Gelse, K.; Pöschl, E.; Aigner, T. Collagens—Structure, function, and biosynthesis. *Adv. Drug Deliv. Rev.* **2003**, *55*, 1531–1546. [CrossRef] [PubMed]
27. Arabpour, Z.; Baradaran-Rafii, A.; Bakhshaiesh, N.L.; Ai, J.; Ebrahimi-Barough, S.; Esmaeili Malekabadi, H.; Nazeri, N.; Vaez, A.; Salehi, M.; Sefat, F. Design and characterization of biodegradable multi layered electrospun nanofibers for corneal tissue engineering applications. *J. Biomed. Mater. Res. A* **2019**, *107*, 2340–2349. [CrossRef]
28. Dedhar, S.; Ruoslahti, E.; Pierschbacher, M.D. A cell surface receptor complex for collagen type I recognizes the Arg-Gly-Asp sequence. *J. Cell Biol.* **1987**, *104*, 585–593. [CrossRef] [PubMed]
29. Mazzoni, E.; D'Agostino, A.; Manfrini, M.; Maniero, S.; Puozzo, A.; Bassi, E.; Marsico, S.; Fortini, C.; Trevisiol, L.; Patergnani, S. Human adipose stem cells induced to osteogenic differentiation by an innovative collagen/hydroxylapatite hybrid scaffold. *FASEB J.* **2017**, *31*, 4555–4565. [CrossRef]
30. Duan, W.; Haque, M.; Kearney, M.T.; Lopez, M.J. Collagen and hydroxyapatite scaffolds activate distinct osteogenesis signaling pathways in adult adipose-derived multipotent stromal cells. *Tissue Eng. Part C Methods* **2017**, *23*, 592–603. [CrossRef]
31. Zhang, D.; Wu, X.; Chen, J.; Lin, K. The development of collagen based composite scaffolds for bone regeneration. *Bioact. Mater.* **2018**, *3*, 129–138. [CrossRef] [PubMed]
32. Sadeghi, A.; Zandi, M.; Pezeshki-Modaress, M.; Rajabi, S. Tough, hybrid chondroitin sulfate nanofibers as a promising scaffold for skin tissue engineering. *Int. J. Biol. Macromol.* **2019**, *132*, 63–75. [CrossRef] [PubMed]
33. Zhang, T.; Chen, H.; Zhang, Y.; Zan, Y.; Ni, T.; Liu, M.; Pei, R. Photo-crosslinkable, bone marrow-derived mesenchymal stem cells-encapsulating hydrogel based on collagen for osteogenic differentiation. *Colloids Surf. B Biointerfaces* **2019**, *174*, 528–535. [CrossRef] [PubMed]
34. Ge, L.; Jiang, M.; Duan, D.; Wang, Z.; Qi, L.; Teng, X.; Zhao, Z.; Wang, L.; Zhuo, Y.; Chen, P. Secretome of olfactory mucosa mesenchymal stem cell, a multiple potential stem cell. *Stem Cells Int.* **2016**, *2016*, 1243659. [CrossRef]
35. Chan, B.P.; Hui, T.; Yeung, C.; Li, J.; Mo, I.; Chan, G. Self-assembled collagen–human mesenchymal stem cell microspheres for regenerative medicine. *Biomaterials* **2007**, *28*, 4652–4666. [CrossRef]
36. Chan, B.P.; Hui, T.Y.; Wong, M.Y.; Yip, K.H.K.; Chan, G.C.F. Mesenchymal stem cell–encapsulated collagen microspheres for bone tissue engineering. *Tissue Eng. Part C Methods* **2010**, *16*, 225–235. [CrossRef]

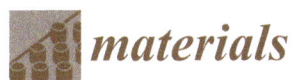

Article

In Vitro Production of Calcified Bone Matrix onto Wool Keratin Scaffolds via Osteogenic Factors and Electromagnetic Stimulus

Nora Bloise [1,2,*], Alessia Patrucco [3], Giovanna Bruni [4], Giulia Montagna [1,5], Rosalinda Caringella [3], Lorenzo Fassina [5], Claudio Tonin [3] and Livia Visai [1,2,*]

1. Department of Molecular Medicine (DMM), Centre for Health Technologies (CHT), UdR INSTM, University of Pavia, Viale Taramelli, 3/B-27100 Pavia, Italy; giulia.montagna04@universitadipavia.it
2. Department of Occupational Medicine, Toxicology and Environmental Risks, Istituti Clinici Scientifici (ICS) Maugeri, IRCCS, Via Boezio, 28-27100 Pavia, Italy
3. Institute of Intelligent Industrial Technologies and Systems for Advanced Manufacturing (STIIMA), Italian National Research Council (CNR), Corso Pella, 16-13900 Biella, Italy; a.patrucco@stiima.cnr.it (A.P.); linda.car87@yahoo.it (R.C.); c.tonin@stiima.cnr.it (C.T.)
4. Center for Colloid and Surface Science (C.S.G.I.), Department of Chemistry, Section of Physical Chemistry, University of Pavia, Viale Taramelli, 16-27100 Pavia, Italy; giovanna.bruni@unipv.it
5. Department of Electrical, Computer and Biomedical Engineering (DIII), Centre for Health Technologies (CHT), University of Pavia, Via Ferrata, 5-27100 Pavia, Italy; lorenzo.fassina@unipv.it

* Correspondence: nora.bloise@unipv.it (N.B.); livia.visai@unipv.it (L.V.); Tel.: +39-0382-987725 (L.V.)

Received: 11 May 2020; Accepted: 4 July 2020; Published: 8 July 2020

Abstract: Pulsed electromagnetic field (PEMF) has drawn attention as a potential tool to improve the ability of bone biomaterials to integrate into the surrounding tissue. We investigated the effects of PEMF (frequency, 75 Hz; magnetic induction amplitude, 2 mT; pulse duration, 1.3 ms) on human osteoblast-like cells (SAOS-2) seeded onto wool keratin scaffolds in terms of proliferation, differentiation, and production of the calcified bone extracellular matrix. The wool keratin scaffold offered a 3D porous architecture for cell guesting and nutrient diffusion, suggesting its possible use as a filler to repair bone defects. Here, the combined approach of applying a daily PEMF exposure with additional osteogenic factors stimulated the cells to increase both the deposition of bone-related proteins and calcified matrix onto the wool keratin scaffolds. Also, the presence of SAOS-2 cells, or PEMF, or osteogenic factors did not influence the compression behavior or the resilience of keratin scaffolds in wet conditions. Besides, ageing tests revealed that wool keratin scaffolds were very stable and showed a lower degradation rate compared to commercial collagen sponges. It is for these reasons that this tissue engineering strategy, which improves the osteointegration properties of the wool keratin scaffold, may have a promising application for long term support of bone formation in vivo.

Keywords: pulsed electromagnetic field; osteogenic factors; wool keratin scaffolds; bone tissue engineering

1. Introduction

In bone tissue engineering (BTE), two fundamental properties that each biomaterial should present are biocompatibility and biodegradability. Other than these properties, most of the materials used as scaffolds for the repair of bone defects offer only a feasible passive support within which the tissue may heal or regenerate. However, an active induction and promotion of the core processes mentioned above would accelerate the tissue healing. In BTE, bioceramic scaffolds (such as calcium phosphates) are widely employed to improve bone regeneration because their chemical similarity to the bony inorganic matrix confers osteoconductive properties, increasing osseointegration.

In general, and within the context of the biodegradable natural polymers, keratin-based materials have changed the field of modern biomaterials due to their distinct properties such as biodegradability, biocompatibility, and mechanical durability. Interestingly, they can be cast as sponges, films, and hydrogels for various biomedical applications [1]. Moreover, keratin constitutes the major components of hair, wool, feathers, and nails, and can be extracted in significant amounts from animal tissues without the need for animal sacrifice [2], something which is not the case for collagen and other animal-derived osteoconductive proteins. In vivo investigation of keratose (water-soluble fraction of the keratin) was studied as a BMP2 carrier for bony regeneration of rat femoral bone defect. Results indicated There was enhanced regeneration of bone along with reduced adipose tissues [3].

This in vitro work of bone-tissue engineering starts from the wool keratin scaffold previously described [4] and aims to enrich the extracellular bone matrix (ECM) components, i.e., the over-wrap of a proteinaceous and, calcified surface, are reveal possible uses in vivo. Herein, we aimed to obtain, directly in vitro, a biomaterial summarizing the characteristics of the compact bone before in vivo implantation. As previously stated [4], wool keratin scaffolds exhibit high level of cell adhesion and proliferation; in particular, the 3D structure of this biomaterial, with controlled-size macro-porosity suitable for cell guesting and nutrient diffusion, provides a suitable environment for bone tissue engineering. In addition, and in order to accelerate and ameliorate ECM deposition we implemented the classical idea of tissue engineering using mechanical stimuli. Theoretically, the growth and development of in vitro tissue substitutes should be supported not only by biomolecules (e.g., growth factors) but also by physical factors provided by the structural context (e.g., geometric and mechanical properties of scaffolds) and by the biophysical context (e.g., the concentrated/distributed, perpendicular/tangential forces acting onto the cell plasma membrane). Fluid shear stress [5], for instance, or ultrasounds [6] or biomaterial features [7] lead to the remodeling of bone matrix in vitro.

Nonetheless, the modulation of the cell behavior on the different biomaterials is clearly proved by the osteoblasts exposed to pulsed electromagnetic field (PEMF) [8,9]. In particular and according to the "tensegrity" theory of Ingber [10], mechanical forces may induce biochemical responses targeting the transcriptional profile via mechanotransduction. The electromagnetic stimulus of this study was demonstrated [8,9] to elicit time varying mechanical forces acting perpendicularly or tangentially onto the cell membrane, in order that these forces were able to modulate the cell behavior via tensile, compressive, and shear deformations.

In this study, the electromagnetic stimulus employed to elicit time-varying mechanical forces acting perpendicularly or tangentially upon the cell membrane [8,9]. In other words, these forces were able to modulate the cell behavior via tensile, compressive and shear deformations. For instance, osteoblasts are susceptible to fluid shear stress and react with an enhanced transcription of bone matrix genes [11,12]. Both traction and compression vary the activities of intracellular signaling molecules such as Rho GTPases, guanine nucleotide exchange factors, GTPase activating proteins, and the MAPK pathway, consequently modulating the expression of transcription factors essential for the homeostasis of bone, cartilage and tooth tissues [13]. As a consequence, we can hypothesize the significance of PEMF application to improve the clinical outcome of numerous regenerative and prosthetic therapies in orthopedics and dentistry fields [14].

In sum our aim was to evaluate the feasibility of wool keratin sponges in supporting osteoblast-like cells viability and ECM deposition. Moreover, we want to verify if PEMFs, with the presence of osteogenic factors, ameliorate osteoblast-like cells responses to wool keratin biomaterial, improving their differentiation and bone matrix enrichment. Such a tissue engineering strategy could be promising for wool keratin scaffold applications in vivo, for example towards a filler for bone defects.

2. Materials and Methods

2.1. Preparation of the Keratin Sponges

Sponges (or scaffolds) were prepared following the previous procedure [4]. Botany wool, 20.3 μm mean fiber diameter, was supplied by The Woolmark Co., Milan, Italy. In brief, 8 g wool fibers snippets were bathed in 400 mL of 0.1 N NaOH, material to liquid ratio 1:50, for 24 h at 60 °C. The snippets were rinsed with tap water until pH neutral, soaked in deionized water and submitted to ultrasonic irradiation for 30 min (600 W, 20 kHz). Coarse fiber fragments were removed from the suspension by filtration with stainless steel 120 mesh sieves. The permeate was centrifuged (12,000 rpm, 15 min), and the supernatant was removed. The solid precipitate was added with deionized water and stirred until the suspension reached 0.05 g/mL. This suspension was added with 1.17 g/mL controlled-size NaCl (400–500 μm), then cast at 50 °C. The resulting material was washed with deionized water in order to remove salt. The sponge was dried at 50 °C, then at 180 °C for 2 h to improve its water stability and increase crosslinks [15].

2.2. Pulsed Electromagnetic Field (PEMF)

Our electromagnetic apparatus (Igea, Carpi, Italy) was used [16]. Cells were exposed to PEMF for 1 h per day at the same moment, adopting the following parameters: magnetic induction amplitude of 2 ± 0.2 mT, frequency of 75 ± 2 Hz, pulse duration of 1.3 ms (Table 1).

Table 1. Experimental set up to investigate the effect of the daily pulsed electromagnetic field (PEMF) treatment on human SAOS-2 osteoblast-like cells seeded onto porous wool keratin scaffold for 21 days.

Experimental Condition	PEMF * Exposure Protocol	In Vitro Investigation
Ctrl (maintenance medium, MM)	not exposure °	Day 7: qRT-PCR bone gene expression Day 21: <ul><li>DNA content</li><li>SEM analysis</li><li>ALP activity</li><li>Phosphate content</li><li>Calcium content</li><li>Bone proteins: qRT-PCR and ELISA</li><li>Confocal Laser Scanning Analysis</li><li>Mechanical characterization</li></ul>
PEMF (MM + PEMF)	1 h per day up to 21 days °	
OF (MM + OF)	not exposure °	
PEMF + OF (MM + OF + PEMF)	1 h per day up to 21 days °	

* The following parameters were adopted: magnetic induction amplitude of 2 ± 0.2 mT, frequency of 75 ± 2 Hz, pulse duration of 1.3 ms. The electromagnetic bioreactor was placed into a standard cell culture incubator in a 37 °C, 5% CO_2 environment. ° The medium was changed every 3 days.

2.3. Cell Cultures

The human osteosarcoma cell line SAOS-2 was cultured in a maintenance medium (MM) constituted of McCoy's 5A modified medium with L-glutamine (Lonza Ltd., Basel, Switzerland) and HEPES (Cambrex Bio Science, Baltimore, MD, USA), supplemented with 15% fetal bovine serum, 1% L-glutamine, 0.4% antibiotics, 2% sodium pyruvate, and 0.2% fungizone. Cells were cultured, routinely trypsinized after confluence, and maintained in an incubator at 37 °C with a 5% CO_2 atmosphere. Before cell seeding, scaffolds (diameter, 0.8 cm; height, 1 cm) were sterilized [4] at 180 °C for 3 h, then washed twice in PBS for 10 min, placed in 48-wells, and incubated O.N. in the maintenance medium. To ensure a maximum number of attached cells for scaffolds a cell suspension of 4×10^5 cells × scaffold was added in two steps onto the top of each scaffold and, after 0.5 h, 1 mL of culture medium was added to cover the scaffolds. After 24 h from seeding, the medium was changed and replaced with MM (control, ctrl) or, to induce osteogenic differentiation, with MM supplemented with osteogenic factors (OF). The osteogenic factors, dexamethasone and β-glycerophosphate were added to the maintenance medium at a concentration of 10^{-8} M and 10 mM, respectively [7]. McCoy's 5A modified medium contains the ascorbic acid, another osteogenic supplement, at a concentration of 0.5 µg/mL. Treatment lasted up to 21 days and the medium was changed every 3 days.

2.4. DNA Content

Total DNA content in SAOS-2 was determined after 21 days of culture using PicoGreen assay (PicoGreen; Molecular Probes, Eugene, OR, USA). Briefly, at the end of incubation, to process material for analysis of DNA content, samples were processed through the three freeze/thaw cycles method in sterile deionized distilled water. Between each freeze/thaw cycle, scaffolds were roughly vortexed. The released DNA content was measured with the fluorometric DNA quantification kit. Samples were diluted 1:100 in 100 µL of working solution (PicoGreen reagent in TE buffer, 1:200) for the measurement. Fluorescence was detected in a dedicated 96-well plate, at 520 nm, after excitation at 480 nm, with CLARIOstar® Plus Multi-mode Microplate Reader (BMG Labtech, Ortenberg, Germany). A DNA standard curve [9], obtained from a known number of osteoblasts, was used to express the results as cell number attached per scaffold.

2.5. Fluorescein Diacetate Assay

At day 21 of culture, live cells were visualized by a vital staining with fluorescein diacetate (FDA) on all experimental groups as described previously [17]. Briefly, 5 mg/mL FDA stock solution (Invitrogen) was prepared in acetone: 40 µL stock solution was diluted in 10 mL phosphate buffer solution (PBS) (137 mM NaCl, 2.7 mM KCl, 4.3 mM Na_2HPO_4, 1.4 mM NaH_2PO_4, pH 7.4) and 250 µL was mixed with 500 µL culture medium. Cells were incubated with a working solution for 10 min. The live cells were examined by a confocal laser scanning microscope model TSC SP5 II (Leica Microsystems, Bensheim, Germany), using a 40× oil immersion objective.

2.6. Scanning Electron Microscopy (SEM)

On day 21 of culture, samples were treated as previously described [16]. The samples were fixed with 2.5% (v/v) glutaraldehyde solution in 0.1 M Na-cacodylate buffer (pH = 7.2) for 1 h at 4 °C, washed with Na-cacodylate buffer, and then dehydrated at room temperature in an ethanol gradient series up to 100%. Scaffolds were then lyophilized 4 h for complete dehydration, and then sputter-coated with gold under high vacuum to render them electrically conductive prior to observation with Zeiss EVO-MA10 scanning electron microscope (Carl Zeiss, Oberkochen, Germany) at accelerating voltage of 20 kV for analysis of cell morphology. An energy dispersive X-ray spectroscopy (EDX) detector (X-max 50 mm^2, Oxford Instruments, Oxford, UK) used coupled with SEM to perform the distribution maps of calcium and phosphorus onto the wool keratin scaffold surfaces. In this case (SEM-EDX analysis), the samples were examined without a conductive coating under low vacuum condition and with an accelerating voltage of 20 kV.

2.7. ALP Activity

ALP activity was estimated using a colorimetric endpoint assay at day 21 as previously reported [7,16]. The assay measures the conversion of the colorless substrate p-nitrophenol phosphate (pNPP) by the enzyme ALP into the yellow product p-nitrophenol (pNP). The rate of color change corresponds to the amount of enzyme present in the solution. Briefly, an aliquot (0.5 mL) of 0.3 M pNPP (dissolved in glycine buffer, pH 10.5) was added to each scaffold at 37 °C. After incubation, the reaction was stopped by the addition of 50 µL 5 M NaOH. Standards of pNPP in concentrations ranging from 0 to 50 µM were freshly prepared from dilutions of a 500 µM stock solution and incubated for 10 min with 7U of ALP (Sigma-Aldrich, St. Louis, MO, United States) previously dissolved in 500 µL of ddH_2O. The optical densities (OD) reading was performed at 415 nm with a microplate reader (BioRad Laboratories, Hercules, California) using 100 µL of standard or samples and placed into individual wells on a 96-well plate. Samples were run in triplicate and optical densities obtained from each sample, after blank subtraction, were compared with the calibration curve of p-nitrophenol standard in order to obtain the ALP activity expressed as µM of p-nitrophenol produced per min per µg of protein.

2.8. Inorganic Phosphate Determination

A commercially available kit (Phosphate Colorimetric Assay Kit, Sigma Aldrich, St. Louis, MO, USA) was used to quantify inorganic phosphate levels. Briefly, the cell-seeded scaffolds were washed with TBS (Tris-buffered saline, 50 mM Tris-Cl, 150 mM NaCl, pH 7.6), and chilled on ice in 1 mL cold TBS for 15 min. TBS buffer containing Tris and NaCl does not interfere with phosphate content in the assay and then not alter the final results. Samples were then sonicated 3 times for 60 s at high setup (one cycle = 30 s sonication—10 s break—10 s sonication—10 s break). The samples were then centrifuged for 15 min at 4 °C at top speed using a cold microcentrifuge to remove any insoluble material. Supernatant was collected and transferred to a clean tube. The supernatant was diluted 1:10 in double-distilled water, and phosphates were determined. At the end of reaction, an absorbance reading was performed at 655 nm with a microplate reader (BioRad Laboratories). Samples were run in triplicate and compared against a standard-solution calibration curve. The amount of phosphate from samples was expressed as pmol/(cells × scaffold).

2.9. Calcium-Cresolphthalein Complexone Method

The calcium content of each sample was assayed to quantify the amount of mineralized matrix present and was measured using a Calcium Fast kit (Mercury S.p.A., Naples, Italy) according to the manufacturer's instructions as previously reported [17]. Samples were run in triplicate and compared with the calibration curve of standards. The colorimetric end point assay measures the amount of purple-colored calcium-cresolphthalein complexone complex formed when cresolphthalein complexone binds to free calcium in an alkaline solution. Briefly, an aliquot (1 mL) of 1 N HCl was added to each sample and incubated for 24 h at RT to release calcium into solution. The sample supernatant was diluted 1/10 with the Assay Working Solution by mixing equal parts of calcium-binding reagent and calcium buffer reagent provided by the kit. Ca^{2+} standards in concentrations ranging from 0 to 10 mg/mL were prepared from dilutions of a 100 mg/mL stock solution of Ca^{2+}. The absorbance reading was performed at 595 nm with a microplate reader (BioRad Laboratories) using 100 µL of standard or sample placed into individual wells of a 96-well plate. Samples were run in triplicate and compared against the standard solution calibration curve. Results are expressed as pg/cell×scaffold and presented as mean ± SD.

2.10. Confocal Laser Scanning Microscopy (CLSM)

For morphological observation, cell-seeded wool fibril sponges were washed for 24 h with PBS, fixed with 4% (w/v) paraformaldehyde solution for 30 min at 4 °C, permeabilized with 0.1% Triton X-100, then stained with Tetramethylrhodamine B isothiocyanate (TRITC) phalloidin conjugate solution (10 µg/mL, EX/EM maxima ca. 540/575, Sigma-Aldrich) in PBS for 40 min at RT, finally incubated with the primary antibody Alexa-Fluor 488 anti-β tubulin and with Hoechst 33342 for nuclei staining (2 µg/mL, Sigma-Aldrich). For osteogenic protein labeling, paraformaldehyde-fixed samples were blocked with PAT [PBS containing 1% (w/v) bovine serum albumin and 0.02% (v/v) Tween 20] for 1 h at RT. Anti-osteocalcin rabbit polyclonal antiserum (provided by Dr. Larry W. Fisher, National Institutes of Health, Bethesda, MD, USA) was used as primary antibody diluted 1:500 in PAT. The incubation with the primary antibody was made overnight at 4 °C, whereas the negative controls were incubated overnight at 4 °C with PAT instead of the primary antibodies. The scaffolds and the negative controls were washed and incubated with Alexa Fluor 488 goat anti-rabbit IgG (Molecular Probes) at a dilution of 1:750 in PAT for 1 h at room temperature. At the end of the incubation, the scaffolds were washed in PBS, counterstained for 5 min with a solution of Hoechst 33342 (2 µg/mL) to target nuclei, and then washed. The images (39 sections, images acquired every 112 µm till 4.4 mm depth) were taken using a confocal laser scanning microscope model TSC SP5 II (Leica Microsystems, Bensheim, Germany), using a 20× oil immersion objective for each sample condition, and the orthogonal projections of images were obtained using Fiji software ((Fiji Is Just) ImageJ 2.0.0-rc-69/1.52p, National Institutes of Health, Bethesda, MA, USA). The fluorescence background of the negative control was almost negligible (Figure S4). Cells seeded and cultured on Tissue Culture Plates (TCPS) after 21 days in MM and with osteogenic factors (OF) were insert as controls (Figure S4).

2.11. qRT-PCR

The total RNA from all samples was extracted on day 7 and 21 of culture with the NucleoSpin® RNA XS kit (MACHEREY-NAGEL GmbH & Co. KG, Düren, Germany) and retro-transcribed to c-DNA with the iScript cDNA Synthesis kit (Thermo Fisher Scientific, Waltham, MA, USA). Quantitative reverse-transcription polymerase chain reaction (qRT-PCR) analysis was performed in a 96-well optical reaction plate using a qPCR Quant3 Studio (Applied BioSystem, Foster City, CA, USA). Analysis was performed in a total volume of 20 µL amplification mixture containing 2× (10 µL) Brilliant SYBR Green QPCR Master Mix (Bio-Rad Laboratories), 2 µL cDNA, 0.4 µL of each primer, and 7.2 µL H_2O. The PCR conditions were as follows: 3 min at 95 °C, 40 cycles of 5 s at 95 °C, and 23 s at 60 °C. The reaction mixture without cDNA was used as a negative control in each run. Gene expression was analyzed in triplicate. GAPDH housekeeping was used as the housekeeping gene and results were analyzed with the $2^{-\Delta\Delta Ct}$ method [18] relative to the expression in the cells at day 0. The primers used are listed in Table S1.

2.12. Extraction of Bone Matrix Proteins and ELISA Assay

To evaluate the amount of extracellular matrix protein constituents onto the keratin scaffold in in all experimental conditions, an enzyme-linked immunosorbent assay (ELISA) was performed as previously described [7]. Briefly, samples were washed extensively with sterile PBS to remove culture medium and then incubated for 24 h at 37 °C with 1 mL of sterile sample buffer (20 mM Tris-HCl, 4 M GuHCl, 10 mM EDTA, 0.066% (*w/v*) sodium dodecyl sulphate (SDS), pH 8.0) At the end of the incubation period, the samples were centrifuged at 4000 rpm for 15 min in order to collect also the sample buffer entrapped inside the pores of the scaffolds. The total protein concentration in the collected sample buffer was evaluated with the BCA Protein Assay kit (Pierce Biotechnology, Inc., Rockford, IL, USA). Calibration curves to measure alkaline phosphatase (ALP), type-I collagen (COL-I), decorin (DCN), osteocalcin (OSC), osteonectin (OSN), and osteopontin (OSP) were prepared as previously described [7]. In order to measure the extracellular matrix amount of each protein the ELISA assay was performed as previously reported [7]. In brief, microtiter wells were coated with increasing concentrations of each purified protein, from 10 ng to 2 µg, in coating buffer (50 mM Na_2CO_3, pH 9.5) overnight at 4 °C. Control wells were coated with bovine serum albumin (BSA) as a negative control. To measure the ECM amount of each protein by ELISA, microtiter wells were coated, overnight at 4 °C, with 100 µL of the previously extracted ECM (20 µg/mL in coating buffer). After three washes with PBS containing 0.1% (*v/v*) Tween 20, the wells were blocked by incubating with 200 µL of PBS containing 2% (*w/v*) BSA for 2 h at 22 °C. The wells were subsequently incubated for 1.5 h at 22 °C with 100 µL with anti-phosphatase (ALP), anti-type-I collagen (COL-I), anti-decorin (DCN), anti-osteocalcin (OSC), anti-osteonectin (OSN), and anti-osteopontin (OSP) polyclonal antisera (1:500 dilution in 1% BSA), kindly provided by Dr. Larry W. Fisher. After washing, the wells were incubated for 1 h at 22 °C with 100 µL of horseradish peroxidase (HRP)-conjugated goat anti-rabbit IgG (1:1000 dilution in 1% BSA). The wells were finally incubated with 10 µL of the development solution (phosphate-citrate buffer with o-phenylenediamine dihydrochloride substrate). The color reaction was stopped with 100 µL of 0.5 M H_2SO_4, and the absorbance values were measured at 490 nm with a microplate reader (BioRad Laboratories). The optical densities from each sample were plotted against a calibration curve containing known amounts of each proteins. An underestimation of the absolute protein deposition is possible because the sample buffer used for matrix extraction contains SDS, which may interfere with protein absorption during the ELISA assay. The amount of extracellular matrix constituents throughout the wool keratin scaffold in the different conditions was expressed as pg/(cells×scaffold).

2.13. Ageing Test

Wool keratin scaffolds and commercial collagen sponges were dried at 105 °C to a constant weight then aged in isotonic fluid (0.02 mg/mL, Ringer's solution, pH 7) at 37 °C, with the fluid replaced every 14 days [19].

2.14. Compression Behavior

Compression properties of the wool keratin scaffolds were determined in conditioned standard atmosphere at 20 °C, 65% RH, with an Instron 5500 R Series IX dynamometer (Instron, Pianezza, Italy). The measurements were performed on the scaffold in the absence or presence of cells in all the conditions (ctrl, PEMF, OF, and OF + PEMF) after 21 days of culture. Six samples (8 mm, diameter; 4 mm, thickness) in conditioned and wet states (bathed in distilled water for 2 h, then drained for testing) were submitted to 10 compression cycles (maximum load of 5 N) at the constant deformation rate of 10 mm/min, in order to evaluate resilience as well. Every compression cycle was stopped on reaching 3 mm stroke, starting from the top of the sponge scaffold. Samples were measured for compression force and deformation, reporting the average and standard deviation of the results.

2.15. Statistics

Three independent experiments (N) (unless otherwise indicated) were performed to get a statistically significant number of events, and in order to test the reproducibility of the results per each type of experiment from 2 to 3 scaffolds (n) were analyzed (as indicated in the figure legends). Results were expressed as mean ± standard deviation. Statistical analysis was carried out using GraphPad Prism 6.0 (GraphPad, Inc., San Diego, CA, USA). Analysis was performed using one-way or two-way ANOVA analysis of variance (ANOVA), followed by Bonferroni post hoc test (significance level of 0.05).

3. Results

To explore the effect of daily treatment with a low-frequency PEMF on human osteoblast-like cells (SAOS-2) seeded onto wool keratin scaffolds on proliferation and bone matrix deposition after 21 days of culture, four conditions were investigated: (a) cells grown in a maintenance medium (MM, control, ctrl); (b) cells grown in MM and daily exposed to PEMF; (c) cells differentiated in medium supplemented with osteogenic factors (OF); and (d) cells differentiated in the presence of OF and treated daily with PEMF (PEMF + OF). The experimental setup was performed as indicated in Table 1. The SAOS-2 cell line was selected because it exhibits several fundamental osteoblast characteristics. Although, this cell line is derived from osteosarcoma and so could display some cellular behavior differences from primary human osteoblasts, it represents an accepted and representative model for in vitro osteogenic study [20], including studies of the multiple osteoblasts responses on new developed biomaterials [21,22].

3.1. Proliferation and Morphology of Osteoblast-Like Cells onto Wool Keratin Scaffold after PEMF Treatment

Firstly, the capability of the 3D fibrous structure of wool to support the cell adhesion and migration into the pore of wool keratin scaffold was confirmed by confocal laser scanning microscopy (Figure S1). Specifically, analysis of the orthogonal projections of CLSM images (Figure S1) displayed that osteoblasts were able to migrate into the pores of wool keratin scaffold after 24 h of incubation, that is a relevant event, since the migration and colonization into the scaffold may favor the bone matrix deposition. We selected PEMF with a frequency of 75 Hz and an intensity of 2 mT based on our previous study, demonstrating that these parameters improve the osteogenic differentiation of human mesenchymal stem cells (MSCs) [23]. The daily treatment with PEMF for 1 h was chosen as an exposure protocol on the basis of viability preliminary studies performed by using a single or daily PEMF dose (Figure S2). Next, cell proliferation on wool keratin scaffolds were assessed after 21 days of culture for the above treatments. The proliferation of SAOS-2 over 21 days was determined through a DNA quantification assay (Figure 1a). According to the data the addition of osteogenic factors, with or without the PEMF exposure resulted in a significant decrease of cell proliferation comparison both with ctrl and PEMF groups (* $p < 0.05$ and § $p < 0.05$, respectively). It can be seen that the proliferation of cells exposed to PEMF and OF simultaneously (PEMF + OF) showed comparable results with OF group ($p > 0.05$). Similarly, no significant difference was observed between ctrl and PEMF stimulated cells ($p > 0.05$). It is important to note that this may be an underestimation of the culture cellularity due to the trapping of DNA within the formed extracellular matrix and fibrous scaffold meshes. The SEM images show that the cells (indicated with red stars in the SEM images) adhered and spread onto the surface of the scaffolds after 21 days (Figure 1b), demonstrating that scaffolds are suitable frameworks for cellular attachment, spreading and proliferation and differentiation. All of these are crucial features for bone healing applications. However, differences were detected among the different experimental conditions. In comparison with ctrl and PEMF, due to OF and PEMF + OF stimuli, cells built their extracellular matrix (ECM) over the scaffold surface, which was tending to be hidden by a dense layer of cell-extracellular matrix (Figure 1b).

3.2. Bone Matrix Production by Human Osteoblast-Like Cells onto Wool Keratin Scaffold after PEMF Treatment

To determine the action of daily PEMF exposure on human osteoblast-like cells cultured onto wool keratin scaffold, at the end of culture and treatment (21 days), all groups were assessed by evaluation of ALP activity, inorganic matrix production, bone-related protein gene expression and deposition. When the ALP activity was examined (Figure 2) it was found that both OF and PEMF + OF groups significantly increased the enzymatic activity over both ctrl and PEMF cultures (* $p < 0.001$ and § $p < 0.001$). The simultaneous treatment with PEMF and OF, however, significantly reduced the ALP activity when compared to the osteogenic factors' sole exposure (° $p < 0.001$).

Next, the quantification of the inorganic matrix produced was performed in all four conditions by the assessment of both phosphate and calcium content (Figure 3a,b). At day 21, the PEMF + OF group had the greatest phosphate content (ctrl, * $p < 0.001$; PEMF, § $p < 0.001$; OF, ° $p < 0.01$). Although no significant differences were detected between ctrl and PEMF samples ($p > 0.05$), a significant increase of phosphate was detected in PEMF + OF group and not in the OF group (° $p < 0.01$). In line with phosphate data, the analysis of calcium content reported that the calcium amount, expressed as pg of calcium per cell × scaffold, was greater in PEMF + OF samples than in the other conditions (* § ° $p < 0.001$). Additionally, the daily PEMF exposure significantly increased the calcium presence over ctrl (PEMF vs. ctrl, * $p < 0.05$) and over OF (PEMF + OF vs. OF, § $p < 0.001$). These quantitative results are corroborated by SEM-EDX elemental mapping (Figure 3c). Inorganic deposits were clearly identified by SEM imaging both in OF and PEMF + OF, but were absent both in ctrl and PEMF groups (Figure 3c). EDX elemental maps, in which calcium and phosphorus concentrations were mapped in green and red, respectively, revealed that the signal of both elements was remarkably higher and localized in specific region onto the wool keratin scaffold surfaces (indicated by the red dotted circles) treated with OF and PEMF + OF than the others (Figure 3c). In these latter conditions, both calcium and phosphorus signals were lower and appeared homogeneously distributed throughout the scaffold's surface.

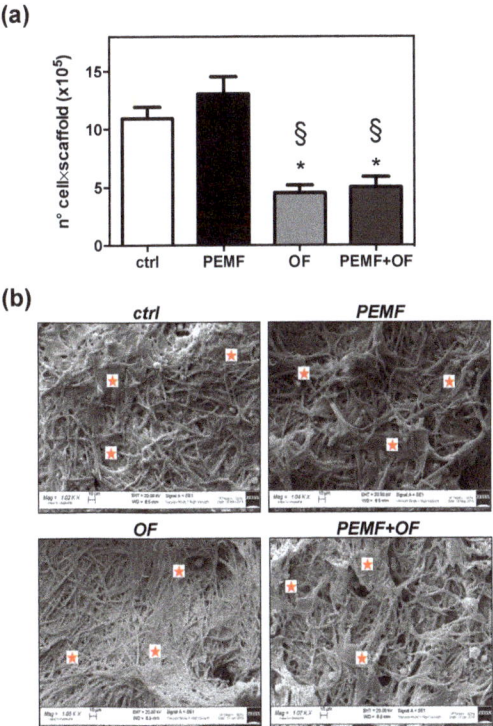

Figure 1. (a) Cell growth evaluation has been assessed by means of DNA quantification at day 21 of culture. Bars represent the mean values ± SD (standard deviation) of results (N = 3; n = 3, symbols indicate statistical significance vs. control (*) and vs. PEMF (§)). (b) Cell morphology assessed by SEM on all samples (scale bars = 10 μm; magnification: ctrl = 1020×; PEMF = 1040×; OF = 1050×; PEMF + OF = 1070×). Red stars indicate cell distribution on the wool keratin scaffolds in all conditions. In OF and PEMF + OF the dense layer of extracellular bone matrix (ECM) made difficult to discriminate a cell from another. Representative live cells visualized by fluorescein diacetate (FDA) staining on the scaffold's surfaces are shown in Figure S3.

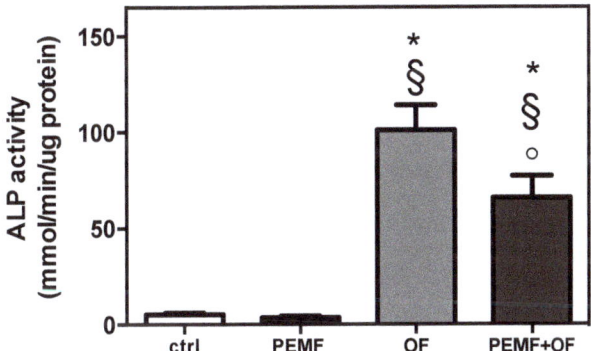

Figure 2. Alkaline phosphatase (ALP) activity after 21 days. ALP activity was colorimetrically determined, corrected for the protein content (measured with the BCA Protein Assay kit), and expressed as mM of p-nitrophenol produced per min per μg of protein. Bars express the mean ± SD (N = 3; n = 2, symbols indicate statistical significance vs. control (*), vs. PEMF (§) and vs. OF (°)).

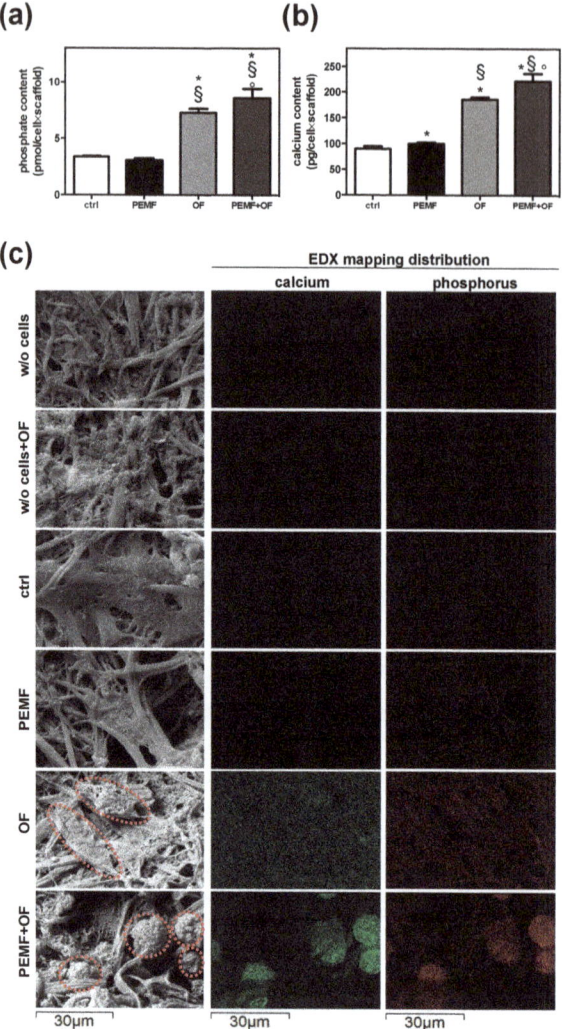

Figure 3. Quantification of inorganic matrix produced for 21 days. (**a**) Quantification of phosphate content by Phosphate Colorimetric Assay kit. Phosphate is measured in pmol/cell×scaffold; results are presented as mean ± SD (N = 3; n = 2; symbols indicate statistical significance vs. control (*), vs. PEMF (§) and vs. OF (°)). (**b**) Quantification of calcium content by the Ca^{2+}/o-cresolphthalein complexone method. Results are expressed as pg/cell×scaffold and presented as mean ± SD (N = 3; n = 2, symbols indicate statistical significance vs. control (*), vs. PEMF (§) and vs. OF (°)). (**c**) Scanning Electron Microscopy with Energy Dispersive X-ray Spectroscopy (SEM-EDX) analysis of calcium and phosphorous deposits. Representative SEM pictures show the presence of inorganic deposits (indicated with red dotted circles) in particular in cells cultured in wool keratin scaffolds and treated for 21 days with PEMF + OF. EDX elemental mapping of calcium (green) and phosphorus (red) relative to the SEM pictures (dimension: 64.68 × 43.12 μm). All EDX analyses were conducted with an accelerating voltage of 20 kV and under low vacuum conditions. Wool keratin scaffolds cultured in maintenance medium in absence of cells (w/o cells) and with OF (w/o cells + OF) for 21 days were included as control. In both these conditions, the calcium and phosphorus signals were negligible.

Subsequently, quantitative real-time PCR (qRT-PCR) analysis of the early and late osteogenic marker expression after 7 and 21 days was performed on the total RNA extracted from cells cultured in different conditions (Figure 4). In general, the addition of osteogenic factors in the maintenance media, with/without PEMF exposure, significantly enhanced osteogenic transcription factors levels in the cells cultured onto wool-keratin scaffold compared to day 0 (+ $p < 0.05$). This increase showed that variations of osteogenic genes were expression time dependent. During the early differentiation (day 1), the osteogenic gene expression was greatly upregulated in OF and PEMF + OF groups compared to ctrl and PEMF condition (* $p < 0.05$; § $p < 0.05$). Notably, expression of OSX, Runx-2, ALP and OSC gene expression was significantly increased by PEMF + OF compared with the OF group (° $p < 0.05$). At the same time, neither the control or PEMF group showed any stimulatory trend for osteogenic markers levels compared to day 0 ($p > 0.05$). Notably, at the end of the experimental procedure (21 days), expression of osteogenic genes declined in OF and PEMF + OF groups, but were still significantly higher than most genes tested on day 0 (+ $p < 0.05$), expect for Runx-2, which reached comparable levels of ctrl and day 0 ($p > 0.05$). Furthermore, on day 21 the stimulatory effect of PEMF in presence of OF was no longer apparent for the above-mentioned genes, with no significant difference between OF and PEM + OF condition ($p > 0.05$). It was interesting to observe that after 21 days of culture, the control group showed an increase of most analyzed genes (OSX, ALP, OSC, DCN, COL-1) in comparison with day 0 (+ $p < 0.05$). A similar trend was observed in PEMF exposure without osteogenic factors, with a strong upregulation of some genes related to the initial phases of osteogenic differentiation, like Runx-2 and ALP, compared with day 0 (+ $p < 0.05$).

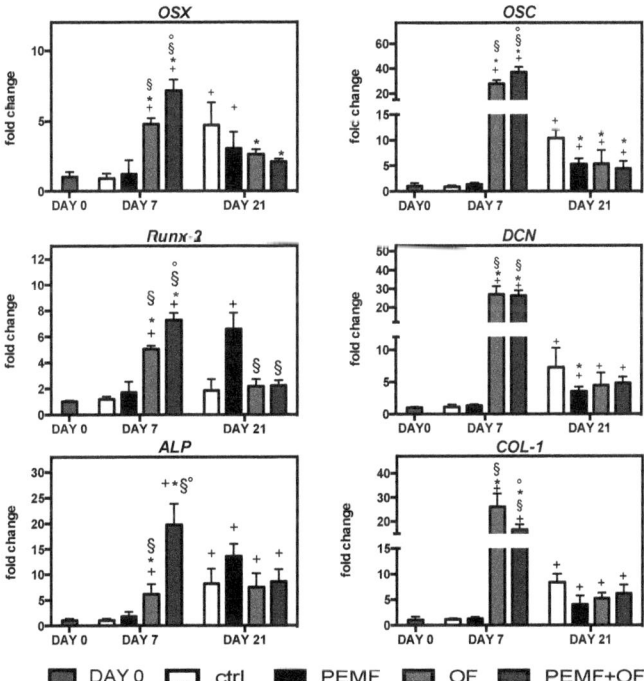

Figure 4. Gene expression of bone-specific markers as determined by quantitative reverse-transcription polymerase chain reaction (qRT-PCR) at day 7 and 21 of culture. Graphs show the fold change of gene expression relative to the expression in the cells at day 0. Symbols indicate statistical significance vs. day 0 (+), vs. control (*), vs. PEMF (§) and vs. OF (°) as determined by two-way ANOVA (N = 2, n = 3). Abbreviations: *OSX*, osterix; *Runx*-2, runt-related transcription factor-2; *ALP*, alkaline phosphatase; *OSC*, osteocalcin; *DCN*, decorin; *COL-I*, type-I collagen.

Furthermore, the extracellular matrix constituents were extracted and quantified by ELISA assay at the end of the culture to characterize the osteogenic process. Remarkably, at the end of the study it emerged that the amount of bone extracellular matrix proteins produced by cells onto wool fibril sponges resulted significantly higher in osteogenic groups (with or without PEMF) than in the control and PEMF-treated cells (* $p < 0.05$ and § $p < 0.05$, Figure 5a). Furthermore, the highest production was detected in cells exposed daily to PEMF with osteogenic factors added in the culture medium (PEMF + OF) over all the other samples. Noteworthy, compared to OF, a significant enhancement of ALP, OSN, DCN, and OSC deposition was found in PEMF + OF samples (° $p < 0.001$, ° $p < 0.01$, ° $p < 0.01$, ° $p < 0.05$, respectively). By contrast, no significant difference was measured between the control and PEMF-treated cells for all bone proteins measured ($p > 0.05$). Lastly, although the thick and intricated structure of the 3D wool keratin scaffolds presented challenges, the orthogonal projections of CLSM images confirmed the presence of cell (nuclei in blue), showing that they were able to migrate and infiltrate into the full depth of the scaffold and colonize its porosities. Agreeing with ELISA data, immunofluorescence images showed a clear and marked osteocalcin fluorescence signal, in particular in cells differentiated in OF and PEMF + OF treatments (Figure 5b).

3.3. Mechanical Properties of Wool Keratin Scaffolds after Cell Growth/Differentiation and PEMF Treatment

During compression cycles carried out in the dry state, wool keratin scaffolds (or sponges) showed a permanent deformation not evident in sponges compressed in wet conditions [4]. Since their application is forecast to be performed in wet conditions (inside body), the compression behavior was evaluated in wet conditions after 21 days of immersion in a culture medium. The compression behavior of sponges submitted to 10 repeated compression cycles in a wet state, after 21 days of immersion in MM with or without cells or PEMF, has been evaluated (Figure 6, Table 2).

Table 2. Mechanical characterization of wool fibril sponges in the wet state after 21 days in different culture conditions.

Experimental Condition	Compression Range (kPa)	Average Modulus (kPa)
without cells in MM	2–8	18.0 ± 5.2
	10–22	11.1 ± 8.3
without cells in PEMF	2–8	14.1 ± 2.2
	10–22	85.2 ± 8.1
without cells in OF	2–8	21.3 ± 3.1
	10–22	80.4 ± 7.4
without cells in PEMF + OF	2–8	22.1 ± 3.1
	10–22	54.4 ± 4.6
with cells in MM (ctrl)	2–8	24.2 ± 2.2
	10–22	102.6 ± 9.1
with cells in PEMF	2–8	16.2 ± 2.7
	10–22	58.3 ± 9.2
with cells in OF	2–8	27.4 ± 30.1
	10–22	90.5 ± 90.2
with cells in PEMF + OF	2–8	25.1± 3.3
	10–22	59.3± 8.1

After 21 days of culture in maintenance (MM) and osteogenic (OF) medium a resilient behavior was still observed: compression traces are almost overlapping each other, and no permanent deformation can be detected (Figure 6). All compression traces display a horizontal line in the load range 22–24 kPa, which is most likely due to reversible crushing deformation of the pore structure of sponges (Figure 6). In other words, water filled the macro- and micro-pores and penetrated into the amorphous keratin domains as well, resulting in increased elasticity of the whole structure. Nevertheless, for compression loads higher than 24 kPa, the structure of the wool fiber assembly would not represent a sponge anymore. Thus, the compression moduli of sponges have been compared in the load ranges 2–8 kPa and 10–22 kPa (Table 2).

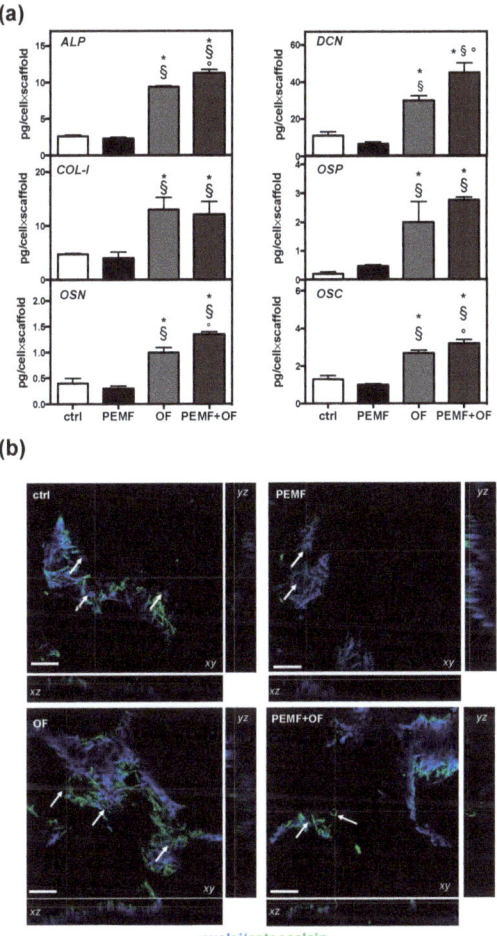

Figure 5. Bone osteogenic protein production by cells onto wool fibril sponges in the different conditions after 21 days of culture. (**a**) Quantification of indicated osteogenic proteins quantified by ELISA assay. Data are expressed as pg/cell×scaffold (N = 3; n = 2, symbols indicate statistical significance vs. control (*), vs. PEMF (§) and vs. OF (°)). (**b**) Representative orthogonal view of Confocal Laser Scanning Microscope (CLSM) images of bone osteocalcin immunolocalization (green) are shown with xy, yz, and xz planes. Nuclei (blue) were counterstained with Hoechst 33342. White arrows indicate the scaffold areas containing cells. Magnification 20×; the scale bar represents 50 µm. Negative control for non-specific staining of the secondary antibody and Tissue Culture Plates (TCPS) controls are shown in Figure S4.

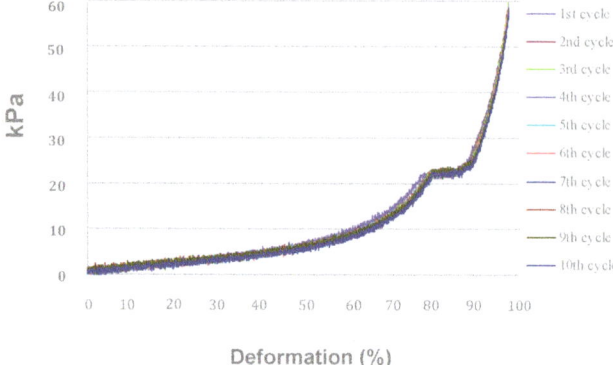

Figure 6. Compression traces of the wool fibril sponges in the wet state after 21 days of culture in MM with cells and PEMF. Similar behavior was obtained for all other conditions tested.

3.4. Ageing Test

Both wool keratin scaffolds and commercial collagen sponges (reference polymeric material) were immersed into the same Ringer's solution (ageing reference solution for bone biomaterials) at 37 °C. The degradation rate of collagen sponges was significantly higher when compared with the degradation rate of the wool scaffolds. The collagen sponges degraded completely in 22 days, whereas the wool sponges exhibited a degradation rate of only 22% only after 180 days (Figure 7).

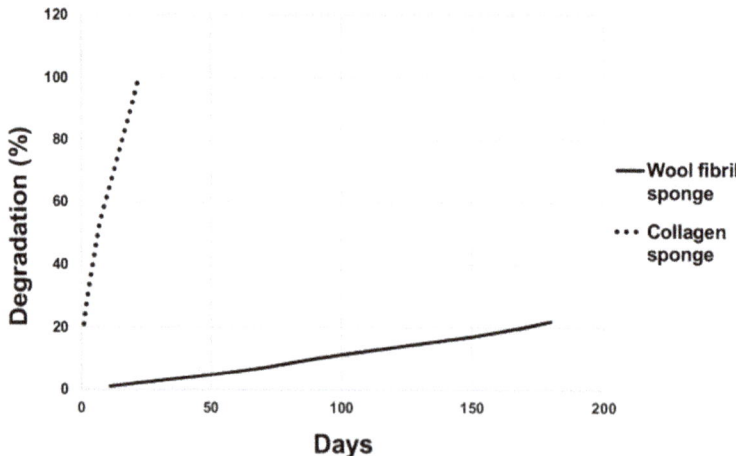

Figure 7. Degradation rate of the commercial collagen sponge vs. wool fibril sponge.

4. Discussion

Our study investigated the effects of electromagnetic stimulation on osteoblasts seeded onto wool keratin scaffolds in terms of growth, differentiation, and bone extracellular matrix production.

Most of the other materials used as scaffolds for the repair of bone defects offer only a feasible structure within which to heal or regenerate and do not induce or boost the regeneration processes. Among the biomaterials, bioceramic scaffolds, mainly from calcium phosphates, are widely employed for bone regeneration because of their chemical similarity to the bony inorganic matrix which confers osteoconductive properties, increasing scaffold integration inside tissue and, as a consequence, leading to the bone healing. A large number of strategies have and are been investigated in order to improve the interaction of biomaterial with bone tissue. The use of PEMF might be a potential adjuvant treatment to enhance the osseointegration process. The effects of PEMF on osteoblasts onto different biomaterials have been investigated in several in vitro and in vivo studies [14]. PEMFs act on osteoblasts, improving their growth, differentiation and expression of a mature phenotype on implanted materials and, as consequence, promote tissue integration [24–26]. Most of these researches were focused on titanium and titanium alloy-based biomaterials [7,23,25,27–30], but similar effects were also achieved after PEMF application on cells cultured onto bioceramic and polymers scaffolds [31–33].

The electromagnetic stimulus of this study was demonstrated [8,9] to elicit time varying mechanical forces acting perpendicularly or tangentially onto the cell membrane. For instance, osteoblasts are susceptible to fluid shear stress and react with an enhanced transcription of bone matrix genes [11,12]. Traction and compression vary the activities of intracellular signaling molecules such as Rho GTPases, guanine nucleotide exchange factors, GTPase activating proteins, and the MAPK pathway, consequently modulating the expression of transcription factors essential for the homeostasis of bone [13]. In addition, several studies demonstrated that the electromagnetic fields are accompanied by increases in cytosolic calcium concentration and might involve calcium/calmodulin pathway [34]. According to Pavalko's diffusion-controlled/solid-state signaling model, the increase of the cytosolic calcium concentration is a starting point of signaling pathways targeting specific genes of the bone matrix [11].

In agreement with this model, our previous findings on human mesenchymal stem cells (hMSCs) showed that the daily PEMF exposure affected cells osteogenesis by interfering with selective calcium-related osteogenic pathways [35], including when they were seeded on TiO_2 nanostructures surfaces [23]. In line with these studies, our previous findings on human mesenchymal stem cells (hMSCs) showed that the daily PEMF exposure affected cells osteogenesis by interfering with selective calcium-related osteogenic pathways [35], including when they were seeded on TiO_2 nanostructures surfaces [23].

We note, however, that though the effects of PEMF stimuli on cells are well documented, the mechanism of action is still unclear. The broad range of settings used for PEMFs stimulation represents an obstacle, making it difficult to compare the results in the literature. It has been demonstrated, for example, that the time of PEMF exposure could be a critical parameter [36]. We previously observed that exposure to PEMF for 10 min per day at the same time increased, on hMSCs, the extracellular matrix secretion as well as enhancing the osteogenic gene expression [23]. Another study on a rat model found that 1 h of exposure significantly improved the bone healing process compared with longer treatment [37]. Moreover, other variables can affect PEMF outcomes, including the types, density, and differentiation stage of cells [38] as well as the medium composition (e.g., serum percentage and osteogenic supplements) [39]. For these reasons, there are contradictory results. PEMF can directly stimulate osteoprogenitor cells towards osteogenic differentiation at the expense of proliferation [40], or enhance both hMSCs osteogenic differentiation and proliferation [41]. Besides, Martino et al. reported that repetitive PEMF exposure increased the SAOS-2 matrix mineralization without affecting cell proliferation [42]. In agreement with Martino et al., in our experimental settings, we observed that, the daily application of pulsed electromagnetic field slightly affected SAOS-2 growth (both with or without osteogenic factors), but that osteogenic differentiation and mineralization significantly increased only in combination with osteogenic agents. The number of proliferated cells and their differentiation should be important parameters to estimate the biological effect of PEMF on cells onto the wool keratin scaffold. According to our results, cell proliferation increased with culture time in all conditions tested (ctrl, PEMF, OF, and PEMF + OF), demonstrating that the scaffold has good biocompatibility. However, at the end of culture, the proliferation resulted lower in the groups cultured in the presence of the osteogenic factors, with or without PEMF, suggesting a link with the osteogenic factors' addition. Commonly, in vitro osteogenic factors (e.g., dexamethasone and β-glycerophosphate) are directly introduced into the culture medium to drive the cells toward osteogenic differentiation: dexamethasone is a synthetic glucocorticoid that activates the osteogenic lineage differentiation and β-glycerophosphate acts as a source of phosphate with an important role in the mineralization process. At the beginning of the osteogenic differentiation, cells undergo a proliferation process that stops when the differentiation starts [43]. Additionally, this phenomenon may clarify the small increase of proliferation found in OF and PEMF + OF groups at the end of the experiments.

Again, because of variables mentioned, the effects of PEMF described in the literature vary considerably, with significant variations in the determination of the peak. Tsai et al. observed an increase of ALP activity on hMSCs after PEMF stimulation on day 7, but not on day 3 and 10 [44], whereas Jansen et al. reported that ALP activity was not significantly affected by PEMF treatment and the peak significantly varied between bone marrow mesenchymal stem cells from different donors [40]. After 21 days, we detected a lower ALP activity in PEMF + OF cultures than the OF samples. During osteogenic differentiation, in the early stages, there is an initial peak in ALP activity, which is followed by a subsequent reduction as the cells mature and lay down mineral [45,46]. Here, it is possible to speculate that the decrease of ALP activity observed in PEMF + OF group over OF may be correlated with the fact that, after 21 days, the cells were in the late stage of differentiation as a consequence of both osteogenic factors and PEMF stimulation, well-known to accelerate and boost the osteogenic differentiation and mineralization [47]. It is probable that we overlooked and missed the PEMF induced stimulation of ALP activity, which could have occurred earlier than 21 days.

The ECM deposition and calcification represent optimal indicators for assessing the in vitro maturation of osteoblastic phenotype [48]. Notably, in our in vitro system, the presence of the osteogenic factors seemed to be critical for the osteogenic commitment in PEMF-treated groups. SAOS-2 cells stimulated by PEMF, without osteogenic factors, clearly displayed comparable levels of mineralization with ctrl groups. By contrast, when cultured in medium containing osteogenic ingredients, PEMF-treated cells increased both phosphate and calcium deposition. SEM images and EDS mapping of the elements Ca, P, and Mg corroborated the idea that the new bone matrix was ultimately deposited onto the surface of the wool keratin scaffold. Also, the osteogenic factors determined an enhancement of both calcium and phosphate contents, but the OF-groups merely presented a homogeneous distribution of both elements onto the scaffold surface. The formation of mineral nodules, mainly in PEMF + OF cases, might be ascribable to the accelerated differentiation exerted by the synergic action of PEMF and OF, a point which was also confirmed by the quantification of bone-related proteins. We observed that PEMF exposure significantly increased the production of some proteins related to the matrix deposition and mineralization (e.g., ALP, OSN, DCN, and OSC), preferentially in osteogenic medium (PEMF + OF group). The enhancement of the proteins implicated in bone formation and remodeling further supports the hypothesis that PEMF, in combination with osteogenic signals, promotes the production of proteins necessary for mineralization (ALP makes the phosphates available for calcification, OSN is a calcium- and collagen-binding ECM glycoprotein acting as a modulator of cell-matrix interactions, DCN orchestrates the correct collagen fibril assembly, OSC is the most specific marker for osteoblasts maturation [49]).

The qRT-PCR analysis appears to confirm the speeding-up effects towards a fully osteoblastic mature state exerted by the simultaneous presence of OF and PEMF. Indeed, during the early differentiation (day 7), we determined an up-regulation of osteogenic markers in both OF and PEMF-treated groups. At day 21 of culture, we found a decrease of the expression of both early (Runx-2, OSX, ALP) and late bone-related genes (COL-I, DCN, OSC) in particular in both PEMF + OF and OF condition than control and PEMF group. These findings strongly suggest that the PEMF + OF exposition seems to accelerate the cells toward the bone differentiation pathway influencing all the proteins involved in terms of transcription and translation in a significant manner. Hypothetically, the bone protein transcription was immediately activated after the osteogenic addition, with or without PEMF exposition, which allowed protein translation. Perhaps the fast reaching of a mature phenotype from the cells in these conditions forced them to downregulate and prematurely stop the protein transcription with respect to protein translation. Interestingly, in the ctrl and PEMF groups, cells could be in an early stage of differentiation, and so result in a higher level of bone gene expression over OF and PEMF + OF, that may be due to spontaneous differentiation of the cells after 21 days of culture in response to the porous topography of the scaffold. In general, similarly to a previous study where PEMF alone did not affect cell mineralization or cell viability in osteoblast-precursor MC3T3-E1 cells [50], we found that SAOS-2 cells matrix mineralization was heavily influenced by the PEMF exposure only when the medium was supplemented with the osteogenic factors. Furthermore, keratin presents peculiar tri-peptide motives relevant for cell binding, such as leucine-aspartic acid-valine (LDV), glutamic acid-aspartic acid-serine (EDS), and arginine-glycine-aspartic acid (RGD). Indeed, these motives are found in several extracellular matrix proteins, like fibronectin [51] and their interaction with cells can elicit different responses [52]. These responses might overlap with the signaling regulation exerted by PEMF and/or osteogenic factors. As reported by Klontzas et al. [53], alginate hydrogels crosslinked with a specific tri-peptide (glycine-histidine-lysine or GHK, characterizing the bone ECM protein osteonectin) significantly induced osteogenic differentiation because of the presence of this GHK peptide. Hence, we can speculate the different mechanical/biochemical stimuli utilized in the present study are acting on the very same or closely interconnected metabolic pathways. To corroborate or refute this hypothesis, further studies should focus on the specific action the individual stimulus has on the osteogenic differentiation pathways. Besides, precise and analytic approaches, such as mass spectrometry-based metabolomics and proteomics could be properly employed for these purposes.

In summary, we have demonstrated the importance of including both physical and biochemical factors for fostering the osteogenic differentiation. PEMF (frequency of 75 Hz, magnetic induction of 2 mT, 1 h of exposure per day) stimulated in the osteogenic cultures the highest production of bone extracellular matrix and, therefore, it could be very useful in combination with osteogenic factors during the cell culture onto wool keratin scaffolds. Finally, no significant differences were detected in mechanical behavior between scaffolds with or without cells, in maintenance or osteogenic medium and with or without PEMF. The presence of SAOS-2 cells influenced neither the compression behavior nor the resilience of keratin scaffolds in wet conditions. As expected, the wool fibril sponges showed high chemical and physical stability after 21 days of culture, despite the fact that they consist of proteins (biodegradable polymers). Ageing tests revealed that wool fibril sponges, characterized by an exceptional number of crosslinks stabilizing the keratin structure are very stable and show a lower degradation rate than commercial collagen sponges. This suggests that these materials have a promising application for long-term support of in vivo bone formation (e.g., as biocompatible, bone-proteins rich, bone-cells rich fillers for bone defects). In the future, experiments involving a higher number of scaffolds may help to study more precisely the not significant results observed in our study.

5. Conclusions

With the awareness that in vivo studies will confirm the feasibility and the bone healing potentiality of the integrated bioengineering approach proposed in this paper, we can conclude by stating that this is the first in vitro evidence of the positive advantages of this approach: the capability of the PEMF to boost the osteogenic differentiation in synergy with osteogenic factors made the 3D wool keratin an osteoconductive biomaterial, which, once tested in in vivo models, may elicit positive bone response and may speed up tissue healing after surgery. Prospectively, this experimental design may be employed to electromagnetically stimulate the differentiation of bone marrow mesenchymal stem cells toward the osteogenic phenotype onto keratin substrates, subsequently leading to a potential application in regenerative medicine.

Supplementary Materials: The following are available online at http://www.mdpi.com/1996-1944/13/14/3052/s1, Figure S1: CLSM morphological analysis of osteoblast-like cells seeded onto the wool fibril sponges, Figure S2: Viability of SAOS-2 cells cultured onto the wool keratin scaffolds and exposed to different PEMF doses, Figure S3: Representative CLSM images of live cells onto wool fibril sponge in the different experimental conditions, Figure S4: Representative CLSM images of negative control for non-specific staining of the secondary antibody and TCPS controls, Table S1: Primers used for qRT-PCR study.

Author Contributions: L.V. conceived the research and was responsible for the correctness of biological analyses and contributed to write and edit the manuscript. C.T., A.P. and R.C. were responsible for the synthesis and characterization of the wool-keratin scaffolds. N.B. performed all the biological experiments and analyses. G.M. contributed to ELISA assays analysis. G.B. performed SEM analysis. L.F. contributed to the PEMF setup. N.B., L.F., and A.P. contributed to write and edit the manuscript. L.V., C.T., and R.C. revised the final manuscript. All authors have read and agreed to the published version of the manuscript.

Funding: The work was supported by Compagnia San Paolo, Turin, project title "Evaluation of the effects of electromagnetic fields on adult stem cells as potential osteoregenerative therapy" (2012) and from an INAIL grant entitled "Effetti dei campi elettromagnetici sulla salute umana: modelli sperimentali in vitro" (2011). We would also like to thank COST Action BM1309 EMF-MED, "European network for innovative uses of EMFs in biomedical applications (2014–2019)" (www.COST-EMF-MED.eu). This research was also supported by a grant of the Italian Ministry of Education, University and Research (MIUR) to the Department of Molecular Medicine of the University of Pavia under the initiative "Dipartimenti di Eccellenza (2018–2022)".

Acknowledgments: The authors wish to thank P. Vaghi (Centro Grandi Strumenti, University of Pavia, Pavia, Italy, https://cgs.unipv.it/) for technical assistance in the CLSM studies. A special thanks to Scott Burgess (University of Pavia) for correcting the English in the manuscript.

Conflicts of Interest: The authors declare no conflict of interest. The funders had no role in the design of the study; in the collection, analyses, or interpretation of data; in the writing of the manuscript, or in the decision to publish the results.

References

1. McLellan, J.; Thornhill, S.G.; Shelton, S.; Kumar, M. *Keratin-Based Biofilms, Hydrogels, and Biofibers*; Chapter 7 of 'Keratin as a Protein Biopolymer'; Springer: Cham, Switzerland, 2019; pp. 187–200.
2. Feroz, S.; Muhammad, N.; Ranayake, J.; Dias, G. Keratin—Based materials for biomedical applications. *Bioact. Mater.* **2020**, *5*, 496–509. [CrossRef]
3. De Guzman, R.C.; Saul, J.M.; Ellenburg, M.D.; Merrill, M.R.; Coan, H.B.; Smith, T.L.; Van Dyke, M.E. Bone regeneration with BMP-2 delivered from keratose scaffolds. *Biomaterials* **2013**, *34*, 1644–1656. [CrossRef] [PubMed]
4. Patrucco, A.; Cristofaro, F.; Simionati, M.; Zoccola, M.; Bruni, G.; Fassina, L.; Visai, L.; Magenes, G.; Mossotti, R.; Montarsolo, A.; et al. Wool fibril sponges with perspective biomedical applications. *Mater. Sci. Eng. C Mater. Biol. Appl.* **2016**, *61*, 42–50. [CrossRef] [PubMed]
5. Fassina, L.; Visai, L.; Asti, L.; Benazzo, F.; Speziale, P.; Tanzi, M.C.; Magenes, G. Calcified matrix production by SAOS-2 cells inside a polyurethane porous scaffold, using a perfusion bioreactor. *Tissue Eng.* **2005**, *11*, 685–700. [CrossRef] [PubMed]
6. Fassina, L.; Saino, E.; Cusella De Angelis, M.G.; Magenes, G.; Benazzo, F.; Visai, L. Low-power ultrasounds as a tool to culture human osteoblasts inside cancellous hydroxyapatite. *Bioinorg. Chem. Appl.* **2010**, *2010*, 456240. [CrossRef]
7. Saino, E.; Maliardi, V.; Quartarone, E.; Fassina, L.; Benedetti, L.; Cusella De Angelis, M.G.; Mustarelli, P.; Facchini, A.; Visai, L. In vitro enhancement of SAOS-2 cell calcified matrix deposition onto radio frequency magnetron sputtered bioglass-coated titanium scaffolds. *Tissue Eng. Part A* **2010**, *16*, 995–1008. [CrossRef]
8. Mognaschi, M.E.; Di Barba, P.; Magenes, G.; Lenzi, A.; Naro, F.; Fassina, L. Field models and numerical dosimetry inside an extremely-low-frequency electromagnetic bioreactor: The theoretical link between the electromagnetically induced mechanical forces and the biological mechanisms of the cell tensegrity. *SpringerPlus* **2014**, *3*, 473. [CrossRef]
9. Fassina, L.; Visai, L.; Benazzo, F.; Benedetti, L.; Calligaro, A.; Cusella De Angelis, M.G.; Farina, A.; Maliardi, V.; Magenes, G. Effects of electromagnetic stimulation on calcified matrix production by SAOS-2 cells over a polyurethane porous scaffold. *Tissue Eng.* **2006**, *12*, 1985–1999. [CrossRef]
10. Mammoto, T.; Ingber, D.E. Mechanical control of tissue and organ development. *Development* **2010**, *137*, 1407–1420. [CrossRef]
11. Pavalko, F.M.; Norvell, S.M.; Burr, D.B.; Turner, C.H.; Duncan, R.L.; Bidwell, J.P. A model for mechanotransduction in bone cells: The load-bearing mechanosomes. *J. Cell. Biochem.* **2003**, *88*, 104–112. [CrossRef]
12. Young, S.R.; Gerard-O'Riley, R.; Kim, J.B.; Pavalko, F.M. Focal adhesion kinase is important for fluid shear stress-induced mechanotransduction in osteoblasts. *J. Bone Miner. Res.* **2009**, *24*, 411–424. [CrossRef] [PubMed]

13. Mammoto, A.; Mammoto, T.; Ingber, D.E. Mechanosensitive mechanisms in transcriptional regulation. *J. Cell Sci.* **2012**, *125*, 3061–3073. [CrossRef]
14. Galli, C.; Pedrazzi, G.; Mattioli-Belmonte, M.; Guizzardi, S. The use of pulsed electromagnetic fields to promote bone responses to biomaterials in vitro and in vivo. *Int. J. Biomater.* **2018**, *2018*, 8935750. [CrossRef]
15. Aluigi, A.; Corbellini, A.; Rombaldoni, F.; Zoccola, M.; Canetti, M. Morphological and structural investigation of wool-derived keratin nanofibres crosslinked by thermal treatment. *Int. J. Biol. Macromol.* **2013**, *57*, 30–37. [CrossRef] [PubMed]
16. Ceccarelli, G.; Bloise, N.; Mantelli, M.; Gastaldi, G.; Fassina, L.; Cusella De Angelis, M.G.; Ferrari, D.; Imbriani, M.; Visai, L. A comparative analysis of the in vitro effects of pulsed electromagnetic field treatment on osteogenic differentiation of two different mesenchymal cell lineages. *Biores. Open Access* **2013**, *2*, 283–294. [CrossRef] [PubMed]
17. Bloise, N.; Ceccarelli, G.; Minzioni, P.; Vercellino, M.; Benedetti, L.; Cusella De Angelis, M.G.; Imbriani, M.; Visai, L. Investigation of low-level laser therapy potentiality on proliferation and differentiation of human osteoblast-like cells in the absence/presence of osteogenic factors. *J. Biomed. Opt.* **2013**, *18*, 128006. [CrossRef] [PubMed]
18. Livak, K.J.; Schmittgen, T.D. Analysis of relative gene expression data using real-time quantitative PCR and the $2^{-\Delta\Delta Ct}$ Method. *Methods* **2001**, *25*, 402–408. [CrossRef]
19. Ayre, W.N.; Denyer, S.P.; Evans, S.L. Ageing and moisture uptake in polymethyl methacrylate (PMMA) bone cements. *J. Mech. Behav. Biomed. Mater.* **2014**, *32*, 76–88. [CrossRef]
20. Anderson, H.C.; Reynolds, P.R.; Hsu, H.H.; Missana, L.; Masuhara, K.; Moylan, P.E.; Roach, H.I. Selective synthesis of bone morphogenetic proteins-1, -3, -4 and bone sialoprotein may be important for osteoinduction by Saos-2 cells. *J. Bone Miner. Metab.* **2002**, *20*, 73–82. [CrossRef]
21. Kitsara, M.; Blanquer, A.; Murillo, G.; Humblot, V.; De Bragança Vieira, S.; Nogués, C.; Ibáñez, E.; Esteve, J.; Barrios, L. Permanently hydrophilic, piezoelectric PVDF nanofibrous scaffolds promoting unaided electromechanical stimulation on osteoblasts. *Nanoscale* **2019**, *11*, 8906–8917. [CrossRef]
22. Saldaña, L.; Bensiamar, F.; Boré, A.; Vilaboa, N. In search of representative models of human bone-forming cells for cytocompatibility studies. *Acta Biomater.* **2011**, *7*, 4210–4221. [CrossRef] [PubMed]
23. Bloise, N.; Petecchia, L.; Ceccarelli, G.; Fassina, L.; Usai, C.; Bertoglio, F.; Balli, M.; Vassalli, M.; Cusella De Angelis, M.G.; Gavazzo, P.; et al. The effect of pulsed electromagnetic field exposure on osteoinduction of human mesenchymal stem cells cultured on nano-TiO_2 surfaces. *PLoS ONE* **2018**, *13*, e0199046. [CrossRef] [PubMed]
24. Bagheri, L.; Pellati, A.; Rizzo, P.; Aquila, G.; Massari, L.; De Mattei, M.; Ongaro, A. Notch pathway is active during osteogenic differentiation of human bone marrow mesenchymal stem cells induced by pulsed electromagnetic fields. *J. Tissue Eng. Regen. Med.* **2018**, *12*, 304–315. [CrossRef]
25. Cai, J.; Li, W.; Sun, T.; Li, X.; Luo, E.; Jing, D. Pulsed electromagnetic fields preserve bone architecture and mechanical properties and stimulate porous implant osseointegration by promoting bone anabolism in type 1 diabetic rabbits. *Osteoporos. Int.* **2018**, *29*, 1177–1191. [CrossRef]
26. Fassina, L.; Bloise, N.; Montagna, G.; Visai, L.; Mognaschi, M.E.; Benazzo, F.; Magenes, G. Biomaterials and biophysical stimuli for bone regeneration. *J. Biol. Regul. Homeost. Agents* **2018**, *32*, 41–49.
27. Fassina, L.; Saino, E.; Sbarra, M.S.; Visai, L.; Cusella De Angelis, M.G.; Mazzini, G.; Benazzo, F.; Magenes, G. Ultrasonic and electromagnetic enhancement of a culture of human SAOS-2 osteoblasts seeded onto a titanium plasma-spray surface. *Tissue Eng. Part. C Methods* **2009**, *15*, 233–242. [CrossRef] [PubMed]
28. Fassina, L.; Saino, E.; Visai, L.; Magenes, G. Electromagnetically enhanced coating of a sintered titanium grid with human SAOS-2 osteoblasts and extracellular matrix. *Conf. Proc. IEEE Eng. Med. Biol. Soc.* **2008**, *2008*, 3582–3585. [PubMed]
29. Fassina, L.; Saino, E.; Visai, L.; Silvani, G.; Cusella De Angelis, M.G.; Mazzini, G.; Benazzo, F.; Magenes, G. Electromagnetic enhancement of a culture of human SAOS-2 osteoblasts seeded onto titanium fiber-mesh scaffolds. *J. Biomed. Mater. Res. A* **2008**, *87*, 750–759. [CrossRef] [PubMed]
30. Fassina, L.; Saino, E.; Visai, L.; Magenes, G. Physically enhanced coating of a titanium plasma-spray surface with human SAOS-2 osteoblasts and extracellular matrix. *Conf. Proc. IEEE Eng. Med. Biol. Soc.* **2007**, *2007*, 6415–6418.

31. Shimizu, T.; Zerwekh, J.E.; Videman, T.; Gill, K.; Mooney, V.; Holmes, R.E.; Hagler, H.K. Bone Ingrowth into Porous Calcium-Phosphate Ceramics—Influence of Pulsing Electromagnetic-Field. *J. Orthop. Res.* **1988**, *6*, 248–258. [CrossRef]
32. Arjmand, M.; Ardeshirylajimi, A.; Maghsoudi, H.; Azadian, E. Osteogenic differentiation potential of mesenchymal stem cells cultured on nanofibrous scaffold improved in the presence of pulsed electromagnetic field. *J. Cell. Physiol.* **2018**, *233*, 1061–1070. [CrossRef] [PubMed]
33. Fassina, L.; Saino, E.; Visai, L.; Schelfhout, J.; Dierick, M.; Van Hoorebeke, L.; Dubruel, P.; Benazzo, F.; Magenes, G.; Van Vlierberghe, S. Electromagnetic stimulation to optimize the bone regeneration capacity of gelatin-based cryogels. *Int. J. Immunopathol. Pharmacol.* **2012**, *25*, 165–174. [CrossRef] [PubMed]
34. Panagopoulos, D.J.; Karabarbounis, A.; Margaritis, L.H. Mechanism for action of electromagnetic fields on cells. *Biochem. Biophys. Res. Commun.* **2002**, *298*, 95–102. [CrossRef]
35. Petecchia, L.; Sbrana, F.; Utzeri, R.; Vercellino, M.; Usai, C.; Visai, L.; Vassalli, M.; Gavazzo, P. Electro-magnetic field promotes osteogenic differentiation of BM-hMSCs through a selective action on Ca^{2+}-related mechanisms. *Sci. Rep.* **2015**, *5*, 13856. [CrossRef] [PubMed]
36. De Mattei, M.; Caruso, A.; Traina, G.C.; Pezzetti, F.; Baroni, T.; Sollazzo, V. Correlation between pulsed electromagnetic fields exposure time and cell proliferation increase in human osteosarcoma cell lines and human normal osteoblast cells in vitro. *Bioelectromagnetics* **1999**, *20*, 177–182. [CrossRef]
37. Huegel, J.; Choi, D.S.; Nuss, C.A.; Minnig, M.C.C.; Tucker, J.J.; Kuntz, A.F.; Waldorff, E.I.; Zhang, N.; Ryaby, J.T.; Soslowsky, L.J. Effects of pulsed electromagnetic field therapy at different frequencies and durations on rotator cuff tendon-to-bone healing in a rat model. *J. Shoulder Elbow Surg.* **2018**, *27*, 553–560. [CrossRef]
38. Diniz, P.; Shomura, K.; Soejima, K.; Ito, G. Effects of pulsed electromagnetic field (PEMF) stimulation on bone tissue like formation are dependent on the maturation stages of the osteoblasts. *Bioelectromagnetics* **2002**, *23*, 398–405. [CrossRef] [PubMed]
39. Chang, W.H.; Chen, L.T.; Sun, J.S.; Lin, F.H. Effect of pulse-burst electromagnetic field stimulation on osteoblast cell activities. *Bioelectromagnetics* **2004**, *25*, 457–465. [CrossRef]
40. Jansen, J.H.; van der Jagt, O.P.; Punt, B.J.; Verhaar, J.A.; van Leeuwen, J.P.; Weinans, H.; Jahr, H. Stimulation of osteogenic differentiation in human osteoprogenitor cells by pulsed electromagnetic fields: An in vitro study. *BMC Musculoskelet. Disord.* **2010**, *11*, 188. [CrossRef]
41. Ferroni, L.; Gardin, C.; Dolkart, O.; Salai, M.; Barak, S.; Piattelli, A.; Amir-Barak, H.; Zavan, B. Pulsed electromagnetic fields increase osteogenetic commitment of MSCs via the mTOR pathway in TNF-α mediated inflammatory conditions: An *in-vitro* study. *Sci. Rep.* **2018**, *8*, 5108. [CrossRef]
42. Martino, C.F.; Belchenko, D.; Ferguson, V.; Nielsen-Preiss, S.; Qi, H.J. The effects of pulsed electromagnetic fields on the cellular activity of SaOS-2 cells. *Bioelectromagnetics* **2008**, *29*, 125–132. [CrossRef] [PubMed]
43. Huang, Z.; Nelson, E.R.; Smith, R.L.; Goodman, S.B. The sequential expression profiles of growth factors from osteoprogenitors to osteoblasts in vitro. *Tissue Eng.* **2007**, *13*, 2311–2320. [CrossRef] [PubMed]
44. Tsai, M.T.; Li, W.J.; Tuan, R.S.; Chang, W.H. Modulation of osteogenesis in human mesenchymal stem cells by specific pulsed electromagnetic field stimulation. *J. Orthop. Res.* **2009**, *27*, 1169–1174. [CrossRef] [PubMed]
45. Aubin, J.E. Regulation of osteoblast formation and function. *Rev. Endocr. Metab. Disord.* **2001**, *2*, 81–94. [CrossRef]
46. Thibault, R.A.; Scott Baggett, L.; Mikos, A.G.; Kasper, F.K. Osteogenic differentiation of mesenchymal stem cells on pregenerated extracellular matrix scaffolds in the absence of osteogenic cell culture supplements. *Tissue Eng. Part A* **2010**, *16*, 431–440. [CrossRef]
47. Ongaro, A.; Pellati, A.; Bagheri, L.; Fortini, C.; Setti, S.; De Mattei, M. Pulsed electromagnetic fields stimulate osteogenic differentiation in human bone marrow and adipose tissue derived mesenchymal stem cells. *Bioelectromagnetics* **2014**, *35*, 426–436. [CrossRef]
48. Alvarez Perez, M.A.; Guarino, V.; Cirillo, V.; Ambrosio, L. In vitro mineralization and bone osteogenesis in poly(ε-caprolactone)/gelatin nanofibers. *J. Biomed. Mater. Res. A* **2012**, *100*, 3008–3019. [CrossRef]
49. Licini, C.; Vitale-Brovarone, C.; Mattioli-Belmonte, M. Collagen and non-collagenous proteins molecular crosstalk in the pathophysiology of osteoporosis. *Cytokine Growth Factor Rev.* **2019**, *49*, 59–69. [CrossRef]
50. Suryani, L.; Too, J.H.; Hassanbhai, A.M.; Wen, F.; Lin, D.J.; Yu, N.; Teoh, S.H. Effects of Electromagnetic Field on Proliferation, Differentiation, and Mineralization of MC3T3 Cells. *Tissue Eng. Part C Methods* **2019**, *25*, 114–125. [CrossRef] [PubMed]

51. Tachibana, A.; Furuta, Y.; Takeshima, H.; Tanabe, T.; Yamauchi, K. Fabrication of wool keratin sponge scaffolds for long-term cell cultivation. *J. Biotechnol.* **2002**, *93*, 165–170. [CrossRef]
52. Sainio, A.; Jarvelainen, H. Extracellular matrix-cell interactions: Focus on therapeutic applications. *Cell. Signal.* **2020**, *66*, 109487. [CrossRef] [PubMed]
53. Klontzas, M.E.; Reakasame, S.; Silva, R.; Morais, J.C.F.; Vernardis, S.; MacFarlane, R.J.; Heliotis, M.; Tsiridis, E.; Panoskaltsis, N.; Boccaccini, A.R.; et al. Oxidized alginate hydrogels with the GHK peptide enhance cord blood mesenchymal stem cell osteogenesis: A paradigm for metabolomics-based evaluation of biomaterial design. *Acta Biomater.* **2019**, *88*, 224–240. [CrossRef] [PubMed]

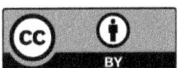

© 2020 by the authors. Licensee MDPI, Basel, Switzerland. This article is an open access article distributed under the terms and conditions of the Creative Commons Attribution (CC BY) license (http://creativecommons.org/licenses/by/4.0/).

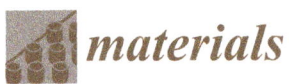

Article

Mineralization in a Critical Size Bone-Gap in Sheep Tibia Improved by a Chitosan-Calcium Phosphate-Based Composite as Compared to Predicate Device

Gissur Örlygsson [1,*], Elín H. Laxdal [2,3], Sigurbergur Kárason [2,4], Atli Dagbjartsson [2], Eggert Gunnarsson [5], Chuen-How Ng [6], Jón M. Einarsson [6], Jóhannes Gíslason [6] and Halldór Jónsson, Jr. [2,7]

1 IceTec, 112 Reykjavík, Iceland
2 Faculty of Medicine, University of Iceland, 101 Reykjavík, Iceland; artvita2@gmail.com (E.H.L.); skarason@landspitali.is (S.K.); ingibjorgsim@internet.is (A.D.); halldor@landspitali.is (H.J.J.)
3 Department of Vascular Surgery, Landspítali University Hospital, 108 Reykjavík, Iceland
4 Department of Anaesthesia and Intensive Care, Landspítali University Hospital, 108 Reykjavík, Iceland
5 Institute for Experimental Pathology, University of Iceland, 112 Reykjavík, Iceland; eggun@hi.is
6 Genis hf., 580 Siglufjörður, Iceland; ngchw@genis.is (C.-H.N.); jon.einarsson@genis.is (J.M.E.); johgisla@gmail.com (J.G.)
7 Department of Orthopaedic Surgery, Landspítali University Hospital, 108 Reykjavík, Iceland
* Correspondence: gissur@taeknisetur.is; Tel.: +354-6983958

Abstract: Deacetylated chitin derivatives have been widely studied for tissue engineering purposes. This study aimed to compare the efficacy of an injectable product containing a 50% deacetylated chitin derivative (BoneReg-Inject™) and an existing product (chronOS Inject®) serving as a predicate device. A sheep model with a critical size drill hole in the tibial plateau was used. Holes of 8 mm diameter and 30 mm length were drilled bilaterally into the proximal area of the tibia and BoneReg-Inject™ or chronOS Inject® were injected into the right leg holes. Comparison of resorption and bone formation in vivo was made by X-ray micro-CT and histological evaluation after a live phase of 12 weeks. Long-term effects of BoneReg-Inject™ were studied using a 13-month live period. Significant differences were observed in (1) amount of new bone within implant ($p < 0.001$), higher in BoneReg-Inject™, (2) signs of cartilage tissue ($p = 0.003$), more pronounced in BoneReg-Inject™, and (3) signs of fibrous tissue ($p < 0.001$), less pronounced in BoneReg-Inject™. Mineral content at 13 months postoperative was significantly higher than at 12 weeks ($p < 0.001$ and $p < 0.05$, for implant core and rim, respectively). The data demonstrate the potential of deacetylated chitin derivatives to stimulate bone formation.

Keywords: bone implant; bone defects; chitosan; degree of deacetylation; bone formation; X-ray micro CT; histology; sheep tibia

1. Introduction

Whenever disease or trauma causes skeletal void or when healing of a fracture is impaired, a common surgical technique is to harvest bone from the iliac crest of the patient and insert it to the injury site to fill the void (autograft). Autografts are regarded as the golden standard in orthopedic surgery. Still, this procedure has a severe drawback, i.e., donor site morbidity such as pain and numbness [1]. Over the last decade, several new products have been introduced, intended to replace bone autografts for filling of skeletal voids and/or for stimulation of bone healing [2,3]. This rapidly growing group of materials is commonly referred to as "synthetic bone graft substitutes". Despite an intensive search for replacement therapies, no single material has been developed with proven properties that would make it suitable for filling skeletal defects as well as for induction or promotion of bone healing [4]. Instead, two major groups of synthetic bone graft materials can be identified where one group has properties intended to provide bone induction, while in

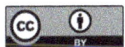

the other group materials have properties that make them suitable to fill bone voids caused by trauma or disease. This second group is by far the larger of the two in terms of product excess, while the group intended for bone induction only consists of a very small number of products. As an example of a material intended for bone induction, synthetic grafts containing bone morphogenic protein (BMP), a recombinant growth factor, are effective in many applications [5]. However they are only approved for a limited number of indications due to safety concerns, such as heterotopic ossification [6,7].

Chitosan is a natural biopolymer that has been shown to promote both differentiation of stem cells into bone-forming osteoblasts and growth of bone colonies in in vitro studies [8–11], suggesting osteogenic properties. Results of in vivo studies indicate that chitosan alone is sufficient to stimulate osteogenesis [10,12,13]. Studies where other materials with osteogenic, osteo-inductive and/or osteoconductive properties were added to chitosan-based composites to further stimulate the bone healing process have also been described in the literature [14,15].

Chitosan is biodegradable and biocompatible and consists of a linear polysaccharide chain comprising randomly distributed β-(1→4)-linked D-glucosamine and N-acetyl-D-glucosamine units. It is derived from chitin, an insoluble linear β-(1→4)-linked N-acetyl-D-glucosamine polysaccharide, by deacetylation. An increased degree of deacetylation increases the solubility of the polymer by exposing positively charged amine groups of the glucosamine units [16]. Chitin itself serves as a structural material in the exoskeleton of arthropods and in the cell walls of fungi and is the second most abundant biopolymer in nature after cellulose.

In a previous study in a rat model the quantitative assessment of osteogenic effect of chitin derivatives was established and used to compare the osteogenic effect of deacetylated chitin derivatives, with degree of deacetylation from 50–96% [17]. The study showed that injectable implants containing 50% and 70% deacetylated highly pure chitin derivatives gave the highest bone volume regeneration of the materials tested. Therefore it was decided to compare the efficacy of a developmental product referred to as BoneReg-Inject™, which contains Chitobiomer™, and an existing, similar and commercially available product, chronOS Inject®, by DePuy Synthes Inc., which served as a predicate device.

BoneReg-Inject™ is a calcium phosphate-based composition comprising tetra-calcium phosphate (TTCP, $Ca_4(PO_4)_2O$) and α-tricalcium phosphate (α-TCP, α-$Ca_3(PO_4)_2$) which reacts in situ to form hydroxyapatite ($Ca_{10}(PO_4)_6(OH)_2$) without excess heat formation. Calcium phosphate based bone cement was chosen as a base for the implants because of its widespread clinical use as well as biocompatible and osteoconductive properties [18]. ChronOS Inject®, however, is based on β-tricalcium phosphate (β-TCP, β-$Ca_3(PO_4)_2$), monocalcium phosphate monohydrate (MCPM, $Ca(H_2PO_4)_2 \cdot H_2O$) and magnesium phosphate ($MgHPO_4 \cdot H_2O$), forming brushite ($CaHPO_4 \cdot 2H_2O$) instead of hydroxyapatite. Both products contain acetylated biopolymers; chronOS Inject® contains sodium hyaluronate and BoneReg-Inject™ contains partially deacetylated chitin.

The aim of the study was to compare the performance of BoneReg-Inject™ and chronOS Inject® in a sheep tibia model with respect to new bone formation, calcification and effect on surrounding tissues on the basis of findings from X-ray micro-CT combined with histology after an observation period of 12 weeks, and to study the long-term effect of the BoneReg-Inject™ implant in a similar model with an observation period of 13 months.

2. Materials and Methods

2.1. Implants

The chitosan polymer used was produced from chitin from the shells of northern Atlantic shrimps (Pandalus borealis). Deacetylation and purification in multiple steps, involving a series of filtration and precipitation steps, was carried out as described earlier [19]. Extensive analytical work was performed to confirm purity and physico-chemical properties of the material [19,20].

Kits of the BoneReg-Inject™ implants were produced and packaged in the laboratories of Genis hf. The implants consisted of 3.0% w/v partially deacetylated chitin (chitosan polymer, 50% DDA) (Genis hf., Siglufjörður, Iceland), 30.9% w/v TTCP/α-TCP (Himed, Old Bethpage, NY, USA), 4.2% w/v sodium glycerol phosphate (Merck, Darmstadt, Germany), 1.9% w/v calcium hydroxide (Sigma-Aldrich, St. Louis, MO, USA), 7.7% w/v phosphoric acid (Merck) and water. These ingredients were packed into a solid and a liquid fraction and sterilized by 20 kGy γ-irradiation. Upon application, solid and liquid components were mixed directly by hand for 3 min; the cement was ready to use 7 min after mixing. The cement was designed to set within 30 min at room temperature but the setting can be delayed up to 2 h by cooling at 2–4 °C. The implant material is soft and injectable, and develops into a non-loadbearing solid (unpublished information) within 24 h, with increasing hydroxyapatite content in the further course of the setting reaction.

The predicate device, ChronOS Inject® (product number 710.066S, Lot No, 2538153), was purchased from Synthes AB, Korta Gatan 9, 171 54 Solna, Sweden.

2.2. Experimental Design

It was decided to use a sheep model and to drill holes (8 mm diameter × 30 mm length) into the proximal epiphyseal area of the tibia to inject a standardized volume of the BoneReg-Inject™ implant or chronOS Inject® into the drill holes in order to compare efficacy, resorption, osteoconductive and bone formation (osteogenic) properties in vivo by these two different injectable implants. One hole was drilled into the right leg and one hole was drilled into the left leg of each sheep. Implants were injected into right leg holes. Left leg holes were left empty to serve as control. This model was intended to serve as a representation of a trabecular bone loss associated with bicondylar fracture of the tibial plateau, involving central impaction and causing substantial loss of trabecular bone. The dimensions of the drill holes were chosen to serve this purpose and at the same time to avoid fracture risk [21,22]. The resulting epiphyseal bone void is typically filled with a bone graft or a bone graft substitute. An important aspect of this model is the involvement of cortical and trabecular bone tissues as well as fat and marrow tissues. The comparison was made by applying X-ray micro-CT and histological evaluation of preserved bone tissue after a live phase of 12 weeks (3 months). During a 13 month live period, the long-term effects of BoneReg-Inject™ were tested using the same model. Long term effects of chronOS Inject® were not assessed in this study which represents a limitation.

For the purpose of the study, 45 healthy female sheep, 5–7 years old and of a pristine Nordic breed, were acquired. Thirty sheep were randomly selected for the comparative 3 months study (15 for BoneReg-Inject™ and 15 for chronOS Inject®) and 15 sheep were randomly selected for the long-term 13 months study on BoneReg-Inject™. The randomization procedure took place before the animals arrived at the surgical facilities, and without the team having seen the sheep. Each sheep already had an identification number. Computer generated random numbers were used to divide the sheep into the 3 test groups, maintaining similar age distribution in all groups. One sheep in the 3 months chronOS Inject® group was diagnosed with *Mycobacterium paratuberculosis* infection in the lower intestines and was euthanized 3 weeks postoperatively. The average age of all animals was 5.9 years; 5.9 years in the BoneReg-Inject™ short term group, 5.9 years in the chronOS Inject® group and 5.8 years in the long term BoneReg-Inject™ group. Bodyweight of the animals ranged from 53–86 kg, with an average of 65.6 kg. Average body weight of animals in the BoneReg-Inject™ and chronOS Inject® group was 64.8 kg and 66.4 kg respectively. The average body weight of animals in the long term BoneReg-Inject™ study was 60.5 kg. Changes in average body weight during the 13 months experiment was +3.24 kg in the BoneReg-Inject™ group, indicating that the animals were in good condition. The changes in body weight in the 3 months comparative study are not available. All 15 sheep in the 3 months BoneReg-Inject™ group, 14 sheep in the 3 months chronOS Inject® group and 15 sheep in the 13 months long term BoneReg-Inject™ group completed the trial alive and without any apparent morbidity.

Before the experiment, sheep were acclimatized for four weeks in the experimental facility (Institute for Experimental Pathology, University of Iceland, Keldur, 112 Reykjavík). During acclimatization and after the operation, animals were kept 3–4 together in a pen. Before the operation, the general health of the animals was confirmed and individual animals assigned to test groups to maintain similar age distribution within the groups. Before the operation the animals were not fed in the afternoon the day before operation and in the morning of the day of operation, but were allowed free access to water. Postoperatively, the sheep were fed hay twice daily (1–2 kg/day) and water ad-libitum.

All experiments were designed and conducted according to the FELASA guidelines. The study protocol was approved by the Icelandic Committee on Animal Experiments with the identification number 0709–0405/2009.

2.3. Surgical Procedure and Sample Preparation

At arrival to the operation theater, the sheep were weighed and injected i.v. with Chanazin 10% and Atropine sulfate. Further medication administered during the procedure is listed in Table 1. The sheep were prepared for surgery by shaving both hind upper legs around the knee and the left side of the neck, to expose the jugular vein. An i.v. catheter was inserted in the jugular vein and a bolus of ketamin 100 mg/50 kg administered. Following that a 3–5 mg/kg bolus of propofol was given. When the animal was anesthetized it was positioned on the right side on the operating table. The sheep breathed spontaneously during the operation receiving 6 L 100% oxygen via mask at the nostrils. Every 5–10 min during the operation a bolus of 1–2 mg/kg propofol was given i.v., more often if there were signs of movement. Continous monitoring of the anaesthesia depth was performed by an assigned person with no other duties during the operation. Monitoring of pulse and oxygenation was carried out with pulse oximetry at the tail after shaving it. The right hind leg was fixed to the table and the left leg fixed in an upright position.

Table 1. Medication and dosages.

Premedication	Chanazin 10% (xylazin) Dosage: 0.1 mL/50 kg Body Weight i.v. and Atropine Sulfate, 1 mL s.c.
General anaesthesia	Narketan Vet. (ketamin 100 mg/mL). Dosage: 1 mL/50 kg i.v. Propofol 10 mg/mL. Bolus at induction 3–5 mg/kg. Maintainance with 1–2 mg/kg every 10 min during the operation and if signs of movement
Local anaesthesia	Xylocain adrenalin 2% and Marcain adrenalin, 5 mg/mL mixed together
Analgesis	Finadyne vet (flunixin) 1 mL/50 kg body weight on day of operation and once a day during the next consecutive 3 days
Antibiotica treatment	Duplocillin LA, 1 mL/10 kg before operation and twice every second day after operation
Euthanasia	T 61, 10 mL/50 kg

The shaved areas on both hind legs were disinfected with Hibiscrub® and subsequently Betadine® solution. The bone surface was accessed through an incision parallel to and over the posterior border of the tibia. The entrance hole was localized centrally between the anterior and posterior borders of the bone at the level of the tuberositas. A hole of 8 mm in diameter was drilled at a right angle through the cortex whereafter the drill was redirected into a 45° upwards direction ending beneath the floor of the tibia plateau. After thorough rinsing of bone debris by flushing with 40–50 mL of sterile, saline water combined with suction, the right leg hole was filled with a standardized amount (1.5 mL) of the experimental test formulation (BoneReg-Inject™ or chronOS Inject®). The drill hole in the left leg was left void for comparison. Prior to application the BoneReg-Inject™ product was mixed according to a procedure described in the "Implants" section above and kept at 2–4 °C until application to delay the setting time. ChronOS Inject® comes with a mixing device which was used to mix the two phases, the liquid and the solid, according to instructions from the manufacturer provided with the product. Within the time frame (3 min) given in product instructions the material was injected to fill the bone void. These materials were injected from a 5 mL sterile syringe mounted with a sterile pipette tip, ensuring that the material would fill the entire space of the drill hole from the tibia plateau down, and outwards, to the opening in the cortex. Thereafter the surgical wounds were closed with 4–0 running Vicryl subcutaneous sutures and the skin with 4–0 Ethilon continuous intracutaneous suture.

After surgery and wake-up, the animals were moved back to the sheep pen for recovery and vital signs monitored until they were ambulatory. All animals survived the anaesthesia and operation without complications.

Postoperatively, the animals received medication according to protocol (Table 1). They were monitored daily concerning behaviour, appearance, and appetite as an expression of general health and well-being. No stabilization such as cast was used and the sheep moved around and loaded their limbs as in normal conditions. In general, a drill hole of this size does not cause instability to the bone or the joint as has been confirmed in the literature [23]. Thus, monitoring through X-ray imaging was not considered necessary. The surgical wounds were regularly evaluated with respect to signs of infection, inflammation and dehiscence.

All animals completing the study appeared healthy and behaved normally throughout the study period. One sheep from the chronOS Inject® group was diagnosed 3 weeks postoperatively with *Mycobacterium paratuberculosis* and was immediately euthanized.

At termination after 3 and 13 months of recovery (short and long term study, respectively), sheep were euthanized by 10 mL/50 kg body weight i.v. injection of T 61. Left and right tibia were explanted at the knee joint and carefully cleaned from soft tissues. The tibia was sawed transversally about 4–5 cm below the proximal end maintaining the entire drill hole within the sample. Samples were placed in plastic jars with a tight lid for fixation in a solution of 3.7% formaldehyde in 50 mM phosphate buffer at pH 7.0. During the period of 11–32 days in the fixation media, samples were scanned in a micro CT-scanner. That is, samples had been between 11 and 32 days in the fixation media when CT-scanning was performed. The sample that had experienced the shortest fixation period had been fixed for 11 days, and the sample that had experienced the longest fixation period had been fixed for 32 days at the timepoint of CT-scanning. After the bones had been kept in the fixation media for 21–35 days and scanning was successfully completed, bone samples were sawed transversely through the epiphysis into 3–4 mm slices with a band saw. That is, the sawing of samples was started at day 21 after initial immersion in fixation media and the sawing was finished at day 35 after initial immersion in fixation media. The slices were photographed and returned into the fixation media and kept there at 22–24 °C under occasional stirring until a total fixation time of 73–94 days from initial immersion into the media. Thereafter, the slices were decalcified in 15% EDTA solution at neutral pH for 13 weeks, with 3 changes of solution during the decalcification period, as explained in the following. Selected sections were further prepared for histological evaluation.

2.4. X-ray Micro CT Analysis

Scanning was performed in an X-ray micro computed tomography (CT)-scanner (nanotom S, General Electric Inspection Technologies, Wunstorf, Germany). The tibia samples were scanned during the period of 11–32 days postmortem. Samples were fixed in a closed plastic cylinder filled with buffered formalin (3.7% formaldehyde in water), which could be mounted on the rotational table in the CT-scanner. Micro CT scanning was performed by transmitting adjusted dosages of X-rays through the sample while the sample was step wise rotated 360° in intervals of 0.5°, collecting 720 2D images from each sample. Magnification was 2.5, voxel size 20 μm/voxel edge, with exposure time of 3000 ms, frame averaging of 3, and 1 frame skipped. X-ray settings were 110 kV and 120 μA, using tube mode 0 and no filter. Volume reconstruction was performed using the Datos-x software accompanying the CT-scanner. Data analysis of X-ray micro CT data was performed using Volume Graphics Studio Max 2.0 from Volume Graphics GmbH, Heidelberg, Germany.

Mineral content was assessed with the help of a hydroxyapatite (HA) phantom from QRM GmbH, Möhrendorf, Germany, which was scanned together with each sample. The phantom has 5 cylindrical inserts of 5 mm diameter with different partial densities of calcium hydroxyapatite of approximately 0, 50, 200, 800 and 1000 mg HA/cm^3. The reconstructed CT-data set from each sample was calibrated according to the HA200 insert, which has a partial HA density of 200.3 mg/cm^3 ± 0.5%. In the following quantitative analysis the HA200 density was chosen as a lower limit, as this was found to include all traces of implanted fillers as well as mineralized tissue. The grayscale value obtained from the calibration for each sample was used to separate the grayscale range into two corresponding density ranges, one of lower density and the other of higher density than the HA200 standard. This value marked the border between mineralized and unmineralized material in the sample and was termed "iso-surface". The volume of all voxels within the defined volume under analysis (sphere or cylinder), having a grayscale value equal to or greater than the iso-surface value, were added up and defined as the "mineral phase volume" within the total volume under analysis. Hence, in the numerical mineral content calculations, the volume of all voxels with a density equal to HA200 or higher, divided by the total volume being analyzed, was defined as "mineral volume ratio" (volume with a density of $\geq$200 mg/cm^3 divided by the total volume).

Mineralization was compared in specific volumes defined by virtual cylinders. A cylinder of 8 mm in length and with a radius of 3 mm was defined and carefully and concentrically orientated with the longitudinal axis in the direction of the drill hole (Figure 1). While keeping the orientation of the cylinder fixed, the radius was increased stepwise to 4, 5 and 6 mm and the mineral phase volume in each cylinder measured. This analysis was repeated in all samples, both empty holes and holes with implant (Figure 1). By subtracting the narrower cylinder from the broader, such as radius 3 mm from radius 4 mm (R4-R3), R5-R4 and R6-R5, mineral phase volume of a 1 mm outer shell (tube) of each cylinder was obtained. Mineral phase volume of the shell of all cylinders was normalized to a standard volume of 1 mm^3, obtaining mineral content with a density higher than that of the hydroxyapatite standard used.

To estimate mineral density inside the implants a virtual sphere with a radius of 2 mm was defined in the center of all implants/drill holes (Figure 1). Mineral phase volume (volume of voxels with a density $\geq$ 200 mg/cm^3) inside the sphere was calculated. Mineral volume ratio was calculated as mineral phase volume/volume of sphere (33.5 mm^3; r = 2 mm). For comparison to initial density of the two implant types (chronOS Inject® and BoneReg-Inject™), samples of implant composites were allowed to harden ex vivo and mineral phase volume measured in triplicates in 2–3 separate spheres in each sample. Mineral phase volume was measured after 24 h of setting ex vivo at 37 °C in saline water and after 18 months of storage in buffered formaldehyde solution at room temperature in order to exclude storage-influenced changes in mineral phase volume.

2.5. Histology

Histological analysis was used for qualitative identification of areas showing dense structures in the micro CT data and to characterize tissue responses to the implant. A ranking system was applied in order to extract statistical data form the histological images.

The medial condyle was sawed off in the sagittal plane, thus forming a plan to lay the tibia on to continue sectioning. Then the tibia plateau was axially (transverse) sawed off (2–3 mm) and subsequently 6–8 axial slices (3–4 mm) were made as far as beyond the cortical entrance of the drill hole. Thereafter all slices were put back into the fixative, carefully ensuring good access of the formaldehyde solution to the entire surface of each slice.

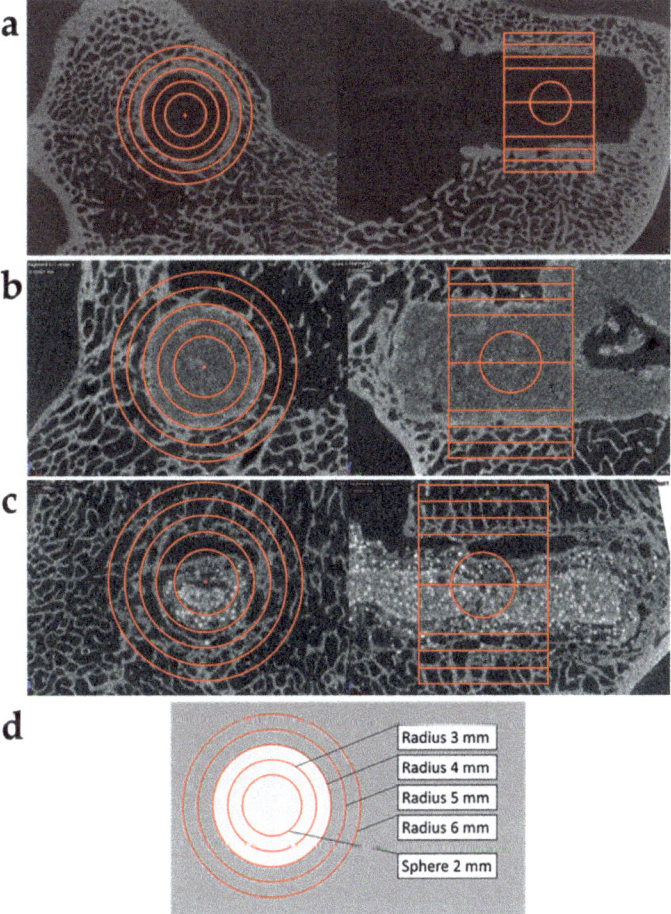

Figure 1. (**a**–**c**) show micro CT constructs in two different planes of samples after 3 months in vivo. (**a**) Sample derived from the left tibia (negative control, empty hole) of an animal receiving BoneReg-Inject™ in right leg drill hole, still essentially void of mineralized tissue. A rim of increased density integrated with the adjacent trabeculum on the edge surrounding the drill hole. The figure shows how virtual cylinders were created, concentric to the drill hole and with different radiuses. (**b**) BoneReg-Inject™ treated sample from the right tibia. A rim of mineralized tissue, well integrated with the adjacent trabecular bone, surrounding the implant, islands of dense material are scattered within the body of the implant. (**c**) chronOS Inject® treated sample from the right tibia. High density granules, characteristic for chronOS Inject® are apparent in the images. Mineralized new tissue is less pronounced in the chronOS Inject® group compared to the BoneReg-Inject™ group. (**d**) Illustration of virtual cylinders created. Length of all cylinders was 8 mm. The largest cylinder has a radius of 6 mm, the smallest has a radius of 3 mm and in the center is a sphere with radius of 2 mm. The cylinder with radius of 4 mm (8 mm in diameter) shows the border of the drill hole.

For further histological preparation, 3 slices were selected from each sample. The most proximal slice was the first slice under the tibial plateau where the implant could be seen macroscopically, containing the greatest amount of trabecular bone surrounding the implant. The most distal slice contained the cortical entrance of the drill hole. The third slice was selected from the slices between the proximal and the distal slices with marrow or fat tissue surrounding the implant. The three slices from each tibia were decalcified in 15%

EDTA (w/v) at pH 7.2–8.0 (EDTA (ethylenediaminetetraacetic acid disodium salt dihydrate), Sigma-Aldrich, St. Louis, MO, USA). The process of decalcification was monitored by micro CT analysis. Decalcification period was about 13 weeks, EDTA-solution was renewed every 3–4 weeks. After complete decalcification, the specimens were dehydrated and embedded in paraffin according to conventional histological protocol. To that end, tissue specimens were put into cassettes and tissue rinsed in running tap water for 30 min. The next step was the conventional method of tissue processing overnight in an automatic tissue processor (Tissue Tek VIP, Sakura Finetek, Inc., Torrance, CA, USA) ending with paraffin embedding where the tissue is embedded in paraffin wax at 63 °C. Paraffin blocks were then moved over to a cooling plate for hardening and after that to a microtome for sectioning (Leica RM2255, Leica Microsystems, Wetzlar, Germany). Disposable blades were used (Accu-Edge Disposable Blades, Sakura) for cutting sections at 3 µm thickness. Sections were mounted on coated microscope slides (Star Frost 76 mm × 26 mm, Knittel Glas GmbH, Braunschweig, Germany), dried in a 60 °C oven for 60 min. Ten sections were taken from each paraffin block at 12 µm intervals each and mounted on 10 Star Frost slides marked with specimen number and Roman numerals from I to X. After drying, H&E staining was performed using Shandon instant Hematoxylin and Eosin solution (Sigma-Aldrich).

For histological ranking samples from 13 sheep from the BoneReg-Inject™ group and samples from 12 sheep from the chronOS Inject® group were used, i.e., 25 sheep in total. Three sections per sample were considered. Two observers blindly examined all samples (25 × 3) separately, a total of 25 × 3 × 2 = 150 observations. This gives 6 observations for each sheep. An average was calculated for each sheep. The average was rounded up to the nearest integer of 0, 1, or 2 and the data analyzed for non-parametrical tests. The ranking (0 = none, 1 = moderate presence or 2 = strong presence) was performed with respect to a bone in implant, signs of cartilage tissue and signs of fibrous tissue.

2.6. Statistical Analysis

For statistical analysis, SigmaPlot 13 (Systat Software, Inc., San Jose, CA, USA) was used. ANOVA and Student's *t*-test (two-tailed) were used for parametrical comparison of groups. For non-parametrical comparison, ANOVA on ranks and Dunn's or Mann-Whitney test was applied. The level of significance was accepted at $p < 0.05$.

3. Results

3.1. Short Term Study, 3 Months In Vivo

3.1.1. Comparison of Mineral Phase Volume inside BoneReg-Inject™ and ChronOS Inject® Implants

Results of mineral phase volume calculations of the 2 mm radius sphere in the center of the implant after 24 h ex vivo and 3 months in vivo, presented in Figure 2a, indicate higher initial mineral phase volume in chronOS Inject® (32.9 mm^3) compared to BoneReg-Inject™ (23.0 mm^3). For comparison, the volume of a full sphere is 33.5 mm^3. However, during 3 months in vivo, the mineral phase volume of chronOS Inject® was reduced to 29.6 mm^3 while the mineral phase volume of BoneReg-Inject™ was reduced to 18.2 mm^3. Figure 2b shows the same data when the initial mineral phase volume has been normalized to 100% for both implants. Hence, during 3 months in vivo, the mineral phase volume of BoneReg-Inject™ was reduced by 21% and chronOS Inject® by 10%. These data suggest that in this model, BoneReg-Inject™ breaks down significantly faster than chronOS Inject® (Student's *t*-test; $p < 0.001$).

3.1.2. Comparison of Mineral Volume Ratio in the Rim of the Implants

Mean mineral volume ratios in concentric virtual cylinders and tubes (1 mm wall thickness) (Figure 1d) represent a gradient of mineral density reaching from the implant and into adjacent tissues (Figure 3). The higher mineral volume ratio of chronOS Inject® in the center of the implants was discussed in the previous section. The same can be observed comparing the mineral volume ratio within cylinders R3. This is reversed for the volume represented by tube R4-R3, forming the rim of the drill hole, where the mineral volume ratio of the BoneReg-Inject™ group was 53% higher than that for chronOS-Inject® group (Student's t-test, $p < 0.001$). On the other hand, no statistical difference was observed between the mineral volume ratio in both materials in the outer cylinders R5-R4 and R6-R5. As expected, the lowest mineral volume ratio was observed in the empty holes (Figure 3). The diameter of the drilling hole is 8 mm (radius 4 mm), suggesting that the BoneReg-Inject™ induced mineralization is a result of bone growth into the drill hole, where the new bone is replacing the implant material as the implant is resolved. A comparison between mineral volume ratio in cylinder R3 on one side and tube R4-R3 on the other side for each type of implant reveals that mineral volume ratio increases on going from R3 to R4-R3 in BoneReg-Inject™, but decreases in chronOS Inject®. This points to increased bone formation in the BoneReg-Inject™ material compared to chronOS Inject®. Histological examination was used to clarify if the mineralized tissue was new bone, as well as possible differences between the groups in terms of tissue response to the two types of implant.

3.1.3. Comparison of Closure of the Cortical Opening of the Drilled Hole

During the 3 months study period, the drill hole through the cortical bone of the tibia was closed to a different degree by bone growth emerging from the edges and striving to fill the hole. Estimated cortical closure of the drilled hole 3 months postoperatively was scored for all samples (0% = no growth, 100% = complete closure of cortical hole). BoneReg-Inject™ group scored highest (94.0%), then chronOS Inject® group (45.0%) and the empty holes had the lowest score (15.0%). However, a statistical difference was revealed between the BoneReg-Inject™ group and the empty hole group ($p < 0.05$), but no difference was found between the ChronOS Inject® and empty hole groups or between the two groups of implant materials (Figure 4).

3.1.4. Histological Examination

Figure 5 shows a series of images selected from two animals from each group representing a characteristic appearance of histological images from BoneReg-Inject™ and chronOS Inject®. Histological images are aligned with the corresponding micro CT sections in order to compare how dense structures in the micro CT data align with newly formed bone tissue. Figure 5e represents samples from each of the treatment groups showing the best case observed of neo-osteoid formation inside the BoneReg-Inject™ implant and the chronOS Inject® implant.

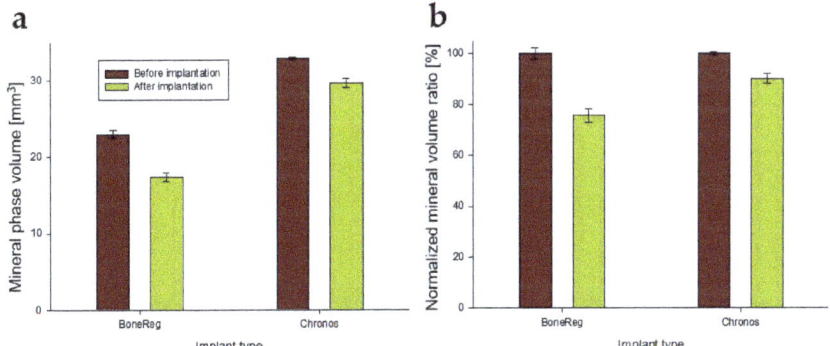

Figure 2. (**a**) Mineral phase volume inside the composites ex vivo (before implantation) and after 3 months in vivo, measured in spheres (radius 2 mm). (**b**) Bars show mineral phase volume before implantation normalized to 100% for both composites and their relative reduction during 3 months in vivo. Mineral phase volume in BoneReg-Inject™ group ($n = 15$) is reduced by 21% and in chronOS Inject® ($n = 14$) by 10%. (Student's t-test; $p < 0.001$). Means and SEM (BoneReg-Inject™ $n = 15$; chronOS Inject® $n = 14$).

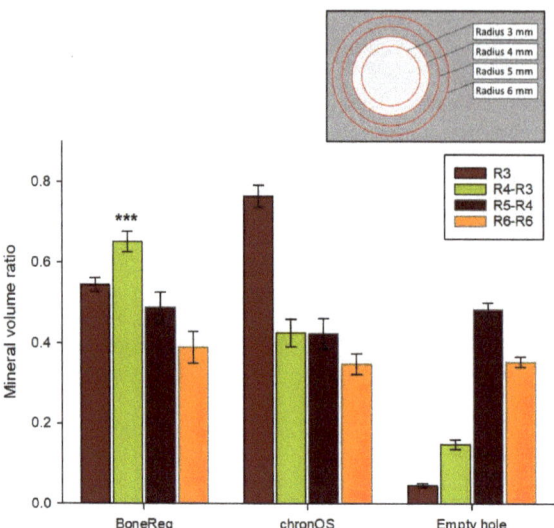

Figure 3. Bars indicate the mean mineral volume ratio in one virtual cylinder and 3 tubes in both experimental groups and the empty holes (negative control). The empty holes in both groups were summed up into a single control group. Results for a cylinder with a 3 mm radius and 3 different tubes with fixed volume are shown; R4-R3, R5-R4, and R6-R5 (see Figure 1 and insert above for location and alignment). The BoneReg-Inject™ group shows a significantly higher mineral volume ratio in a 1 mm rim of the implant (R4-R3) compared to the chronOS Inject® group (Student's t-test $p < 0.001$, indicated by three asterisks in the figure). Values are means and bars are standard error of the mean (SEM). R3 = radius 3 mm, R4 = radius 4 mm, etc. (BoneReg-Inject™ $n = 15$; chronOS Inject® $n = 14$).

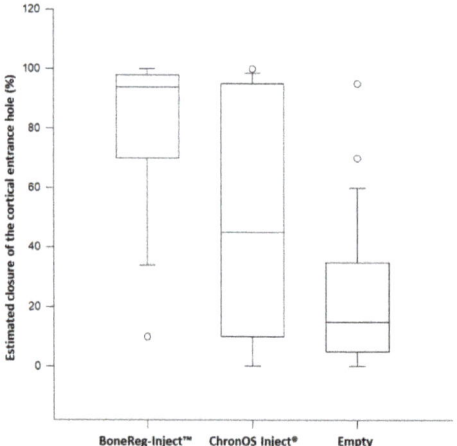

Figure 4. Scoring of percentage closure of cortical entrance hole in the two test groups and the empty holes in both groups 3 months postoperatively shown as box plot based on results from ANOVA on ranks, and only showing a significant difference between BoneReg-Inject™ and empty hole (Empty), Dunn's Method, $p < 0.05$. Boxes show a 50% confidence limit and bars show a 90% confidence limit. The median is indicated by the horizontal line within the boxes. (BoneReg-Inject™ $n = 15$; chronOS Inject® $n = 14$; Control $n = 29$).

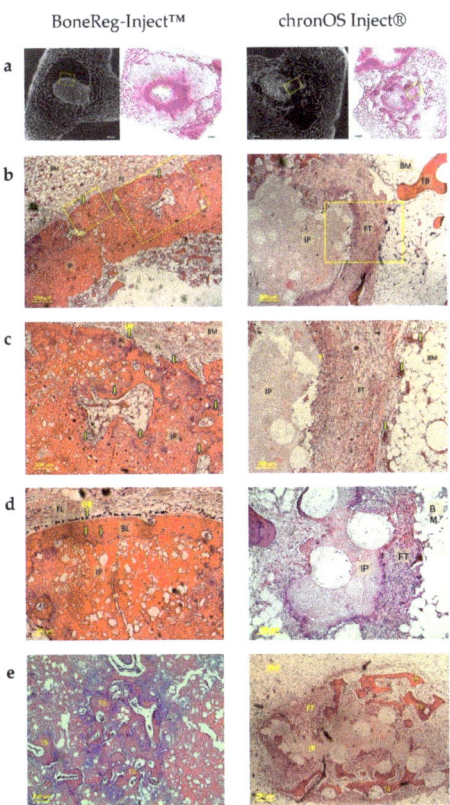

Figure 5. 3 months postoperative. (**a**) An alignment of histological sections with two-dimensional cross-sections of micro CT constructs in a bone marrow/trabecular bone area in the right legs of sheep with BoneReg-Inject™ implant (left column) and chronOS Inject® implant (right column). The left images in each column show the two-dimensional micro CT cross sections in the plane aligned with the histological section in the right image. The scale bars are 2 mm. BoneReg-Inject™ column: (**b**) Histological section, a close up of the area of the yellow frame shown. (**a**). The rim of neo-osteoid covering the implant is clearly visible (yellow arrows). BM: Bone marrow, FL: Fibrous layer, IP: Implant. (**c**) A close up of the right yellow frame in (**b**). New bone, connected to the bone shell covering the implant, has grown into the implant (yellow arrows). Characteristic blue deposits seen on the interface between new bone and the implant indicate areas of calcification. Osteoblast-like cells (OB) visible on the outer layer of the new bone shell. (**d**) A close up of the left yellow frame in (**b**). The rim of neo-osteoid covering the implant is evident (BL) and individual osteocytes are visible (yellow arrows). Osteoblast-like cells (OB) are visible on the outer layer of the bone shell. (**e**) Trabecular-like neo-osteoid formation inside the BoneReg-Inject™ implant. Blue indicates regions of on-going calcification. chronOS Inject® column: (**b**) A close up of the yellow frame area shown in (**a**). The fibrous tissue covering the implant is characteristic of the chronOS Inject® group. The characteristic granules are apparent in the implant. FT: Fibrous tissue, TB: Trabecular bone. (**c**) A close up of the yellow framed area in (**b**) showing the implant surrounded by fibrous tissue and bone marrow. It is characteristic for the chronOS Inject® group to see this layer of fibrous tissue surrounding the implant (*). Blood vessels with red blood cells are evident both in the bone marrow and fibrous tissue layer (yellow arrows). (**d**) Implant surrounded by fibrous tissue. (**e**) Trabecular-like neo-osteoid (TB) formed inside the layer of fibrous tissue replacing the chronOS Inject® implant (IP), as it resolves. This formation of new bone was generally rare in the chronOS Inject® group and was poorly integrated with the existing surrounding trabecular bone.

A qualitative pathological evaluation, based on three sections from the right leg of each animal. revealed differences between BoneReg-Inject™ and the predicate device.

BoneReg-Inject™ Group: The implanted material was intensely eosinophilic and finely granular. Around the implant was a rim of neo-osteoid, its thickness approximately that of a normal bony trabecula. In some cases, there were signs of the inner border of the new osteoid undergoing calcification. The outer periphery of the rim was lined by a row of osteoblasts, osteoclasts being virtually absent. In some cases, neo-osteoid at the periphery of the rim was seen to connect with adjacent preexistent bone. No foreign body reaction was noted around the implant.

ChronOS Inject® Group: The implanted material was homogenous, weakly eosinophilic and punctuated by large perfectly round defects. Around the implant, most cases demonstrated signs of marked tissue reaction, consisting of granulation tissue, i.e., newly formed vessels, fibroblasts, and lymphocytes, as well as foreign body reaction, including epithelioid histiocytes and multinucleated giant cells of the foreign body type. No cytoplasmic inclusions were noted in giant cells. Neo-osteoid was inconspicuous, seen only in a minority of cases. Where seen, neo-osteoid was haphazardly present, without an apparent connection to preexistent bone trabeculae.

A histological ranking was used for comparison of samples from both groups. Samples were rated from 0–2 in terms of parameters of interest regarding group differences in the histological images. Significant differences between the two groups were revealed concerning: (1) amount of new bone within the implant ($p < 0.001$), (2) signs of cartilage tissue ($p = 0.003$) and (3) signs of fibrous tissue ($p < 0.001$). Table 2 shows the ranking outcome. The histological ranking showed more bone in implant, more signs of cartilage tissue and less fibrous tissue for BoneReg-Inject™ implants compared to the predicate device.

Table 2. Mann-Whitney rank sum test results. A total comparison of 25 sheep tibia, 13 of BoneReg-Inject™ and 12 of chronOS Inject® implants. When ranking histological samples (0, 1 or 2) with respect to a bone in implant, signs of cartilage tissue and signs of fibrous tissue, a statistical evaluation showed significant differences between the two groups. 0 = none; 1 = moderate presence; 2 = strong presence.

	BoneReg Median	BoneReg 25%	BoneReg 75%	ChronOS Median	ChronOS 25%	ChronOS 75%	p
Bone in implant	1	0	1	0	0	0	<0.001
Cartilage	0	0	1	0	0	0	0.003
Fibrous tissue	0	0	0	1	0.5	2	<0.001

3.2. Long Term Effect of BoneReg-Inject™, 13 Months In Vivo

3.2.1. X-ray Micro CT Analysis

Comparison of micro CT data of BoneReg-Inject™ implants at 3 and 13 months postoperative revealed continuous mineralization during the 10 months period. The new mineralized tissue appeared well integrated with the adjacent trabecular bone and appeared to be increasingly migrating into the implanted material.

Mineral volumes obtained using virtual cylinders defining specific volumes inside and surrounding the BoneReg-Inject™ implants were used to compare 3 and 13 months postoperatively (Figure 6).

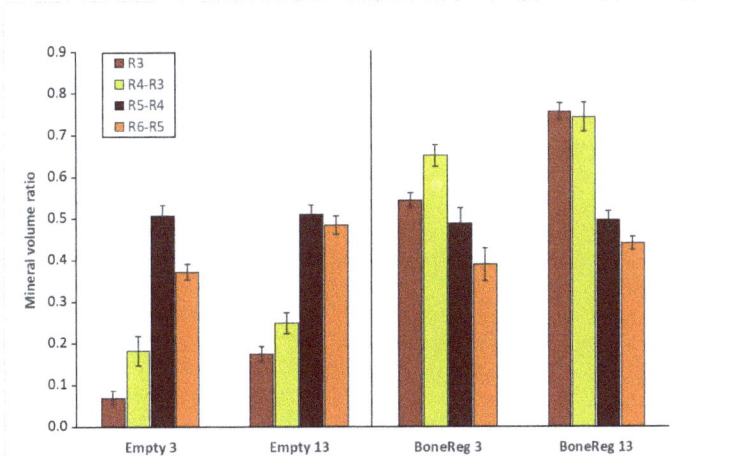

Figure 6. Mineral volume ratio in a virtual cylinder (R3) and tubes R4-R3, R5-R4 and R6-R5 in BoneReg-Inject™ samples after 3 months (BoneReg 3) and 13 months (BoneReg 13) and in the empty control (Empty 3 and Empty 13). Mean and SEM (n = 15 for each treatment). Mineral content within the implanted scaffold at 13 months postoperatively was significantly higher than at 3 months postoperatively (R3 t-test, $p < 0.001$ and R4-R3 t-test, $p < 0.05$). In the empty drill holes, mineral content within R3 was significantly higher after 13 months (t-test, $p < 0.001$). A significant increase in mineral content was also observed in the trabecular bone outside the empty holes (R6-R5, t-test, $p < 0.001$), potentially reflecting a response to counteract weakening of the bone due to the drill hole.

When comparing the empty holes (Empty 3 and Empty 13), a significant increase is observed in the innermost cylinder (R3) during the 10 month period (t-test, $p < 0.001$). No significant difference is observed in the rim of the drill hole (R4-R3 or R5-R4) but there is a significant increase in the trabecular bone density in R6-R5 during the 10 months period (t-test, $p < 0.001$). This might reflect a response to a weakening of the tissue structure imposed by the drill hole.

Comparing short and long term effect of BoneReg-Inject™ implants (BoneReg 3 versus BoneReg 13, Figure 6), there is a significant increase in mineral content of the R3 cylinders (t-test, $p < 0.001$) as well as for the R4-R3 tubes (t-test, $p < 0.05$). The mineral content of the adjacent outer trabecular bone tissue, R5-R4, and R6-R5, is not increased over time. This suggests that the implant possesses both osteoconductive and osteogenic activities, leading to the formation of new mineralized bone tissue in the implanted material, remodeling the implanted scaffold into a new mineralized bone tissue.

3.2.2. Histological Evaluation

In the long-term 13 month group, the BoneReg-Inject™ implant is eosinophilic and finely granular in appearance. Around the implant is a rim of new bone with a trabecular structure. Trabecular spaces are filled with non-reactive bone marrow. The outer periphery of the new bone is lined by osteoblasts and in some cases connects with adjacent preexistent bone. Bone in-growth is observed in the implanted material, in many cases including its central part. The border between the implant and the new osteoid is often covered with blue deposits indicating calcification. There were no histological signs of inflammation. An example of a series of histological images is shown in Figure 7.

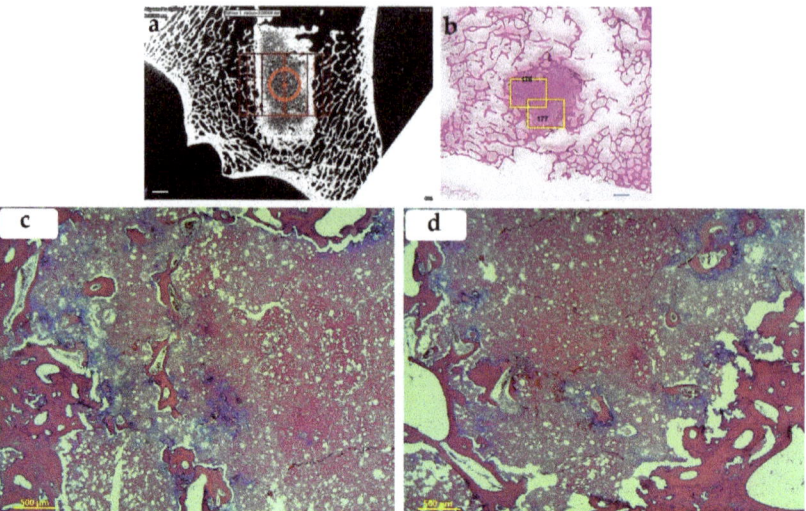

Figure 7. BoneReg-Inject™. (**a**) Micro CT image (scale bar = 2 mm) and (**b**) a histological slide showing BoneReg-Inject™ implant at 13 months postoperative (scale bar = 2 mm). New bone is well integrated with the surrounding trabecular bone. Yellow frames on the histological slide refer to regions in focus in (**c**) (176) and (**d**) (177). In this animal, the micro CT image shows relatively well-developed colonization of mineralized tissue inside the implant. The histological slide indicates trabecular-like neo-osteoid replacing the resolved outer rim of the implant and integrating into the surrounding trabecular bone. (**c**,**d**) show neo-osteoid replacing the resolved surface of the implant and forming islands scattered inside the mass of the implant. Blue indicates calcification. Samples stained with hematoxylin and eosin.

4. Discussion

A significant difference was observed between the two experimental groups, BoneReg-Inject™ and chronOS Inject®, with more bone regeneration in the BoneReg-Inject™ group.

The BoneReg-Inject™ group was characterized by the formation of a dense mineralized new bone tissue, surrounding the entire implant with scattered islands of new bone formation throughout the interior of the implant.

Quantitative analysis of mineral volume ratio revealed that the BoneReg-Inject™ implant underwent more rapid resolution compared to the chronOS Inject® implant. Higher mineral volume ratio was measured on the periphery of the BoneReg-Inject™ implant pointing to a more pronounced formation of new bone. Histological ranking results supported this finding.

In the long term group implanted with BoneReg-Inject™, a continuing resolution of the implant was apparent and a continuous bone formation within the implant was observed. This indicates that the BoneReg-Inject™ bone void filler comprises a sustained stimulation of bone formation and is replaced by new bone tissue as the implant is resolved with time.

The results obtained here can be viewed in the light of results from experiments that our group performed in rat mandibular bone [17]. It was found that implants containing 50–70% DDA chitosan polymer may stimulate new bone growth. The main increase in bone volume took place in bone tissue surrounding the drill hole in the mandibular bone. The findings suggested that the increase in bone volume was the combined result of biomechanical stresses around the drill hole, and the implant material or components thereof. In the current experiment the same 50% DDA chitosan polymer was used. Here, a significant difference in mineral volume ratio outside the BoneReg-Inject™ implants compared to the chronOS Inject® implants was not observed, but a non-significant trend towards an increased mineral volume ratio outside the BoneReg-Inject™ implants could be identified. Less biomechanical stress is expected around the drill hole in the current study as compared to the rat study, as the ratio between the hole and the surrounding bone is lower, thus displaying relatively lower levels of mechanical stress. This might lead to a lower factor of biomechanical stimulation of bone growth. However, extensive formation of new bone was observed within the implant in the current study. This might reflect the better containment of the implant, so that biomechanical stimulation through the implant is more effective than in the rat mandibular model. Another explanation may be found in the differences in the biological nature of the mandibular bone compared to the tibial bone (intramembranous ossification vs. endochondral ossification) leading to different conditions for the evolvement of the effect of the chitosan polymer and thus bone formation within the implant in the tibia.

Various chitosan composites and chitosan coatings for bone tissue engineering materials have been tested and reported. A common feature of the research is that the chitosan used is highly deacetylated, as opposed to the chitosan employed in the current research. Chitosan preparation and dissolution strategies vary and different composite components are used, all potentially influencing the biological properties and activity of the chitosan. This often makes the comparison between results from different research groups complicated. Some researchers have observed a neutral effect of the use of chitosan in bone implants [24,25]. Several recent papers indicate a positive influence of chitosan on bone regeneration. A chitosan/dicarboxylic acid scaffold was shown in vivo to be an effective bone regeneration material with good osteoinductive and osteoconductive properties [26]. In a review paper, titanium surfaces functionalized with chitosan were concluded to have greater osseointegration capacity than uncoated controls [27]. Thitiset et al. [28], used chitoologosaccharide for preparation of composites that did show promising results in cell culture, as well as for new bone formation in vivo. The results from Thitiset et al. are remarkable in the light of our ideas on the mechanism of action of chitosan in bone regeneration where chitooligosachharides play a central role [17].

5. Conclusions

Our overall conclusion is that, in this non-weightbearing sheep tibia model, BoneReg-Inject™ showed osteogenic and osteoconductive properties without identifiable foreign body reaction. In the same model chronOS Inject® provokes foreign body reactions surrounding the implant with significantly less signs of new bone tissue formation. A long-term study indicates that the BoneReg-Inject™ implant stimulates sustained bone formation and is replaced by normal-looking new bone tissue.

For clinical use in bone defects, the current results point to an opportunity for the application of implant materials containing specific, partially deacetylated chitin derivatives, as an active component. The materials stimulate bone formation within the defect over an extended period and, while slowly degrading, facilitate bone ingrowth into the defect.

Author Contributions: Conceptualization, J.G. and H.J.J.; Methodology, E.H.L., S.K., A.D., C.-H.N., J.M.E., J.G. and H.J.J.; Validation, A.D. and J.G.; Formal Analysis, J.M.E.; Investigation, G.Ö., E.H.L., S.K., A.D., E.G., C.-H.N., J.M.E., J.G. and H.J.J.; Resources, E.G., C.-H.N., G.Ö., E.H.L., S.K., H.J.J. and J.G.; Data Curation, J.M.E. and G.Ö.; Writing—Original Draft Preparation, G.Ö., J.G. and J.M.E.; Writing—Review & Editing, G.Ö., E.H.L., S.K. and H.J.J.; Visualization, J.M.E. and G.Ö.; Supervision, J.G. and H.J.J.; Project Administration, J.G.; Funding Acquisition, J.G. All authors have read and agreed to the published version of the manuscript.

Funding: This work was supported by the Technology Development Fund, managed by the Icelandic Centre for Research [RAN 090303-0246].

Institutional Review Board Statement: The animal study protocol was approved by the Committee on Animal Experiments of the Icelandic Food and Veterinary Authority (protocol code: 0709-0405; date of approval: 13 June 2009).

Informed Consent Statement: Not applicable.

Data Availability Statement: The data presented in this study are available on request from the corresponding author. The data are not publicly available due to the size of the X-ray microCT datasets.

Acknowledgments: We thank Jóhannes Björnsson and Kristrún Ólafsdóttir at the Department of Pathology, Landspítali University Hospital, Reykjavík, Iceland, for assistance with microscopical sectioning, staining, and analysis of histological samples.

Conflicts of Interest: Jóhannes Gíslason, Jón M. Einarsson and Chuen-How Ng are employees of Genis hf.

References

1. Dennis, S.C.; Berkland, C.J.; Bonewald, L.F.; Detamore, M.S. Endochondral ossification for enhancing bone regeneration: Converging native extracellular matrix biomaterials and developmental engineering in vivo. *Tissue Eng. Part B Rev.* **2015**, *21*, 247–266. [CrossRef]
2. Oryan, A.; Alidadi, S.; Moshiri, A.; Maffulli, N. Bone regenerative medicine: Classic options, novel strategies, and future directions. *J. Orthop. Surg. Res.* **2014**, *9*, 18. [CrossRef]
3. Dimitriou, R.; Jones, E.; McGonagle, D.; Giannoudis, P.V. Bone regeneration: Current concepts and future directions. *BMC Med.* **2011**, *9*, 66. [CrossRef]
4. Collignon, A.M.; Lesieur, J.; Vacher, C.; Chaussain, C.; Rochefort, G.Y. Strategies developed to induce, direct, and potentiate bone healing. *Front. Physiol.* **2017**, *8*, 927. [CrossRef]
5. Sheikh, Z.; Javaid, M.A.; Hamdan, N.; Hashmi, R. Bone regeneration using bone morphogenetic proteins and various biomaterial carriers. *Materials* **2015**, *8*, 1778–1816. [CrossRef] [PubMed]
6. Ramly, E.P.; Alfonso, A.R.; Kantar, R.S.; Wang, M.M.; Siso, J.R.D.; Ibrahim, A.; Coelho, P.G.; Flores, R.L. Safety and efficacy of recombinant human bone morphogenetic protein-2 (rhBMP-2) in craniofacial surgery. *Plast Reconstr. Surg. Glob. Open* **2019**, *7*, e2347. [CrossRef] [PubMed]
7. Niu, S.; Anastasio, A.T.; Faraj, R.R.; Rhee, J.M. Evaluation of heterotopic ossification after using recombinant human bone morphogenetic protein–2 in transforaminal lumbar interbody fusion: A computed tomography review of 996 disc levels. *Glob. Spine J.* **2019**, *10*, 280–285. [CrossRef] [PubMed]
8. Venkatesan, J.; Vinodhini, P.A.; Sudha, P.N.; Kim, S.K. Chitin and chitosan composites for bone tissue regeneration. *Adv. Food Nutr. Res.* **2014**, *73*, 59–81. [CrossRef]
9. Klokkevold, P.R.; Vandemark, L.; Kenney, E.B.; Bernard, G.W. Osteogenesis enhanced by chitosan (poly-N-acetyl glucosaminoglycan) in vitro. *J. Periodontol.* **1996**, *67*, 1170–1175. [CrossRef]
10. Tan, M.L.; Shao, P.; Friedhuber, A.M.; Moorst, M.; Elahy, M.; Indumathy, S.; Dunstan, D.E.; Wei, Y.; Dass, C.R. The potential role of free chitosan in bone trauma and bone cancer management. *Biomaterials* **2014**, *35*, 7828–7838. [CrossRef]
11. Ahsan, S.M.; Thomas, M.; Reddy, K.K.; Sooraparaju, S.G.; Asthana, A.; Bhatnagar, I. Chitosan as biomaterial in drug delivery and tissue engineering. *Int. J. Biol. Macromol.* **2018**, *110*, 97–109. [CrossRef] [PubMed]
12. Pang, Y.; Qin, A.; Lin, X.; Yang, L.; Wang, Q.; Wang, Z.; Shan, Z.; Li, S.; Wang, J.; Fan, S.; et al. Biodegradable and biocompatible high elastic chitosan scaffold is cell-friendly both in vitro and in vivo. *Oncotarget* **2017**, *8*, 35583–35591. [CrossRef] [PubMed]
13. Ho, M.H.; Yao, C.J.; Liao, M.H.; Lin, P.I.; Liu, S.H.; Chen, R.M. Chitosan nanofiber scaffold improves bone healing via stimulating trabecular bone production due to upregulation of the Runx2/osteocalcin/alkaline phosphatase signaling pathway. *Int. J. Nanomed.* **2015**, *10*, 5941–5954.
14. Levengood, S.L.; Zhang, M. Chitosan-based scaffolds for bone tissue engineering. *J. Mater. Chem B Mater. Biol Med.* **2014**, *2*, 3161–3184. [CrossRef]
15. Oryan, A.; Sahvieh, S. Effectiveness of chitosan scaffold in skin, bone and cartilage healing. *Int. J. Biol. Macromol.* **2017**, *104*, 1003–1011. [CrossRef] [PubMed]
16. Younes, I.; Rinaudo, M. Chitin and chitosan preparation from marine sources. Structure, properties and applications. *Mar. Drugs* **2015**, *13*, 1133–1174. [CrossRef]
17. Kjalarsdóttir, L.; Dýrfjörð, A.; Dagbjartsson, A.; Laxdal, E.H.; Örlygsson, G.; Gíslason, J.; Einarsson, J.M.; Ng, C.H.; Jónsson, H., Jr. Bone remodeling effect of a chitosan and calcium phosphate based composite. *Regen. Biomater.* **2019**, *6*, 231–240. [CrossRef]
18. Eliaz, N.; Metoki, N. Calcium phosphate bioceramics: A review of their history, structure, properties, coating technologies and biomedical applications. *Materials* **2017**, *10*, 334. [CrossRef]
19. Gíslason, J.; Einarsson, J.M.; Ng, C.-H.; Bahrke, S. Compositions of Partially Deacetylated Chitin Derivatives. U.S. Patent US9078949B2, 14 July 2015.
20. Lieder, R.; Darai, M.; Thor, M.B.; Ng, C.-H.; Einarsson, J.M.; Gudmundsson, S.; Helgason, B.; Gaware, V.S.; Másson, M.; Gíslason, J.; et al. In vitro bioactivity of different degree of deacetylation chitosan, a potential coating material for titanium implants. *J. Biomed. Mater. Res. Part A* **2012**, *100A*, 3392–3399. [CrossRef]
21. Pobloth, A.M.; Johnson, K.A.; Schell, H.; Kolarczik, N.; Wulsten, D.; Duda, G.N.; Schmidt-Bleek, K. Establishment of a preclinical ovine screening model for the investigation of bone tissue engineering strategies in cancellous and cortical bone defects. *BMC Musculoskelet. Disord.* **2016**, *17*, 111. [CrossRef]

22. Edgerton, B.C.; An, K.N.; Morrey, B.F. Torsional strength reduction due to cortical defects in bone. *J. Orthop. Res.* **1990**, *8*, 851–855. [CrossRef] [PubMed]
23. Malhotra, A.; Pelletier, M.H.; Yu, Y.; Christou, C.; Walsh, W.R. A sheep model for cancellous bone healing. *Front. Surg.* **2014**, *1*, 37. [CrossRef]
24. Jin, H.H.; Kim, D.H.; Kim, T.W.; Shin, K.K.; Jung, J.S.; Park, H.C.; Yoon, S.Y. In vivo evaluation of porous hydroxyapatite/chitosan–alginate composite scaffolds for bone tissue engineering. *Int. J. Biol. Macromol.* **2012**, *51*, 1079–1085. [CrossRef] [PubMed]
25. Khoshakhlagh, P.; Rabiee, S.M.; Kiaee, G.; Heidari, P.; Miri, A.K.; Moradi, R.; Moztarzadeh, F.; Ravarian, R. Development and characterization of a bioglass/chitosan composite as an injectable bone substitute. *Carbohydr. Polym.* **2017**, *157*, 1261–1271. [CrossRef] [PubMed]
26. Sukpaita, T.; Chirachanchai, S.; Suwattanachai, P.; Everts, V.; Pimkhaokham, A.; Ampornaramveth, R.S. In vivo bone regeneration induced by a scaffold of chitosan/dicarboxylic acid seeded with human periodontal ligament cells. *Int. J. Mol. Sci.* **2019**, *20*, 4883. [CrossRef]
27. López-Valverde, N.; López-Valverde, A.; Ramírez, J.M. Systematic review of effectiveness of chitosan as a biofunctionalizer of titanium implants. *Biology* **2021**, *10*, 102. [CrossRef]
28. Thitiset, T.; Damrongsakkul, S.; Yodmuang, S.; Leeanansaksiri, W.; Apinun, J.; Honsawek, S. A novel gelatin/chitooligosaccharide/demineralized bone matrix composite scaffold and periosteum-derived mesenchymal stem cells for bone tissue engineering. *Biomater. Res.* **2021**, *25*, 19. [CrossRef] [PubMed]

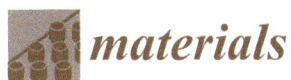

Article

Evaluation of Osteoconduction of a Synthetic Hydroxyapatite/β-Tricalcium Phosphate Block Fixed in Rabbit Mandibles

Luis Carlos de Almeida Pires [1], Rodrigo Capalbo da Silva [2], Pier Paolo Poli [3,*], Fernando Ruas Esgalha [1], Henrique Hadad [2], Letícia Pitol Palin [2], Ana Flávia Piquera Santos [2], Luara Teixiera Colombo [2], Laís Kawamata de Jesus [2], Ana Paula Farnezi Bassi [2], Carlo Maiorana [3], Roberta Okamoto [4], Paulo Sérgio Perri de Carvalho [1] and Francisley Ávila Souza [2]

1. Implant Dentistry Post-Graduation Program, São Leopoldo Mandic School of Dentistry and Research Center, Campinas, SP 13 045 755, São Paulo, Brazil; luiscapires@hotmail.com (L.C.d.A.P.); fernandoesgalha@uol.com.br (F.R.E.); paulo.perri@unesp.br (P.S.P.d.C.)
2. Department of Diagnosis and Surgery, Araçatuba Dental School, São Paulo State University Júlio de Mesquita Filho—UNESP, Araçatuba, SP 16 015 050, São Paulo, Brazil; capalbo.rodrigo@gmail.com (R.C.d.S.); henriquehadad@gmail.com (H.H.); leticiappalin@gmail.com (L.P.P.); anaflaviaps_06@hotmail.com (A.F.P.S.); luara_colombo@hotmail.com (L.T.C.); kawamata_lais@hotmail.com (L.K.d.J.); ana.bassi@unesp.br (A.P.F.B.); francisley.avila@unesp.br (F.Á.S.)
3. Implant Center for Edentulism and Jawbone Atrophies, Maxillofacial Surgery and Odontostomatology Unit, Fondazione IRCSS Cà Granda Ospedale Maggiore Policlinico, University of Milan, 20122 Milan, Italy; carlo.maiorana@unimi.it
4. Department of Basic Science, Araçatuba Dental School, São Paulo State University Júlio de Mesquita Filho—UNESP, Araçatuba, SP 16 015 050, São Paulo, Brazil; roberta.okamoto@unesp.br
* Correspondence: pierpaolo_poli@fastwebnet.it; Tel.: +39-02-55032621

Received: 16 September 2020; Accepted: 29 October 2020; Published: 31 October 2020

Abstract: (1) Background: This study aimed to evaluate the incorporation of hydroxyapatite/β tricalcium phosphate blocks grafted in rabbit mandibles. (2) Methods: Topographic characterization of biomaterial was performed through scanning electron microscopy coupled with energy-dispersive X-ray spectroscopy (SEM-EDX). Ten rabbits randomly received autogenous bone graft harvested from the tibia (Autogenous Group—AG) or synthetic biomaterial manufactured in β-tricalcium phosphate (Biomaterial Group—BG) at their right and left mandibular angles. Euthanasia was performed at 30 and 60 postoperative days; (3) Results: SEM-EDX showed a surface with the formation of crystals clusters. Histological analyses in BG at 30 days showed a slower process of incorporation than AG. At 60 days, BG showed remnants of biomaterial enveloped by bone tissue in the anabolic modeling phase. Histometric analysis showed that mean values of newly formed bone-like tissue in the AG (6.56%/9.70%) were statistically higher compared to BG (3.14%/6.43%) in both periods, respectively. Immunohistochemical analysis demonstrated early bone formation and maturation in the AG with more intense osteopontin and osteocalcin staining. (4) Conclusions: The biomaterial proved to be a possible bone substitute, being incorporated into the receiving bed; however, it showed delayed bone incorporation compared to autogenous bone.

Keywords: biocompatibility; biomaterials; bone augmentation; bone conduction; bone grafting; calcium hydroxyapatite; tissue regeneration

1. Introduction

The results of alveolar bone remodeling after tooth loss, dentoalveolar trauma, and infections may promote an unfavorable site for dental implant rehabilitation with proper prosthetic planning [1]. Bone defects have different patterns and sizes, and their reconstruction can be classified into vertical and horizontal augmentation [2]. Several techniques have been proposed to treat bone defects, including bone substitutes from different origins such as autogenous, heterologous, and alloplastic materials [3,4].

In particular, block grafting is a recommended treatment in cases of horizontal defects, associated with severe atrophy of the alveolar bone [5–8]. In order to recreate the proper anatomy of the alveolar ridge, autogenous bone is considered the gold standard, being the only graft material that presents osteogenic, osteoinductive, and osteoconductive characteristics simultaneously [9]. On the other hand, the harvesting procedure is not free from drawbacks, including the risk of neurovascular injuries at the donor site, the need for an additional surgical site, an extended surgical time, an increasing post-operative patient morbidity, and a prolonged recovery time occasionally associated with hospitalization of the patient for extraoral donor sites [10]. Thus, research has been directed towards the use of biomaterials as autogenous bone substitutes when reconstructive surgery is needed. Currently, a wide range of synthetic or biological biomaterials is commercially available.

Among the different biomaterials, beta-tricalcium phosphate (β-TCP) ceramic has been introduced as a bone substitute [11]. β-TCP acting as a scaffold promotes bone formation through osteoconduction. As a result of its biocompatibility, bioactivity, favorable incorporation, and osteoconductive properties, synthetic β-TCP has been generally accepted and evaluated as a grafting material [12–14]. Its structural characteristic resembling the mineral phase of bone tissue is another factor that promotes great expectations for this material as a bone substitute [15]. As a disadvantage, biomaterials based on β-TCP present high solubility, which makes them unsuitable in reconstructions that need to maintain and create bone volume [16]. In order to reduce its rapid absorption, the association of β-TCP with hydroxyapatite (HA) in different proportions has been studied [17]. It was found that the biphasic composition consisting of HA and β-TCP provides better osteoconductive capabilities when compared to monophasic ceramics, decreasing osteoclastic activity allowing the formation of a framework for osteoconduction [18]. The search for the ideal ratio of HA and β-TCP, although controversial, is considered important because it modifies the solubility of the biomaterial and influences the resorption time. In a biocompatibility and biomechanical study, the association of 60%/40% HA/β-TCP has been tested and suggested as the ideal proportion of these components [19]. The combination of 60% HA/40% β-TCP has been used in a study to lift maxillary sinus in humans, obtaining favorable results for bone neoformation, proving to be an interesting ratio [20]. Different experimental studies in animals and clinical trials have demonstrated the favorable incorporation of such biphasic composition in the filling of critical defects in the calvarium, maxillary sinus, and alveolar socket preservation after dental extraction [14,21,22]. However, most studies employing β-TCP were performed in the reconstruction of two or more walls filled with cements or granular biomaterials, which may promote bone neoformation by taking advantage of the osteoconductive potential of the material. On the contrary, few studies are currently available that evaluate the incorporation of this biomaterial in the form of blocks for horizontal alveolar ridge augmentation [23,24].

In view of the above, the purpose of the present study was to analyze and compare the process of bone incorporation of autogenous bone graft and 60% HA/40% β-TCP blocks fixed by means of bicortical screws to the mandibular angles of rabbits.

2. Materials and Methods

2.1. Study Design

The study protocol was approved by the local Animal Experimentation Ethical Committee (CEEA) with the identification number 00999/2011. The sample size calculation was based on histometric and immunohistochemistry values retrieved from the authors' pilot analyses (unpublished data) before the commencement of the study. New bone formation was determined as the primary outcome. Thus, a significant difference of 5% (standard deviation of 2%) was considered, and for 80% power and setting alpha at 0.05, five grafts per group were necessary in order to compare two different groups.

The sample consisted of 10 male New Zealand white adult rabbits with a weight ranging from 3 to 4 kg. The animals were kept in individual cages in a humidity- and temperature-controlled environment, on a light-dark cycle (12:12 h), and fed with water and rabbit chow (Procoelho-Primor, São Paulo, SP, Brazil) ad libitum. The surgical procedures were made at the local Rabbit Experimentation Center. After randomization using computer-generated lists on the website Research Randomizer (https://www.randomizer.org/), the animals received the bone blocks in their mandibles according to a split-mouth model as described below.

In the autogenous group (AG), an autogenous bone block harvested from the medial portion of the left tibial metaphysis was randomly grafted into the left or right mandibular angle. In the biomaterial group (BG), the synthetic biphasic calcium phosphate biomaterial (Grafts® BCP, Smart Bone Substitute, Aix-En-Provence, France) in the form of blocks was randomly grafted into the contralateral mandibular angle. The biomaterial was composed of a stable component (HA) and a bioactive bioabsorbable component (β-TCP) in a 60:40 ratio, respectively. The rationale was to provide a good balance between support for cell growth and graft absorption. The pores greater than 100 μm distributed over the entire surface of the material provided a degree of porosity of 70%. The relationship between porosity and the HA/TCP ratio represented a novelty that could provide greater cellular activity and maintenance of the trabecular architecture of the biomaterial.

2.2. Topographic Characterization of the Biomaterial

After covering the biomaterial with a thin layer of carbon, the surface topography of the biomaterial was analyzed using an electron microscope (SEM ZEISS, model EVO LS15, Oberkochen, Germany) to analyze the biomaterial surface morphology and its porosity, coupled with the X-ray dispersive energy spectroscopy system (Oxford model EDX microanalysis detector, Inca X-act, Oxford instruments, Abingdon, UK), for semi-quantitative analysis of the chemical composition of surfaces.

2.3. Experimental Surgery

General anesthesia was induced by intramuscular injections of ketamine hydrochloride (Vetaset—Fort Dodge Saúde Animal Ltd., Campinas, São Paulo, Brazil) at a dose of 50 mg/kg body weight associated with xylazine hydrochloride (Dopaser—Laboratório Calier do Brasil Ltd., Osasco, São Paulo, Brazil) at a dose of 5 mg/kg body weight. Subsequently, trichotomy and topical antisepsis were performed in both mandibular angle regions and in the left tibia with iodine solution (PVPI 10%, Riodeine, Rioquímica, São José do Rio Preto, Brazil). In addition, local infiltration of 0.3 mL/kg of mepivacaine hydrochloride (Scandicaine 2% with epinephrine 1:100,000, Septodont, Saint Maur des Fossés, France) was used as local anesthesia. A 2-cm dermal incision was made with a #15 scalpel blade (Feather Industries Ltd., Tokyo, Japan) mounted on a #3 scalpel handle in correspondence with each mandibular angle. Soft tissues were dissected respecting tissue planes reaching the periosteum. The periosteal tissue was finally incised in order to expose the bone tissue of the recipient area (Figure 1a). Bone decortication of the lateral plate of the mandibular angle was performed with a #701 rotary drill (Maillefer Instruments, Ballaigues, Switzerland), mounted on a straight surgical handpiece (Kavo do Brasil, Joinvile, Brazil), under constant irrigation of 0.9% sterile saline solution (Darrow, Rio de Janeiro, Brazil). In the AG, following the exposure of the recipient area, autogenous bone was harvested from the tibia. A 2-cm linear incision was made in correspondence with the left tibial metaphysis. A full-thickness skin flap, including skin, muscle, and periosteum, was raised exposing the surface of the bone. A circular osteotomy was performed (Figure 1b) by means of 8-mm internal diameter trephine bur (Neodent®, Curitiba, Paraná, Brazil) mounted on a contra-angle handpiece with a 20:1 reduction (Kavo® do Brasil, Joinvile, Brazil) at a speed of 1500 rpm under constant irrigation with 0.9% sodium chloride (Darrow, Rio de Janeiro, Brazil). The bone was carefully removed from the trephine and preserved in a sterile saline solution. In the BG, biphasic calcium phosphate ceramic blocks were harvested using the same trephine size, in order to collect grafts of the same diameter in both experimental groups. Autogenous (Figure 1c) or synthetic block grafts (Figure 1d) were subsequently perforated with a 1.2 mm-diameter drill under copious irrigation with sterile saline approximately in their central portion, and randomly fixed to the left or right mandibular angle by means of compressive 1.6 × 8 mm osteosynthesis bicortical screws (SIN, Sistema de Implante Nacional, São Paulo, Brazil) resulting in appositional onlay-like block graft. The recipient bed was perforated with a 1.0 mm-diameter drill cooled with sterile saline in order to favor nourishment and revascularization of the block graft.

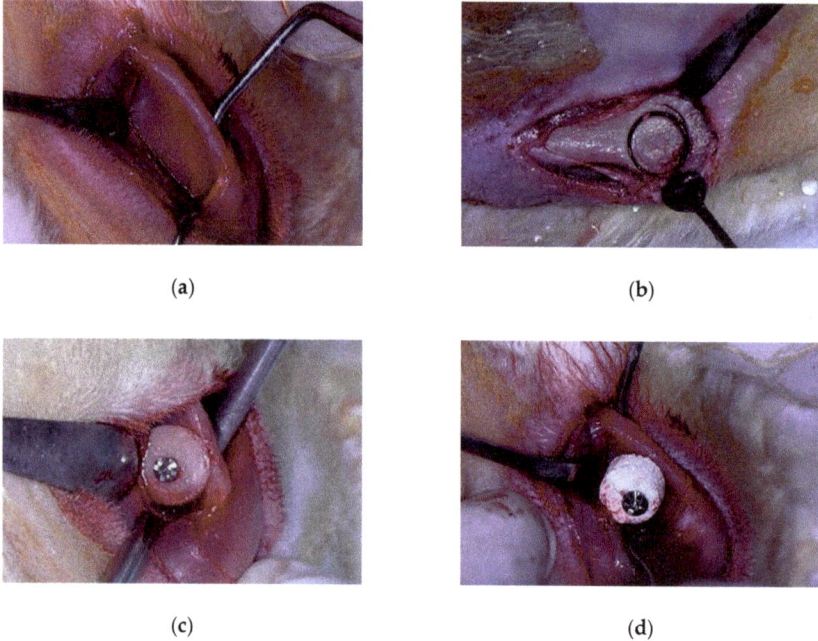

Figure 1. Experimental surgery procedure: (**a**) Surgical exposure of the recipient bed; (**b**) Autogenous bone block grafting procedure; (**c**) Autogenous block grafted in the autogenous group; (**d**) Biomaterial block grafted in the biomaterial group.

Soft tissues were carefully repositioned and sutured in different layers for primary wound closure using an absorbable suture (Polyglactin 910—Vicryl 4.0, Ethicon, Johnson Prod., São José dos Campos, SP, Brazil), while a non-resorbable monofilament suture (Nylon 4.0, Ethicon, Johnson, São José dos Campos, SP, Brazil) was used for interrupted skin suturing. Additional antisepsis with PVPI was conducted after the suturing. Intramuscular pentabiotic (0.1 mL/kg, Fort Dodge Saúde Animal Ltd., SP, Brazil) was injected immediately after the surgery. A single dose of sodic dipyrone (1 mg/kg/day, Ariston Indústrias Químicas e Farmacêuticas Ltd., São Paulo, SP, Brazil) was also administered. Neither food nor movement restriction was applied to the animals that remained in individual cages during the experimental period. At 30 and 60 postoperative days, 5 animals in each group, respectively, were sacrificed by a lethal dose of pentobarbital (200 mg/kg). The soft tissues were then dissected, and the mandible of each rabbit was extracted. Osteotomies were performed on each mandible to obtain bone samples with at least 3 cm of margins circumferentially around the grafted area. All samples were immersion-fixed in 10% neutral buffered formalin (Reagentes Analíticos®, Dinâmica Odonto-Hospitalar Ltd., Catanduva, SP, Brazil).

2.4. Histological Laboratorial Processing

After fixing and washing for 24 h in running water, the descaled were decalcified in 20% EDTA (ethylenediaminetetraacetic acid, Merck, Darmstadt, Germany) dissolved in Milli-Q water, replaced weekly for a period of 6 weeks, at room temperature. Following decalcification, the osteosynthesis screws were carefully removed. The samples were then dehydrated in an ascending series of alcohol concentrations (70, 90, 95, and absolute alcohol), changing the solutions every hour in an orbital shaker (KLine CT—150®, Cientec—Equipamentos para Laboratório, Piracicaba, SP, Brazil). The samples were successively cleared in xylol, paraffin-embedded, and prepared using a precision saw to obtain 5 μm thick sections. The sections were mounted onto slides and stained with hematoxylin eosin (HE Merck & Co., Inc., Kenilworth, NJ, USA) for qualitative and histometric analysis, and stained by osteopontin (OP), osteocalcin (OC), and Tartrate-resistant Acid Phosphatase (TRAP) for the immunohistochemical analysis.

2.5. Qualitative Histological Analysis

Five slides of each sample were obtained for hematoxylin and eosin staining in the most central region of the piece. The qualitative evaluation was performed by a researcher, blinded with respect to the experimentation through a binocular optical microscope JENAMED 2 (Carl-Zeiss, Oberkochen, Germany), considering the internal part of the bone graft, the interface between the bone graft and the recipient bed, and the newly formed tissue.

2.6. Histometric Analysis

The capture of the region of interest involving the bone substitute/autogenous bone block, the interface between the graft and the recipient bed, and the recipient bed, was performed with a 40× magnification, considering the most central region identified by the contour of the fixation screw and the limits of the graft. The capture generated an image of the bone substitute, the recipient bed, and their interface. After obtaining the images, the quantitative analysis was performed using dedicated software (Image J version 1.53, NIH Image, Bethesda, MD, USA). The image and respective percentage value generated by the capture using the "rectangle" tool was considered as the total area to be evaluated. After that, through the integrated tool "polygon", the bone substitute, connective tissue, and newly formed bone tissue areas were delimited and the respective percentage areas proportional to the total area were calculated and submitted to statistical tests.

2.7. Immunohistochemical Analysis

The immunohistochemical analysis was performed in the Department of Basic Sciences, Araçatuba Dental School—UNESP (FAPESP, 2015/14688-0). The histological slices obtained after 30 and 60 days from the surgical procedure were used.

The immunohistochemical procedure started by deparaffinization and rehydration of the slices, and then endogenous peroxidase activity was inhibited with hydrogen peroxide. Endogenous biotin was blocked with skimmed milk. The primary antibodies (Santa Cruz Biotechnology, Inc., 10410 Finnell Street, Dallas, TX 75220 USA) were used against Osteopontin (OP—SC10593), Osteocalcin (OC—SC18319), and Tartrate-resistant Acid Phosphatase (TRAP—SC30832). OP and OC proteins are expressed during the mineralization process, where OP marks osteoblasts at the beginning of the mineralization process and OC is expressed in the late stages of the mineralization process. TRAP, on the other hand, is expressed by osteoclast activity, allowing the evaluation of the resorption process. The rabbit anti-goat IgG (H+L) secondary antibody, Biotin (Pierce Biotechnology, Waltham, MA, USA) was used and the reaction signal was amplified by streptavidin (Dako North America, Inc., 6392 Via Real Carpinteria, CA 93013, USA). The Diaminobenzidine (Dako North America, Inc., 6392 Via Real Carpinteria, CA 93013, USA) ends the reaction and then the slices were counterstained with Meyer Hematoxylin.

For each antibody used, the expression of proteins was evaluated semi-quantitatively by assigning different "scores" in accordance with the immunostained cells in the wound-healing process. The analysis was performed with an optical microscope (LeicaR DMLB, Heerbrugg, Switzerland) by means of scores (ordinal qualitative analysis); when the scores were light labeling (++), moderate labeling (+++), and intense labeling (++++) it was considered positive for diaminobenzidine, taking care to hold negative controls to evaluate the specificity of the antibodies. These scores and the methodology were established according to previous studies [25–27], where light labeling represented about 25% of the immunolabeling area in the blades, moderate labeling represented about 50%, and intense labeling represented about 75%.

2.8. Statistical Analysis

An independent statistician performed the statistical analysis using IBM SPSS Statistics 24.0 (IBM Corp., Armonk, NY, USA). The results were initially submitted to the Shapiro–Wilk test to assess data distribution. After testing for normality, Student's *t*-test was performed for parametric data, while the Mann–Whitney U test was applied in cases of non-parametric data. A significance level of 0.05 was adopted for all tests.

3. Results

3.1. Topographic Characterization of Biomaterial

The SEM-EDX analysis evidenced a surface with the formation of crystals clusters and high macroporosity > 100 μm between it. The pores showed a crater shape and approximately 100 μm to 200 μm in diameter in multidirectional ways (Figure 2a). It was possible to observe regions with different heights on the same block surface (Figure 2b). The biomaterial base showed irregularities of the surface accompanied by its porosity, as well as the crystal clusters in different shapes and sizes (Figure 2c–e). The X-ray Dispersive Energy Spectroscopy analysis showed the amount of phosphorus (467), oxygen (372), and calcium (365) ions present, respectively, followed by a low percentage of magnesium (Figure 2f).

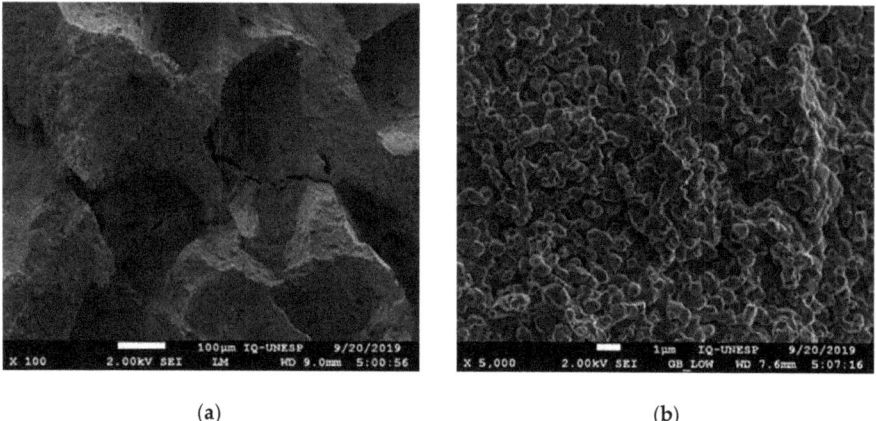

Figure 2. *Cont.*

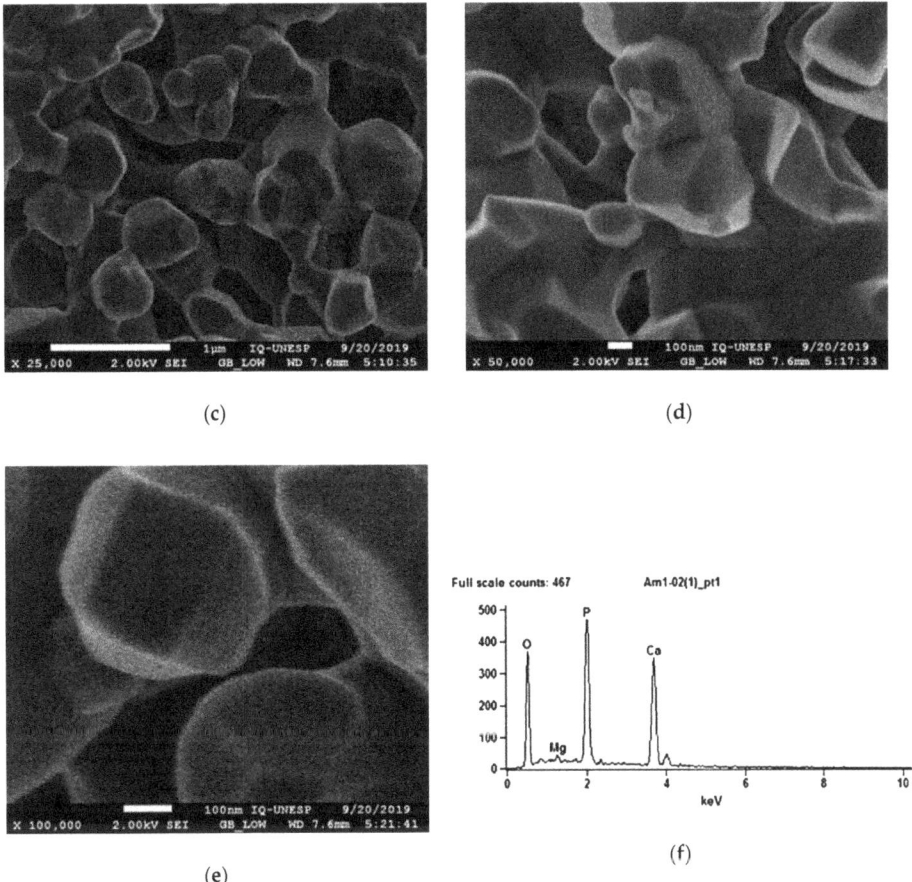

Figure 2. SEM-EDX analysis: (a–e) SEM views of the biomaterial surface at ×100, ×5000, ×25,000, ×50,000, and ×100,000 magnifications, respectively. (f) EDX spectrometry values obtained before the surgery. The elements found were phosphorus, oxygen, calcium, and magnesium.

3.2. Qualitative Histological Analysis

- Autogenous group

In the AG, after 30 healing days (Figure 3a), it was possible to observe the autogenous bone graft (A), and bone trabeculae under the receiving bed (B). The space between the graft and the recipient bed was occupied by bone tissue with a relevant number of trabeculae in the maturation stage with high cellular activity and good vascularization (C). Focusing on the graft (Figure 3b), autogenous bone (A) and newly formed bone (B) could be identified. In the inner part of the autogenous bone graft, small areas of resorption (black arrows) might indicate a phase of remodeling.

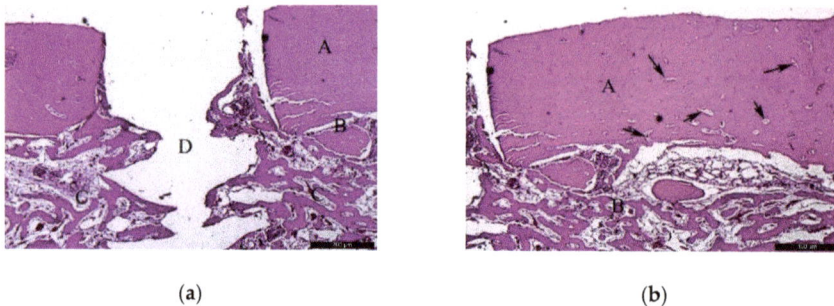

Figure 3. Histological analysis of the autogenous group (AG) at 30 days. (**a**) Autogenous bone graft (A) positioned over the recipient bed (B), trabeculae in maturation stage and good vascularization (C); space previously occupied by the osteosynthesis screw is recognizable in (D). Hematoxylin and eosin stain at a magnification 40×; (**b**) Autogenous bone (A) newly formed bone (B), and small areas of resorption (black arrows). Hematoxylin and eosin stain at a magnification 125×.

In the AG, after 60 post-operative days (Figure 4a), it was possible to observe the autogenous bone graft (A) in contact with the newly formed bone (B). Internally, the presence of connective tissue areas might suggest a remodeling phase of the bone. The identification of anucleated cells could suggest the presence of osteoblasts (red arrows). At the microscopic examination (Figure 4b), it was possible to distinguish the autogenous bone graft (A) and newly formed bone (B) separated by a cement line (black arrow). In the inner part of the autogenous bone graft, connective tissue areas were noticed, confirming the remodeling phase of the bone. Osteocytes were clearly visible (red arrows).

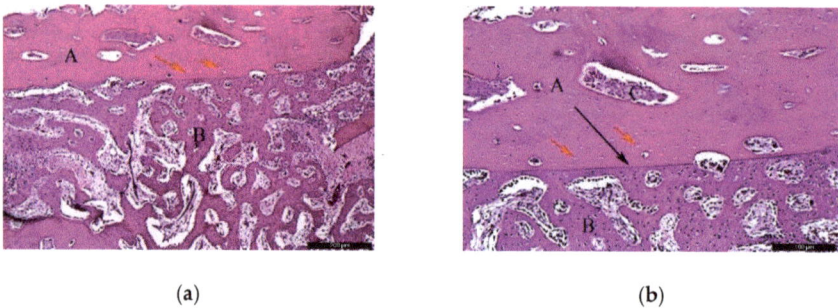

Figure 4. Histological analysis of the AG at 60 days. (**a**) Autogenous bone graft (A) in contact with the newly formed bone (B), and anucleated cells suggesting the presence of osteoblasts (red arrows). Hematoxylin and eosin stain at a magnification 40×; (**b**) Autogenous bone graft (A) and newly formed bone (B) separated by a cement line (black arrow) and osteocytes (red arrows). Hematoxylin and eosin stain at a magnification 125×.

- Biomaterial group

In the BG, after 30 healing days (Figure 5a), it was possible to observe the biomaterial (A) in close contact with the newly formed bone (B), and the residual recipient site (C). In the surrounding areas of the neoformed bone, it was possible to identify a high number of lining cells compatible with osteoblasts (blue arrows) suggesting a phase of matrix synthesis. At higher magnification (Figure 5b), the contiguous contact between the biomaterial (A) and the neoformed bone (B) was appreciated. Lining osteoblast cells were identified in the periphery of the newly formed bone (blue arrows).

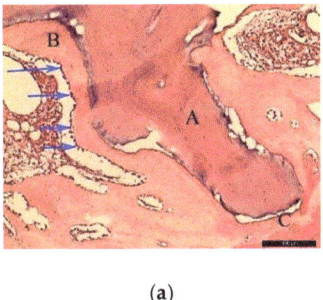 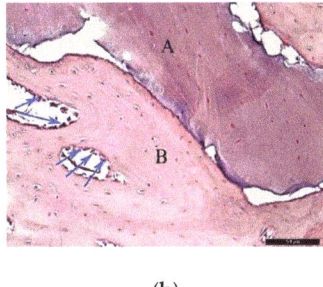

(a) (b)

Figure 5. Histological analysis of the biomaterial group (BG) at 30 days. (**a**) Biomaterial (A) in close contact with the newly formed bone (B), and the residual recipient site (C); osteoblast-like lining cells are indicated with blue arrows. Hematoxylin and eosin stain at a magnification 40×; (**b**) Biomaterial (A), newly formed bone (B), and lining osteoblast cells in the periphery of the newly formed bone (blue arrows). Hematoxylin and eosin stain at a magnification 125×.

In the BG, after 60 post-operative days (Figure 6a), the biomaterial (A) was enwrapped by neoformed bone (B). In the inner part of the biomaterial, it was possible to observe islands of newly formed bone, highlighting the osteoconductivity capability of the bone substitute. At the same time, areas of resorption associated with volume loss were noticed, indicating high solubility of the biomaterial. At higher magnification (Figure 6b), it was possible to observe the bone substitute (A) on the recipient bed (B), and neoformed bone tissue (C).

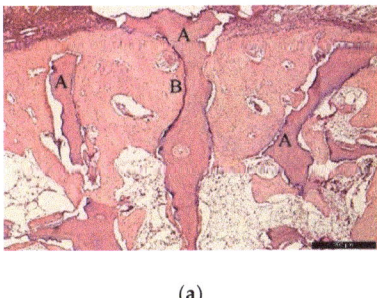 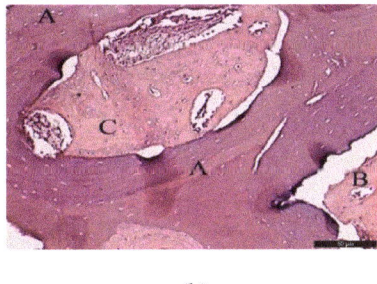

(a) (b)

Figure 6. Histological analysis of the BG at 60 days. (**a**) Biomaterial (A) enwrapped by newly formed bone (B). Hematoxylin and eosin stain at a magnification 40×; (**b**) Biomaterial (A) on the recipient bed (B), and newly formed bone (C). Hematoxylin and eosin stain at a magnification 125×.

3.3. Histometric Analysis

The mean values of the neoformed bone tissue in the AG were 6.56% and 9.70% at 30 and 60 postoperative days, respectively, while the mean values of connective tissue were 47.83% and 45.34% in the same periods evaluated. Additionally, the mean values of autogenous graft remnants were 45.61% and 44.96%, respectively. For the BG, the mean values of newly formed bone tissue were 3.14% and 6.43% at 30 and 60 postoperative days, respectively, while the mean values of connective tissue were 41.58% and 45.34% in the same periods analyzed. The mean remaining values of the synthetic biomaterial based on β-tricalcium phosphate were 55.28% and 40.26%, respectively. The registered data were submitted to statistical analysis, namely *t*-test for parametric data (neoformed bone tissue, and bone substitute in both periods of analysis, and connective tissue at 60 days period), and Mann–Whitney test for non-parametric data (connective tissue at 30 days period). The mean values of neoformed bone tissue in the AG were statistically higher when compared to the mean values of neoformed bone tissue in the BG at both experimental periods. Conversely, there was no statistically significant difference between groups in the amount of connective tissue and bone substitute in both experimental periods. The data of newly formed bone tissue, connective tissue, and remnants of autogenous graft and biomaterial for both groups are reported in Table 1.

Table 1. Analysis of the comparison between the biomaterial and autogenous bone at each experimental period.

Period	Group	Bone Substitute	Connective Tissue	Newly Formed Bone
30 days	Biomaterial	55.28%	41.58%	3.14% *
	Autogenous	4.61%	47.83%	6.56% *
60 days	Biomaterial	40.26%	53.31%	6.43% *
	Autogenous	44.96%	45.34%	9.70% *

* Statistically significant difference between BG and AG.

3.4. Immunohistochemical Analysis

At 30 postoperative days, in both groups, it was possible to observe bone tissue in the ongoing maturation phase, with neoformed bone trabeculae, and the presence of osteoblastic lineage cells. Already at 60 days, in both groups, organized, mature bone tissue, with the presence of osteocytes inside the gaps surrounded by a mineralized bone matrix, was noticed.

In the AG, at 30 days, it was possible to observe an intense osteopontin staining, showing a very intense (++++) initial bone mineralization activity, with positivity for the cells (osteoblasts) around the trabeculated bone, as well as the staining itself in the mineralized extracellular matrix (Figure 7a). In contrast, in the same period, in the BG, a light marking (++) was observed (Figure 7d), with a scarce mineralized extracellular matrix.

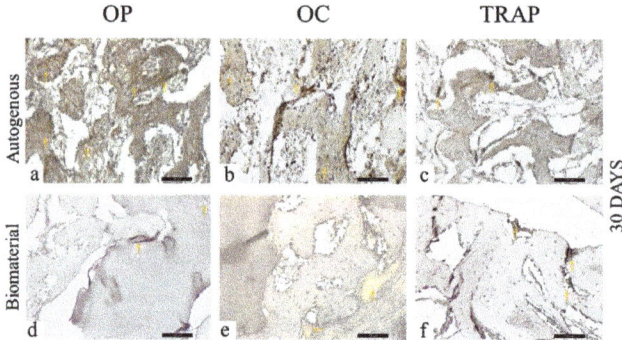

Figure 7. Osteopontin (OP), Osteocalcin (OC), and Tartrate-resistant Acid Phosphatase (TRAP) immunostaining at 30 days for the experimental groups. Immunolabeling is indicated by orange arrows. (a) OP immunostaining at 30 days in the AG; (b) OC immunostaining at 30 days in the AG; (c) TRAP immunostaining at 30 days in the AG; (d) OP immunostaining at 30 days in the BG; (e) OC immunostaining at 30 days in the BG; (f) TRAP immunostaining at 30 days in the BG.

Regarding osteocalcin, a protein related to the late stage of mineralization of the extracellular matrix, a moderate (+++) staining was observed in the AG (Figure 7b), with cells of the osteoblastic lineage and the extracellular matrix presenting positive immunostaining for this protein. When the osteopontin and osteocalcin marking was correlated for this experimental group, it was observed that the bone mineralization activity was in the initial stages, compatible with the evaluation period

(30 days). In the BG, it was possible to notice positive osteocalcin light (++) staining in the pre-existing bone tissue, with osteoblast lineage cells and a positively stained extracellular matrix (Figure 7e).

The TRAP expression, showing osteoclasts in bone resorption activity, was light (++) in the AG (Figure 7c), with low osteoclast activity, and was moderate (+++) for the BG (Figure 7f), indicating resorption activity.

At 60 days, in the AG, a moderate (+++) osteopontin staining was observed (Figure 8a), with the presence of positively stained cells adjacent to the bone tissue. It is worth noting the organization of the bone tissue visible in the region of interest. At the same time, osteocalcin was markedly intense (++++), with areas of precipitation on mature bone tissue (Figure 8b). Positively marked osteocytes were noted, characterizing the maturity of the bone tissue in this period. TRAP protein was lightly (++) marked, with few osteoclasts in resorption activity (Figure 8c).

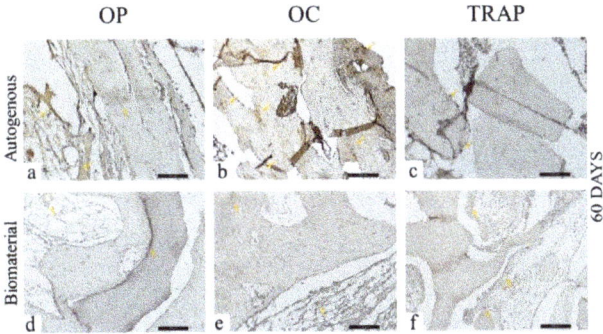

Figure 8. Osteopontin (OP), Osteocalcin (OC), and Tartrate-resistant Acid Phosphatase (TRAP) immunostaining at 60 days for the experimental groups. Immunolabeling is indicated by orange arrows. (**a**) OP immunostaining at 60 days in the AG; (**b**) OC immunostaining at 60 days in the AG; (**c**) TRAP immunostaining at 60 days in the AG; (**d**) OP immunostaining at 60 days in the BG; (**e**) OC immunostaining at 60 days in the BG; (**f**) TRAP immunostaining at 60 days in the BG.

For the BG, light (++) staining was observed for osteopontin, osteocalcin, and TRAP, showing few cells stained for each of these proteins (Figure 8d–f). Regarding osteopontin and osteocalcin, which are extracellular matrix proteins presenting staining on the mineralized matrix, the low mineralization activity for both proteins in this later period stands out. There were also few TRAP stained in the region of interest.

The scores obtained from the immunohistochemical analysis in the periods of 30 and 60 days are listed in Tables 2 and 3, respectively.

Table 2. Osteopontin (OP), Osteocalcin (OC), and Tartrate-resistant Acid Phosphatase (TRAP) immunostaining at 30 days for the experimental groups.

30 Days	Autogenous Group	Biomaterial Group
OP	++++	++
OC	+++	++
TRAP	++	+++

Table 3. Osteopontin (OP), Osteocalcin (OC), and Tartrate-resistant Acid Phosphatase (TRAP) immunostaining at 60 days for the experimental groups.

30 Days	Autogenous Group	Biomaterial Group
OP	+++	++
OC	++++	++
TRAP	++	++

4. Discussion

The ability of bioceramics to interact with osteoblastic cells is essentially related to their structural properties. Synthetic β-calcium-phosphate-based biomaterials present a porosity of approximately 70%. This type of conformation provides a considerable surface area supplied with several protein-binding sites available for a stable adhesion with a high number of osteoblasts [28]. Another factor that must be considered is the pore diameter. A previous study showed that wide pores with an accessible volume (>200 μm) exhibited an incremented proliferation and differentiation of osteoblasts within the scaffold, as a result of the revascularization process supplying oxygen and nourishment [29]. The same concept can be applied to calcium-phosphate-based biomaterials, in which the presence of pores allows the migration and proliferation of osteoblasts and mesenchymal cells along with the revascularization process needed to promote bone formation. In addition, a porous surface enhances the interconnection between the biomaterial and the surrounding bone tissue, creating high mechanical stability in the recipient bone–biomaterial interface [30]. The SEM showed a macroporosity > 100 μm of the synthetic biomaterial employed in the present study, which constitutes approximately 45% of its composition, thus facilitating the biological exchanges needed for the osteogenic process. Conversely, such porosity led to technical difficulties during the stabilization of the graft to the recipient bed during the experimental surgery. Higher strength was needed to tighten the screws while fixing the graft, with the risk of developing cracks and fractures of the blocks. Consequently, special attention was paid while fixing the biomaterial to the recipient bone in order to prevent block fractures during the intra- and post-operative periods. Indeed, the drilling technique in cases of such small-sized blocks is extremely challenging, especially for the biomaterial group, as the bone substitute is very friable. In addition, from an anatomical standpoint, the mandibular angle is particularly fragile, and requires care to obtain an effective fixation. Thus, the perforations were made in a direction that guaranteed the preservation of the block and the recipient bed in order to avoid complications such as the fracture of the block or the loss of stability in the fixation. This, however, often resulted in a non-centered position of the osteosynthesis screw, which may be considered a technical limitation during the histomorphometric analysis, as a central position of the screw would have been more helpful by serving as a reference guide during the cutting process. Energy-dispersive X-ray spectroscopy showed the presence of a low percentage of magnesium on the biomaterial surface. This component can promote the osteoimmunomodulatory properties, by improving osteoinduction by BMP signaling [31], being considered essential for bone tissue [32,33].

Autogenous bone graft is characterized by a relevant number of advantages with respect to most of the bone substitutes, particularly in terms of biocompatibility and regenerating potential. Autogenous bone is considered the gold standard due to its osteogenic properties, in addition to osteoinductive and osteoconductive capabilities, promoting the apposition of new bone tissue from the pre-existing bone as a model for new bone formation. In the present study, such properties have been validated when analyzing the microscopic images of the autogenous block graft at 60 post-operative days. Close contact between the recipient bed and the grafted autogenous block was observed, together with the presence of cement lines, newly formed bone associated with a high number of trabeculae, and vital osteocytes populating the inner portions of the graft. These biological events were promoted by the bone matrix, which induced the differentiation of osteoprogenitor cells of the recipient region into osteoblasts in order to stimulate bone formation. Those advantages and characteristics are supported by the expected results of the histometric analysis, where the AG presented a statistically significant difference in bone neoformation when compared to the BG. However, the autogenous graft needs a donor site, which contributed to the development of biomaterials, such as the HA-β-TCP used in the present experimental study, and although the histometric findings showed a greater amount of newly formed bone (bone incorporation) for the AG, the biomaterial was incorporated into the recipient bed and allowed bone formation by osteoconduction, which was expected. A previous study compared autogenous bone grafts with allogeneic grafts in block form through histological, histometric, and immunohistochemistry analyzes, showing the superiority of the autogenous bone in new bone formation and maturation of bone tissue during the incorporation process [34]. This highlights the need to search for an ideal biomaterial as an alternative to autogenous grafts.

Histological findings were confirmed by the immunostaining of OP and OC proteins. The marking of OP was intense at 30 days in the AG and light in the BG, showing earlier osteoblastic activity in the former. A delayed incorporation is confirmed within 60 days, when AG showed intense osteocalcin expression indicating bone maturation, whereas BG showed light expression of this protein, which represents the formation of an immature tissue in this period. In a previous study assessing critical-size defects in rat calvaria filled with autogenous bone or beta-tricalcium phosphate biomaterial, the authors evaluated the immunostaining of osteocalcin at 30 and 60 postoperative days [13]. It was observed that the AG showed higher protein expression at 60 days, indicating a greater maturation of the bone tissue formed compared to the biomaterial, which is in agreement with the results obtained herein.

Considering the donor site, the rabbit tibia was used to collect the autogenous graft. The reason is related to low post-operative morbidity, and ease of the surgical technique with respect to other donor sites. Harvesting bone from the rabbit calvaria leaves the dura-mater exposed due to an inability to separate the external and the internal cortical plates. The tibia is mainly characterized by cortical bone, with the presence of an intra-medullary canal. Hence, due to its composition, the tibia could be safely used to retrieve bone tissue in the form of blocks, with an adequate thickness for bone reconstructions [35]. On the other hand, in order to reduce the morbidity associated with the harvesting procedure, the research has been directed toward the use of bone substitutes. Among the wide range of biomaterials, synthetic bioceramics are gaining space in clinical scenarios as an alternative to autogenous bone grafts in maxillo-facial reconstructions. This study evaluated the incorporation of a biomaterial based on beta-tricalcium phosphate with hydroxyapatite compared to autogenous bone grafted in rabbit mandibles, in order to simulate critical clinical situations requiring horizontal augmentation in mandibular alveolar ridges, in which the use of biomaterial blocks may be indicated. However, for vertical defects, as an alternative to autogenous bone grafts, these biomaterials may not be the best clinical choice, or even contraindicated.

The biocompatibility and bifunctionality of calcium phosphate bioceramics in the substitution of bone tissue have been evaluated in vivo [36]. It was concluded that HA and β-TCP were progressively resorbed and substituted with newly formed bone, acting as a scaffold that could be favorably colonized by osteogenic cells. β-TCP has been compared to biphasic calcium phosphate ceramic containing HA/β-TCP in a 75:25 ratio in the process of trabecular bone repair in an animal model [30]. The histomorphometric analysis demonstrated that 36% of β-TCP, used alone, underwent resorption in 26 weeks, whereas the HA/β-TCP group healed undisturbed. Bone neoformation occurred in both groups; however, a higher amount of peripheral bone volume was observed in the biphasic ceramic group. Therefore, it was concluded that both bone substitutes were biocompatible and were characterized by a satisfying osteoconductive potential; nevertheless, the biodegradation of β-TCP was faster, losing the volume that should be maintained. A previous study evaluated β-TCP as a bone substitute in preserving the alveolar ridge for subsequent implant insertion in humans [37]. The ridge dimensions were measured before the grafting procedure and after a 6-month healing period at the second stage surgery for tissue sample harvesting and implant placement. Resorption of approximately 9% occurred during the healing time. After 6 months, the histological evaluation showed a complete resorption of the biomaterial, replaced by vital bone of good quality and quantity, which allowed a proper implant insertion. This might underline the osteoconductive properties of the biomaterial associated with a high level of solubility. Accordingly, the same pattern has been observed during the histological analysis of the present study. However, it must be noticed that the biomaterial has been used in a more challenging clinical situation in the present study, namely, as an appositional block graft to increase the bone thickness, and not as a filling material in self-containing defects during socket preservation procedures. In addition, a recent study evaluated HA/β-TCP in the form of blocks [38]. The study assessed and compared qualitatively autogenous bone grafts versus a synthetic biomaterial based on HA/β-TCP in a 60:40 proportion. The biomaterial underwent gradual resorption followed by the apposition of bone tissue. Nonetheless, even at 60 post-operative days, it was possible to detect a certain amount of bone substitute in contact with newly formed bone and the recipient bed.

5. Conclusions

In conclusion, the biomaterial based on β-tricalcium phosphate combined with hydroxyapatite evaluated in the present experimental study served as a scaffold, promoting bone formation in the grafted area and highlighting its osteoconductive property. However, there was a delay in the incorporation process when compared to the autogenous block graft.

Author Contributions: Conceptualization, F.A.S., A.P.F.B., P.S.P.d.C., R.O., C.M.; methodology, L.C.d.A.P., R.C.d.S., L.K.d.J., P.P.P., F.R.E., L.T.C., R.O.; validation, H.H., L.P.P., F.R.E., A.F.P.S.; formal analysis, L.C.d.A.P., R.C.d.S., L.K.d.J., F.Á.S., A.P.F.B., R.O.; investigation, P.S.P.d.C., C.M., H.H., F.R.E., F.Á.S.; resources, P.P.P., L.P.P., A.F.P.S., L.T.C.; data curation, H.H., P.P.P., L.C.d.A.P., R.C.d.S., L.K.d.J., L.P.P., A.F.P.S., L.T.C., R.O.; writing—original draft preparation, L.C.d.A.P., R.C.d.S., L.K.d.J., H.H., L.P.P., A.F.P.S., F.R.E., P.S.P.d.C.; writing—review and editing, P.P.P., L.T.C., C.M., F.Á.S., A.P.F.B., R.O.; visualization, L.C.d.A.P., R.C.d.S., L.K.d.J., H.H., A.F.P.S., L.P.P.; supervision, P.P.P., L.T.C., C.M., R.O.; project administration, F.Á.S., A.P.F.B., and P.S.P.d.C. All authors have read and agreed to the published version of the manuscript.

Funding: This research received no external funding.

Conflicts of Interest: The authors declare no conflict of interest.

References

1. Araujo, M.G.; Lindhe, J. Dimensional ridge alterations following tooth extraction. An experimental study in the dog. *J. Clin. Periodontol.* **2005**, *32*, 212–218. [CrossRef] [PubMed]
2. Esposito, M.; Grusovin, M.G.; Felice, P.; Karatzopoulos, G.; Worthington, H.V.; Coulthard, P. The efficacy of horizontal and vertical bone augmentation procedures for dental implants—A Cochrane systematic review. *Eur. J. Oral Implantol.* **2009**, *2*, 167–184. [CrossRef] [PubMed]
3. Beretta, M.; Cicciù, M.; Poli, P.P.; Rancitelli, D.; Bassi, G.; Grossi, G.B.; Maiorana, C. A Retrospective Evaluation of 192 Implants Placed in Augmented Bone: Long-Term Follow-Up Study. *J. Oral Implant.* **2015**, *41*, 669–674. [CrossRef]
4. Yamada, M.; Egusa, H. Current bone substitutes for implant dentistry. *J. Prosthodont. Res.* **2018**, *62*, 152–161. [CrossRef]
5. Garcia-Júnior, I.R.; Souza, F.Á.; Figueiredo, A.A.S.; Poli, P.P.; Benetti, F.; Ferreira, S.; De Melo, W.M.; Rahal, S. Maxillary Alveolar Ridge Atrophy Reconstructed with Autogenous Bone Graft Harvested From the Proximal Ulna. *J. Craniofac. Surg.* **2018**, *29*, 2304–2306. [CrossRef]
6. Maiorana, C.; Ferrario, S.; Poli, P.P.; Manfredini, M. Autogenous Chin Block Grafts in the Aesthetic Zone: A 20-Year Follow-Up Case Report. *Case Rep. Dent.* **2020**, *2020*, 6525797. [CrossRef]
7. Maiorana, C.; Poli, P.P.; Borgonovo, A.E.; Rancitelli, D.; Frigo, A.C.; Pieroni, S.; Santoro, F. Long-Term Retrospective Evaluation of Dental Implants Placed in Resorbed Jaws Reconstructed With Appositional Fresh-Frozen Bone Allografts. *Implant. Dent.* **2016**, *25*, 400–408. [CrossRef]
8. Maiorana, C.; Poli, P.P.; Mascellaro, A.; Ferrario, S.; Beretta, M. Dental implants placed in resorbed alveolar ridges reconstructed with iliac crest autogenous onlay grafts: A 26-year median follow-up retrospective study. *J. Cranio-Maxillofac. Surg.* **2019**, *47*, 805–814. [CrossRef]
9. Sakkas, A.; Wilde, F.; Heufelder, M.; Winter, K.; Schramm, A. Autogenous bone grafts in oral implantology—Is it still a "gold standard"? A consecutive review of 279 patients with 456 clinical procedures. *Int. J. Implant. Dent.* **2017**, *3*, 1–17. [CrossRef] [PubMed]

10. Myeroff, C.; Archdeacon, M. Autogenous Bone Graft: Donor Sites and Techniques. *J. Bone Jt. Surg. Am. Vol.* **2011**, *93*, 2227–2236. [CrossRef] [PubMed]
11. Piattelli, A.; Scarano, A.; Mangano, C. Clinical and histologic aspects of biphasic calcium phosphate ceramic (BCP) used in connection with implant placement. *Biomaterials* **1996**, *17*, 1767–1770. [CrossRef]
12. Guillaume, B. Filling bone defects with β-TCP in maxillofacial surgery: A review. *Morphologie* **2017**, *101*, 113–119. [CrossRef] [PubMed]
13. De Freitas Silva, L.; de Carvalho Reis, E.N.R.; Barbara, T.A.; Bonardi, J.P.; Garcia Junior, I.R.; de Carvalho, P.S.P.; Ponzoni, D. Assessment of bone repair in critical-size defect in the calvarium of rats after the implantation of tricalcium phosphate beta (β-TCP). *Acta Histochem.* **2017**, *119*, 624–631. [CrossRef]
14. Schmidt, L.E.; Hadad, H.; De Vasconcelos, I.R.; Colombo, L.T.; Capalbo-Da-Silva, R.; Santos, A.F.P.; Cervantes, L.C.C.; Poli, P.P.; Signorino, F.; Maiorana, C.; et al. Critical Defect Healing Assessment in Rat Calvaria Filled with Injectable Calcium Phosphate Cement. *J. Funct. Biomater.* **2019**, *10*, 21. [CrossRef]
15. Tebyanian, H.; Norahan, M.H.; Eyni, H.; Movahedin, M.; Mortazavi, S.J.; Karami, A.; Nourani, M.R.; Baheiraei, N. Effects of collagen/β-tricalcium phosphate bone graft to regenerate bone in critically sized rabbit calvarial defects. *J. Appl. Biomater. Funct. Mater.* **2019**, *17*. [CrossRef] [PubMed]
16. Gallinetti, S.; Canal, C.; Ginebra, M.-P. Development and Characterization of Biphasic Hydroxyapatite/β-TCP Cements. *J. Am. Ceram. Soc.* **2014**, *97*, 1065–1073. [CrossRef]
17. Kim, S.E.; Park, K. Recent Advances of Biphasic Calcium Phosphate Bioceramics for Bone Tissue Regeneration. *Adv. Exp. Med. Biol.* **2020**, *1250*, 177–188. [CrossRef] [PubMed]
18. Yamada, S.; Heymann, D.; Bouler, J.M.; Daculsi, G. Osteoclastic resorption of calcium phosphate ceramics with different hydroxyapatite/beta-tricalcium phosphate ratios. *Biomaterials* **1997**, *18*, 1037–1041. [CrossRef]
19. Wang, Y.; Wang, K.; Li, X.; Wei, Q.; Chai, W.; Wang, S.; Che, Y.; Lu, T.; Zhang, B. 3D fabrication and characterization of phosphoric acid scaffold with a HA/β-TCP weight ratio of 60:40 for bone tissue engineering applications. *PLoS ONE* **2017**, *12*, e0174870. [CrossRef]
20. Ohayon, L. Maxillary sinus floor augmentation using biphasic calcium phosphate: A histologic and histomorphometric study. *Int. J. Oral Maxillofac. Implant.* **2014**, *29*, 1143–1148. [CrossRef]
21. Kakar, A.; Rao, B.H.S.; Hegde, S.; Deshpande, N.; Lindner, A.; Nagursky, H.; Patney, A.; Mahajan, H. Ridge preservation using an in situ hardening biphasic calcium phosphate (β-TCP/HA) bone graft substitute—A clinical, radiological, and histological study. *Int. J. Implants Dent.* **2017**, *3*, 25. [CrossRef] [PubMed]
22. Olaechea, A.; Mendoza-Azpur, G.; O'Valle, F.; Padial-Molina, M.; Martin-Morales, N.; Galindo-Moreno, P. Biphasic hydroxyapatite and ß-tricalcium phosphate biomaterial behavior in a case series of maxillary sinus augmentation in humans. *Clin. Oral Implants Res.* **2019**, *30*, 336–343. [CrossRef] [PubMed]
23. Kakar, A.; Kakar, K.; Rao, B.H.S.; Lindner, A.; Nagursky, H.; Jain, G.; Patney, A. Lateral alveolar ridge augmentation procedure using subperiosteal tunneling technique: A pilot study. *Maxillofac. Plast. Reconstr. Surg.* **2018**, *40*, 3. [CrossRef] [PubMed]
24. Jensen, S.S.; Broggini, N.; Hjorting-Hansen, E.; Schenk, R.K.; Buser, D. Bone healing and graft resorption of autograft, anorganic bovine bone and beta-tricalcium phosphate. A histologic and histomorphometric study in the mandibles of minipigs. *Clin. Oral Implants Res.* **2006**, *17*, 237–243. [CrossRef] [PubMed]
25. Pedrosa, W.F., Jr.; Okamoto, R.; Faria, P.E.P.; Arnez, M.F.M.; Xavier, S.P.; Salata, L.A. Immunohistochemical, tomographic and histological study on onlay bone graft remodeling. Part II: Calvarial bone. *Clin. Oral Implants Res.* **2009**, *20*, 1254–1264. [CrossRef] [PubMed]
26. Manrique, N.; Pereira, C.C.S.; Luvizuto, E.R.; Sánchez, M.R.; Okamoto, T.; Okamoto, R.; Sumida, D.H.; Antoniali, C. Hypertension modifies OPG, RANK, and RANKL expression during the dental socket bone healing process in spontaneously hypertensive rats. *Clin. Oral Investig.* **2015**, *19*, 1319–1327. [CrossRef]
27. Palin, L.P.; Polo, T.O.B.; Batista, F.R.D.S.; Gomes-Ferreira, P.H.S.; Júnior, I.R.G.; Rossi, A.C.; Freire, A.; Faverani, L.; Sumida, D.H.; Okamoto, R. Daily melatonin administration improves osseointegration in pinealectomized rats. *J. Appl. Oral Sci.* **2018**, *26*, e20170470. [CrossRef]
28. Antunes, A.A.; Oliveira Neto, P.; de Santis, E.; Caneva, M.; Botticelli, D.; Salata, L.A. Comparisons between Bio-Oss(®) and Straumann(®) Bone Ceramic in immediate and staged implant placement in dogs mandible bone defects. *Clin. Oral Implants Res.* **2013**, *24*, 135–142. [CrossRef]
29. Yuan, H.; Doel, M.V.D.; Li, S.; Van Blitterswijk, C.A.; De Groot, K.; De Bruijn, J.D. A comparison of the osteoinductive potential of two calcium phosphate ceramics implanted intramuscularly in goats. *J. Mater. Sci. Mater. Electron.* **2002**, *13*, 1271–1275. [CrossRef]

30. Bodde, E.W.H.; Wolke, J.G.C.; Kowalski, R.S.Z.; Jansen, J.A. Bone regeneration of porous beta-tricalcium phosphate (Conduit TCP) and of biphasic calcium phosphate ceramic (Biosel) in trabecular defects in sheep. *J. Biomed. Mater. Res. A* **2007**, *82*, 711–722. [CrossRef]
31. Houshmand, B.; Shamsoddin, E.; Golabgiran, M. Biomaterial selection for bone augmentation in implant dentistry: A systematic review. *J. Adv. Pharm. Technol. Res.* **2019**, *10*, 46–50. [CrossRef]
32. Zhang, X.; Chen, Q.; Mao, X. Magnesium Enhances Osteogenesis of BMSCs by Tuning Osteoimmunomodulation. *BioMed. Res. Int.* **2019**, *2019*, 7908205. [CrossRef]
33. Rude, R.K.; Gruber, H.; Wei, L.; Frausto, A.; Mills, B. Magnesium Deficiency: Effect on Bone and Mineral Metabolism in the Mouse. *Calcif. Tissue Int.* **2003**, *72*, 32–41. [CrossRef] [PubMed]
34. Junior, E.G.; De Lima, V.; Momesso, G.; Mello-Neto, J.; Érnica, N.; Filho, O.M. Potential of autogenous or fresh-frozen allogeneic bone block grafts for bone remodelling: A histological, histometrical, and immunohistochemical analysis in rabbits. *Br. J. Oral Maxillofac. Surg.* **2017**, *55*, 589–593. [CrossRef] [PubMed]
35. Miceli, A.L.C.; Pereira, L.C.; Torres, T.D.S.; Calasans-Maia, M.D.; Louro, R.S. Mandibular Reconstruction with Lateral Tibial Bone Graft: An Excellent Option for Oral and Maxillofacial Surgery. *Craniomaxillofac. Trauma Reconstr.* **2017**, *10*, 292–298. [CrossRef]
36. Ghanaati, S.; Barbeck, M.; Detsch, R.; Deisinger, U.; Hilbig, U.; Rausch, V.; Sader, R.; E Unger, R.; Ziegler, G.; Kirkpatrick, C.J. The chemical composition of synthetic bone substitutes influences tissue reactions in vivo: Histological and histomorphometrical analysis of the cellular inflammatory response to hydroxyapatite, beta-tricalcium phosphate and biphasic calcium phosphate ceramics. *Biomed. Mater.* **2012**, *7*, 015005. [CrossRef] [PubMed]
37. A Horowitz, R.; Mazor, Z.; Miller, R.J.; Krauser, J.; Prasad, H.S.; Rohrer, M.D. Clinical evaluation alveolar ridge preservation with a beta-tricalcium phosphate socket graft. *Compend. Contin. Educ. Dent.* **2009**, *30*, 588–590.
38. Lee, J.-T.; Cha, J.-K.; Kim, S.; Jung, U.-W.; Thoma, D.S.; Jung, R.E. Lateral onlay grafting using different combinations of soft-type synthetic block grafts and resorbable collagen membranes: An experimental in vivo study. *Clin. Oral Implants Res.* **2020**, *31*, 303–314. [CrossRef]

Publisher's Note: MDPI stays neutral with regard to jurisdictional claims in published maps and institutional affiliations.

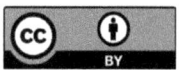

© 2020 by the authors. Licensee MDPI, Basel, Switzerland. This article is an open access article distributed under the terms and conditions of the Creative Commons Attribution (CC BY) license (http://creativecommons.org/licenses/by/4.0/).

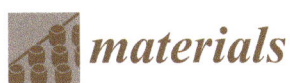

Article

Sol–Gel Synthesis and Characterization of a Quaternary Bioglass for Bone Regeneration and Tissue Engineering

Ricardo Bento [1], Anuraag Gaddam [1,2] and José M. F. Ferreira [1,*]

1 CICECO—Aveiro Institute of Materials, Department of Materials and Ceramic Engineering, University of Aveiro, Santiago University Campus, 3810-193 Aveiro, Portugal; ricardobento@ua.pt (R.B.); anuraagg@ua.pt (A.G.)
2 Instituto de Física de São Carlos, Universidade de São Paulo, São Carlos 13566-590, SP, Brazil
* Correspondence: jmf@ua.pt; Tel.: +351-234-370-242

Abstract: Sol–gel synthesis using inorganic and/or organic precursors that undergo hydrolysis and condensation at room temperature is a very attractive and less energetic method for preparing bioactive glass (BG) compositions, as an alternative to the melt-quenching process. When properly conducted, sol–gel synthesis might result in amorphous structures, with all of the components intimately mixed at the atomic scale. Moreover, developing new and better performing materials for bone tissue engineering is a growing concern, as the aging of the world's population leads to lower bone density and osteoporosis. This work describes the sol–gel synthesis of a novel quaternary silicate-based BG with the composition 60 SiO_2–34 CaO–4 MgO–2 P_2O_5 (mol%), which was prepared using acidified distilled water as a single solvent. By controlling the kinetics of the hydrolysis and condensation steps, an amorphous glass structure could be obtained. The XRD results of samples calcined within the temperature range of 600–900 °C demonstrated that the amorphous nature was maintained until 800 °C, followed by partial crystallization at 900 °C. The specific surface area—an important factor in osteoconduction—was also evaluated over different temperatures, ranging from 160.6 ± 0.8 m^2/g at 600 °C to 2.2 ± 0.1 m^2/g at 900 °C, accompanied by consistent changes in average pore size and pore size distribution. The immersion of the BG particles in simulated body fluid (SBF) led to the formation of an extensive apatite layer on its surface. These overall results indicate that the proposed material is very promising for biomedical applications in bone regeneration and tissue engineering.

Keywords: bioactive glasses; alkali-free; sol–gel; bone regeneration; tissue engineering

Citation: Bento, R.; Gaddam, A.; Ferreira, J.M.F. Sol–Gel Synthesis and Characterization of a Quaternary Bioglass for Bone Regeneration and Tissue Engineering. *Materials* **2021**, *14*, 4515. https://doi.org/10.3390/ma14164515

Academic Editor: Gigliola Lusvardi

Received: 30 June 2021
Accepted: 4 August 2021
Published: 11 August 2021

Publisher's Note: MDPI stays neutral with regard to jurisdictional claims in published maps and institutional affiliations.

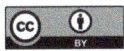

Copyright: © 2021 by the authors. Licensee MDPI, Basel, Switzerland. This article is an open access article distributed under the terms and conditions of the Creative Commons Attribution (CC BY) license (https://creativecommons.org/licenses/by/4.0/).

1. Introduction

Noticeable increases in life expectancy have been achieved over the past two centuries, as well documented in several literature reports [1,2]. The overall scientific progress made in the medical field, especially over the most recent decades, has greatly contributed to an increase in the population's quality of life and life expectancy. Such progresses together brought an unavoidable increase in the average age of the population, with social, economic, and medical consequences [3,4]. Older people are less capable of physical exertion, and the reduction of the mechanical stimuli of the bones, along with the degradation of the tissues due to a lifetime of use, increases the risk of fractures [5,6]. The consequent increased incidence of bone-related diseases (e.g., osteoporosis, trauma fractures, removal of tumours, etc.) challenges researchers to provide new therapeutic solutions to prevent the onset of osteopathy, and to develop bone grafts to treat these ailments. Autografts, although still considered the gold standard due to their optimal osteogenic, osteoinductive, and osteoconductive properties, have multiple drawbacks, including the donor site morbidity and their limited availability [7]. On the other hand, allografts are often associated with risk of infection and a high non-union rate with host tissue [8,9]. Therefore, tissue engineering—and bone tissue engineering in particular—presents itself as a most promising alternative solution to the current bone grafting approaches [10].

Several materials have been tried, and have achieved some success. Among these materials, bioceramics and bioglasses are promising candidates for bone regeneration, owing to their natural properties—such as biocompatibility, osteoinduction, and osteoconduction—adding to their composition, which is similar to that of bone [11]. Dense ceramics, such as alumina [12,13] or zirconia [14–16], have found a wide use in load-bearing applications due to their excellent mechanical properties and low in vivo toxicity. However, the paradigm changed with the discovery of bioactive glasses (BGs) by Larry Hench et al., due to their ability to bond to living tissues through the formation of an interfacial bone-like hydroxyapatite layer when the bioglass is put in contact with biological fluids in vivo. Among a number of tested compositions, the one exhibiting the highest bioactivity index became well known, and has been trademarked as 45S5 Bioglass® since 1985 [17]. Since then, the topic has received increasing attention, inspiring many other investigations aimed at further exploring the in vitro and in vivo performances of this BG, or gradually developing other related BG compositions [18–20]. Even though these glasses possess excellent affinity with native bone, their commercial success has so far been relatively limited. Their drawbacks include inadequate mechanical properties and high dissolution rates of alkaline ions in biological conditions, which may have a harmful impact on cells [21–26], along with several other shortcomings, as well summarized elsewhere [27]. Conversely, it has been demonstrated that well-designed alkali-free bioactive glass compositions offer a great number of advantages, including the ability to achieve full densification before the onset of crystallization, a fast biomineralization capability, with the formation of a crystalline surface apatite layer after immersion in SBF solution for 1 h [28,29], and good in vivo performances [30].

Traditionally, bioactive glasses are produced by melt-quenching. However, this technique incurs higher energy costs, and often results in partial devitrification with the formation of crystalline phases, which have reduced biological properties and are unsuitable for producing porous scaffolds [11]. Due to this, the sol–gel method has been regarded as a favourable alternative, as it yields glasses with higher purity, requiring low densification temperatures and allowing the production of a varied amount of compositions [31,32]. This technique does, however, exhibit some drawbacks—namely, the high cost of the precursors, and the difficulty in producing dense, monolithic pieces [33]. The present work aims at using water as a single solvent in the sol–gel synthesis of a novel, well-balanced, and thermally stable alkali-free BG composition intended for biomedical applications in bone regeneration and tissue engineering.

2. Materials and Methods
2.1. Bioglass Synthesis

A quaternary bioactive glass with a composition consisting of 60 SiO_2–34 CaO–4 MgO–2 P_2O_5 (mol%) was prepared via the sol–gel method, following a detailed procedure described elsewhere [32]. Briefly, tetraethyl orthosilicate (TEOS, $Si(O_2H_5)$, ≥98%), supplied by Sigma-Aldrich, and triethyl phosphate (TEP, $O_4P(C_2H_5O)$, ≥98%), supplied by Merck Schuchardt, were used as Si and P network precursors, respectively, while calcium nitrate tetrahydrate ($Ca(NO_3)_2 \cdot 4 H_2O$), supplied by Panreac, and magnesium nitrate hexahydrate ($Mg(NO_3)_2 \cdot 6 H_2O$), supplied by Scharlab, were selected as Ca and Mg network modifiers, respectively. Nitric acid ($HNO_3 \geq 65\%$) supplied by Labkem was used as a catalyst to promote the hydrolysis of network precursors. Each preparation was planned to yield 0.2 mol of bioactive glass by mixing 1.46 g of TEP, 25.00 g of TEOS, 2.05 g of magnesium nitrate, and 16.06 g of calcium nitrate. Two separate aqueous solutions were initially prepared: one containing the network precursors, and the other the network modifiers. In brief, the required amounts of TEOS and TEP were added together to 20 mL of deionized water acidified with two drops of concentrated nitric acid, under magnetic stirring for 30 min, until obtaining a transparent sol. The solution of the network modifiers was prepared in parallel by simply adding the required amounts Ca(NO$_3$)$_2$·4 H$_2$O and Mg(NO$_3$)$_2$·6 H$_2$O to 20 mL of deionized water under magnetic stirring for 30 min. Due to their high solubility, this solution soon became transparent. Afterwards, both solutions were mixed together and magnetically stirred for a further 60 min, before being poured into Petri dishes and stored in an oven for 24 h at 100 °C to promote a relatively rapid sol–gel transition and drying. After 24 h, the xerogel was crushed with an agate pestle and mortar into a fine powder, and then heat treated at different temperatures.

2.2. Thermal Treatment

Ground xerogel powder was calcined for 2 h at temperatures of 600, 700, 800, and 900 °C, with a heating rate of 0.5 °C min^{-1}, and the powders' properties were assessed through several characterization techniques, as described below.

2.2.1. XRD Characterization

The powders' crystalline phase content was determined by X-ray diffraction (XRD, Rigaku Geigerflex D/Mac, C Series, Tokyo, Japan) using Cu K$_\alpha$ radiation with 2θ varying from 5–70° in steps of 0.026 s^{-1}.

2.2.2. FTIR Characterization

The functional groups of the samples were analysed by FTIR (FTIR Bruker Tensor 27) over the wavenumber range of 2000–300 cm^{-1}, with 256 scans and 4 cm^{-1} resolution.

2.2.3. SEM Imaging

Specimens were covered with a thin (15-nm) carbon layer using a thin film deposition system (PVD 75, Kurt J. Lesker Co., Jefferson Hills, PA, USA) before being examined using a Hitachi S4100 scanning electron microscope with a 15.0-kV accelerating voltage.

2.2.4. Specific Surface Area Analysis

Specific surface area (SAA) and pore analyses were carried out with the BET, BJH, and t-plot methods (Micrometric Gemini M-2380); N$_2$ was used as an adsorbate, and samples were previously degassed at 200 °C.

2.2.5. SBF Immersion Assays

Powder samples were immersed in SBF for a period of 28 days. Every 7 days, the sample's reaction with the SBF was halted by filtering, rinsing with deionized water, and drying.

3. Results and Discussion

3.1. Bioglass Synthesis—Effect of Mixing Time

The XRD patterns of the bioglasses prepared according to previous works [32] displayed an unexpected crystalline phase upon calcining at 600 °C. Since the synthesis experiments were carried out in the winter, an explanatory hypothesis for this was the relatively low room temperatures (15–17 °C) prevailing in the lab, which might have delayed the reaction kinetics. Therefore, the duration of the mixing step was increased from 30 to 60 min in order to allow complete hydrolysis. This longer mixing period successfully produced amorphous glasses, as shown in Figure 1.

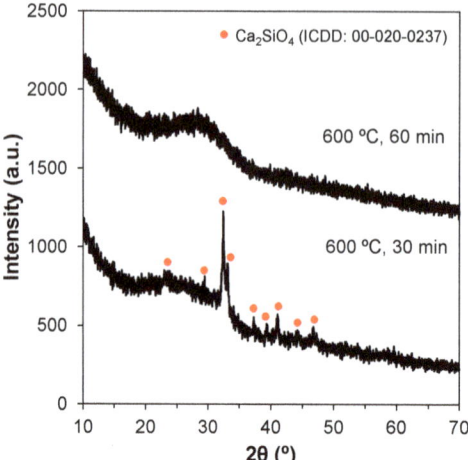

Figure 1. XRD patterns showing the effect of mixing times on the production of amorphous glasses via the sol–gel method. Changing the mixing period from 30 to 60 min produced amorphous glasses.

3.2. Effect of Heat Treatment Temperature on the Relevant Properties of Bioactive Glass Samples

Heat treating the sol–gel-derived bioactive glasses is important to burn off the organics and release the nitrate ions from the Ca and Mg precursors. Increasing the heat treatment temperature enhances the densification of the material, affecting its overall physical properties.

3.2.1. Crystalline Phase Assemblage

Heat treatment beyond a certain temperature level is likely to promote devitrification. Therefore, the ideal heat treatment temperature for the sintering step can be assessed by XRD. Figure 2 shows that the samples calcined within the temperature range 600–800 °C remain amorphous.

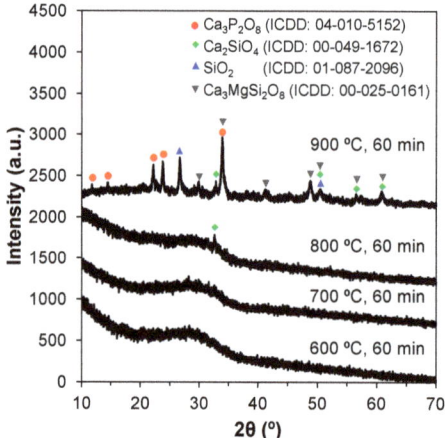

Figure 2. Effect of calcination temperature on glasses produced via the sol–gel method. Crystalline phases appear at 900 °C.

However, relatively well-defined crystalline peaks appear in the XRD pattern of the sample heat-treated at 900 °C. The crystalline phases were identified as silicon oxide (SiO_2), calcium silicate (Ca_2SiO_4), calcium phosphate ($Ca_3(PO_4)_2$), and calcium magnesium nitrate ($Ca_3Mg(SiO_4)_2$). These results suggest that if an amorphous material is envisaged, the calcination temperature should not go much beyond 800 °C.

3.2.2. Specific Surface Area

The impact of calcination temperature on the specific surface area (SSA) of the powders was assessed by resorting to gas adsorption of N_2, using the BET technique. The evolution of SSA as a function of temperature is shown in Figure 3.

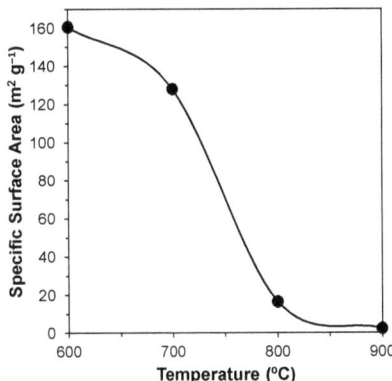

Figure 3. Effect of temperature on the specific surface area of the powders.

It can be seen that the SSA after calcination at 600 °C is still relatively high (~160 m^2 g^{-1}), and gradually decreases (to ~130 m^2 g^{-1}) with temperature increasing to 700 °C. This is followed by a drastic change (to 16 m^2 g^{-1}) with a further increase in the calcination temperature to 800 °C, and then by a more gradual decrease to ~2–3 m^2 g^{-1} upon heat treatment at 900 °C.

3.2.3. Adsorption and Desorption Isotherms

The porous structure profiles of the samples were initially investigated by analysing their respective adsorption and desorption isotherms. These plots are shown in Figure 4. After an initial intersection between adsorption and desorption curves at relatively low pressures, associated with the formation of the N_2 monolayer, a hysteresis loop can be observed due to the condensation of the N_2 at higher pressures within the finer pores, creating multilayers. Such curves are classified as type IV according to IUPAC. At 900 °C, the curves do not intersect, producing an isothermal profile without a classification in IUPAC. It is known that the finer pores are the first to be eliminated due to their high driving force for densification. Accordingly, the average pore size tends to increase with an increase in the heat treatment temperature. On the other hand, some pores might have shrunk into the microporous scale and become less accessible (more impervious) to gas exchanges. This explains why condensation is less evident for the sample calcined at 900 °C, rendering the BET method ineffective at these ranges, and producing an isotherm with an apparently open loop.

Regarding the different hysteresis loops found in these type IV isotherms, at 600 and 700 °C, an H5 loop—characterized by a slight delay in desorption before a descending curve—can be observed, pointing towards a structure where both open and partially blocked mesopores are present. For the powder sample calcined at 800 °C, an H2 (Figure 4c) hysteresis can be observed, indicated by the larger delay before desorption, with a steeper, quasilinear, descending curve. This loop also correlates to pore blocking, but with a greater range of pore neck widths.

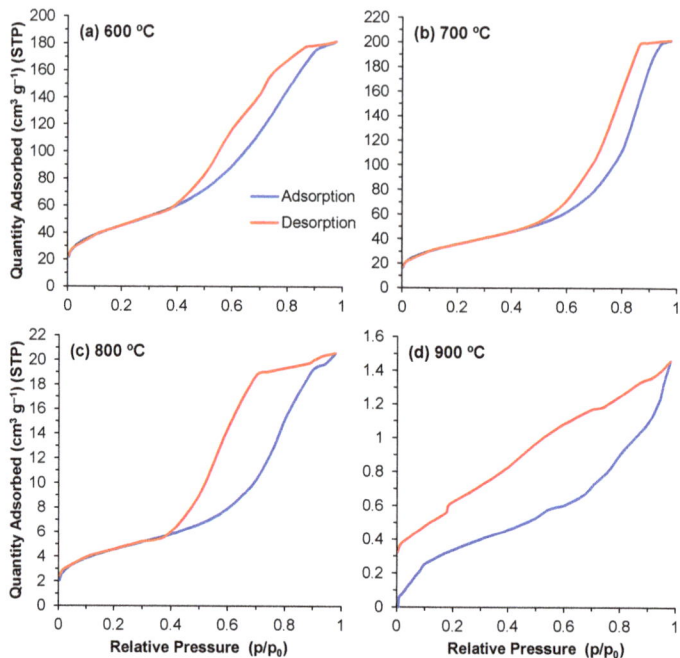

Figure 4. (a–d) Isotherm curves for powders calcined at temperatures of 600–900 °C.

3.2.4. Pore Size Distribution

The pore distribution profiles obtained through the BJH method describe the surface area of these powders in even greater detail. The contributions of the different pore sizes to the overall surface area (dA/dlog(w)) and pore volume (dV/dlog(w)) are displayed in Figures 5 and 6, respectively. For all of the powders, the majority of the contribution to the total area and pore volume came from pores within the 18–200 Å range. The data depict the aforementioned decrease in total surface area and volume; however, the same data also depict an interesting trend regarding the porous evolution of these samples. Comparing the samples calcined at 600 °C with those calcined at 700 °C, the decrease in surface area is paired with a shift of the relative contribution to the total area from the smaller pores to larger ones. From 700 °C to 900 °C, this trend is reversed, and we observe that the major contribution to the total values comes from increasingly smaller pore ranges, highlighting the transition from a mesoporous to a microporous material. This shift is likely derived from the closure of the smaller pores in the 600–700 °C transition, which means that the larger pores, which are still open, are the main responsible factor for the measured surface area. With further increases in temperature, these pores will continue shrinking, resulting in smaller pores in the 800 and 900 °C samples.

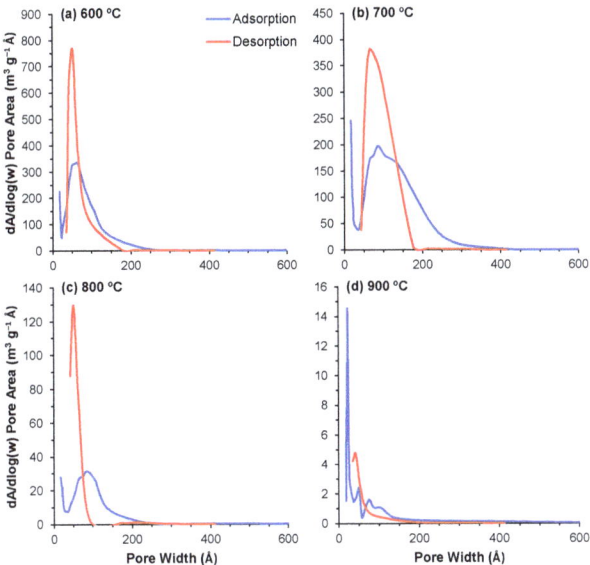

Figure 5. (a–d) Contribution of the different pore sizes to the overall surface area for the powders calcined at temperatures of 600–900 °C.

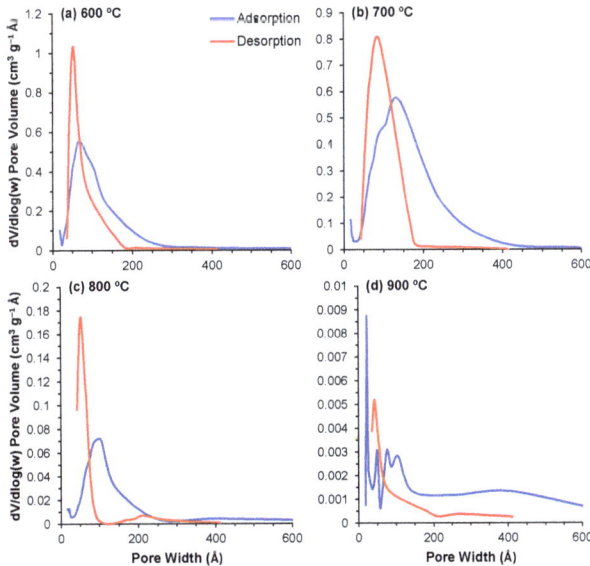

Figure 6. (a–d) Contribution of the different pore sizes to the overall pore volume for the powders calcined at temperatures of 600–900 °C.

3.3. Bioactivity Assessment through SBF Immersion Assays

The bioactivity of the bioactive glass powders was assessed by immersion in simulated body fluid (SBF) over a period of 28 days. Considering the generally high SSA values of the samples, the amount of powder that was added per mL of the SBF solution was double compared to the standard ratio of 0.5 cm² mL⁻¹ proposed by Popa et al. [34] for bulk samples, calculated according to the following equation:

$$SM = \frac{\rho \cdot SA \cdot D}{6} \quad (1)$$

where SM is the sample mass in grams, ρ is the density in grams per cubic centimetre, SA is the sample area in square centimetres exposed to the SBF solution, and D is the average particle diameter in centimetres. The tested powders were assumed to be perfect spheres with a diameter of ~1.25×10^{-2} cm (~125 µm, the average aperture size of the two sieves used, 150 µm and 100 µm). For 20 mL of SBF, 0.06 g of bioglass powder was added. Samples were retrieved every 7 days, and the reaction halted, and were then analysed via XRD and FTIR measurements, as well as through scanning electron microscopy.

3.3.1. XRD Patterns

The XRD patterns for the SBF-treated glass powders can be seen in Figure 7. Calcium phosphate and calcite were the two phases formed on the surface of the particles. Peaks at 24 and 32° were present for all tested timepoints, and can be associated with apatite reflections. Other peaks in the regions around 29, 40, 47, and 50° can be attributed to apatite reflections as well. These crystalline peaks indicate the presence of a hydroxyapatite layer on the powders' surface. Both crystalline phases formed are bioactive and prone to binding between the implant material and the living tissues.

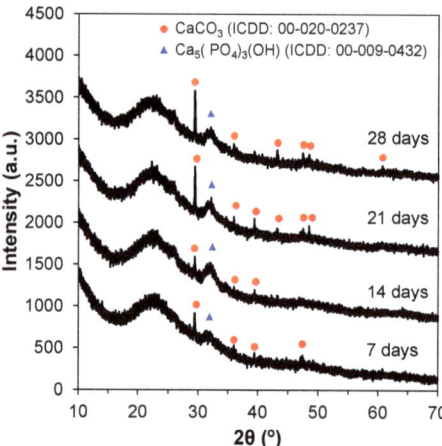

Figure 7. XRD patterns of powders (calcined at 600 °C) immersed in SBF from 7 to 28 days.

3.3.2. FTIR Spectra

The FTIR spectra further point towards the formation of a hydroxyapatite layer, as seen in Figure 8a. The spectra reveal the three main vibrational modes of the Si–O–Si groups—namely, the peaks in the 1000–1100 cm⁻¹ range are associated with the stretching vibration of the Si–O–Si groups, with the bridging oxygens moving opposite of the silicone; at ~780 cm⁻¹, a peak associated with the bending vibration of the Si–O–Si group, characterized by the oxygen atom moving at right angles; and finally, at 500 cm⁻¹, the rocking vibration of the Si–O–Si is observed. Phosphate groups can also be identified by the peak at 600 cm⁻¹ assigned to asymmetric bending. The peak at the ~1500–1550 cm⁻¹ range is associated with a C–O stretch, indicating that carbon from the atmosphere may have reacted with calcium from the powders to form carbonates. Another carbonate stretching vibration can be observed at ~1300 cm⁻¹, related to unhydrolysed residual organics from the sol–gel step. Finally, the band located at ~1600 cm⁻¹ is attributed to the hydrogen bonded to water that was absorbed in the sample [35–37]. To better understand the formation of hydroxyapatite due to SBF, the spectra were subtracted from the base glass, corresponding to 0 days, as seen in Figure 8b. The subtracted spectra reveal peaks at 1384, 1147, 968, 854, 744, 669, and 518 cm^{-1}, which correspond to the following vibrational modes: asymmetric stretching of CO_3^{2-}, asymmetric stretching of PO_4^{3-}, symmetric stretching of PO_4^{3-}, asymmetric bending of CO_3^{2-}, symmetric bending of CO_3^{2-}, stretching of PO_4^{3-}, and bending of PO_4^{3-}, respectively [37]. The spectra show that with the increasing number of days, the amount hydroxyapatite also increases.

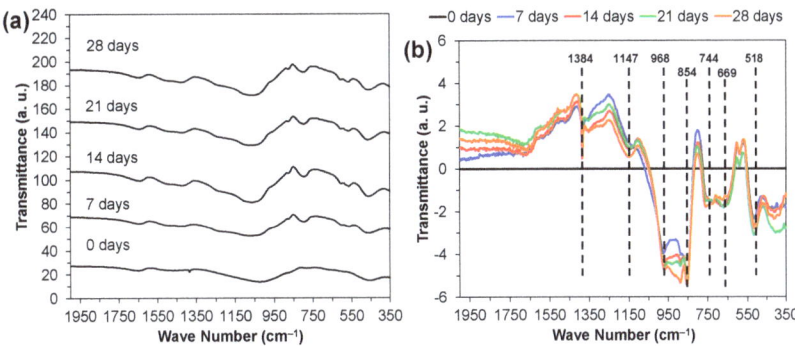

Figure 8. (a) FTIR spectra for powders that were calcined at 600 °C before immersion in SBF for different durations; (b) FTIR spectra with the 0-day sample baseline subtracted.

3.3.3. SEM Images

SEM observations further sustain the previous data by showing a relatively smooth surface for the control powder samples (0 days, calcined at 600 °C), whereas after 28 days, a rugged apatite surface with small circular apatite crystals can be observed (Figure 9).

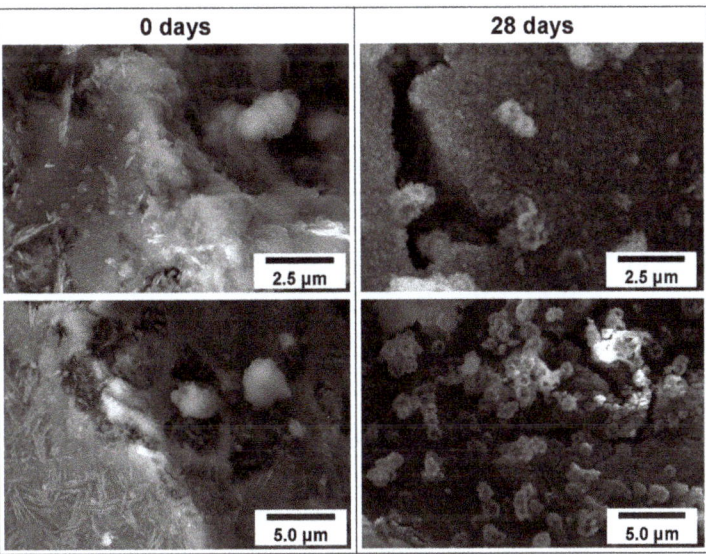

Figure 9. SEM images of powder (calcined at 600 °C) surfaces before (0 days) and after immersion in SBF for 28 days, confirming the formation of a carbonated hydroxyapatite layer.

4. Conclusions

This work reports on the fabrication and processing of a new bioactive glass belonging to the SiO_2–CaO–MgO–P_2O_5 system via the sol–gel method. The effects of calcination temperature on the crystalline phase assemblage and on the specific surface area of these powders was studied. The results show an accentuated decreasing trend in the surface area with increasing temperature. At temperatures >> 800 °C, the samples undergo crystallization. According to BET results, the sample calcined at 600 °C shows the highest surface area, thus being suitable for biological applications, including the storage and release of pharmaceutical drugs. This sample also shows the formation of a hydroxyapatite layer after only 7 days of SBF treatment, and is therefore a promising material for future applications in bone regeneration and tissue engineering.

Author Contributions: Conceptualization, J.M.F.F. and R.B.; methodology, R.B.; software, R.B. and A.G.; validation, J.M.F.F., A.G. and R.B.; formal analysis, R.B. and A.G.; investigation, R.B.; resources, J.M.F.F.; data curation, J.M.F.F. and A.G.; writing—original draft preparation, R.B.; writing—review and editing, J.M.F.F. and A.G.; visualization, A.G.; supervision, J.M.F.F.; project administration, J.M.F.F.; funding acquisition, J.M.F.F. All authors have read and agreed to the published version of the manuscript.

Funding: This research received no external funding.

Institutional Review Board Statement: Not applicable.

Informed Consent Statement: Not applicable.

Data Availability Statement: Not applicable.

Acknowledgments: This work was developed within the scope of the project CICECO-Aveiro Institute of Materials, FCT Ref. UID/CTM/50011/2019, financed by national funds through the Portuguese Foundation for Science and Technology (FCT/MCTES).

Conflicts of Interest: The authors declare no conflict of interest.

References

1. Biggs, B.; King, L.; Basu, S.; Stuckler, D. Is wealthier always healthier? The impact of national income level, inequality, and poverty on public health in Latin America. *Soc. Sci. Med.* **2010**, *71*, 266–273. [CrossRef]
2. Clark, R. World health inequality: Convergence, divergence, and development. *Soc. Sci. Med.* **2011**, *72*, 617–624. [CrossRef]
3. Galasso, V.; Profeta, P. The political economy of social security: A survey. *Eur. J. Polit. Econ.* **2002**, *18*, 1–29. [CrossRef]
4. Orlická, E. Impact of Population Ageing and Elderly Poverty on Macroeconomic Aggregates. *Procedia Econ. Financ.* **2015**, *30*, 598–605. [CrossRef]
5. Wilson, R.T.; Chase, G.A.; Chrischilles, E.A.; Wallace, R.B. Hip Fracture Risk Among Community-Dwelling Elderly People in the United States: A Prospective Study of Physical, Cognitive, and Socioeconomic Indicators. *Am. J. Public Health* **2006**, *96*, 1210–1218. [CrossRef]
6. Ngugyen, T.V.; Eisman, J.A.; Kelly, P.J.; Sambroak, P.N. Risk Factors for Osteoporotic Fractures in Elderly Men. *Am. J. Epidemiol.* **1996**, *144*, 255–263. [CrossRef]
7. Sen, M.K.; Miclau, T. Autologous iliac crest bone graft: Should it still be the gold standard for treating nonunions? *Injury* **2007**, *38*, S75–S80. [CrossRef]
8. Nandi, S.K.; Roy, S.; Mukherjee, P.; Kundu, B.; De, D.K.; Basu, D. Orthopaedic applications of bone graft & graft substitutes: A review. *Indian J. Med. Res.* **2010**, *132*, 15–30. [PubMed]
9. Greenwald, M.A.; Kuehnert, M.J.; Fishman, J.A. Infectious disease transmission during organ and tissue transplantation. *Emerg. Infect. Dis.* **2012**, *18*, e1. [CrossRef] [PubMed]
10. Roseti, L.; Parisi, V.; Petretta, M.; Cavallo, C.; Desando, G.; Bartolotti, I.; Grigolo, B. Scaffolds for Bone Tissue Engineering: State of the art and new perspectives. *Mater. Sci. Eng. C* **2017**, *78*, 1246–1262. [CrossRef]
11. Jones, J.R. Review of bioactive glass: From Hench to hybrids. *Acta Biomater.* **2013**, *9*, 4457–4486. [CrossRef]
12. Mohanty, M. Medical Applications of Alumina Ceramics. *Trans. Indian Ceram. Soc.* **1995**, *54*, 200–204. [CrossRef]
13. Rahmati, M.; Mozafari, M. Biocompatibility of alumina-based biomaterials—A review. *J. Cell. Physiol.* **2019**, *234*, 3321–3335. [CrossRef] [PubMed]
14. Li, K.; Chen, J.; Peng, J.; Koppala, S.; Omran, M.; Chen, G. One-step preparation of CaO-doped partially stabilized zirconia from fused zirconia. *Ceram. Int.* **2020**, *46*, 6484–6490. [CrossRef]
15. Manicone, P.F.; Rossi Iommetti, P.; Raffaelli, L. An overview of zirconia ceramics: Basic properties and clinical applications. *J. Dent.* **2007**, *35*, 819–826. [CrossRef] [PubMed]

16. Chen, Y.-W.; Moussi, J.; Drury, J.L.; Wataha, J.C. Zirconia in biomedical applications. *Expert Rev. Med. Devices* **2016**, *13*, 945–963. [CrossRef]
17. Hench, L.L. Bioceramics: From Concept to Clinic. *J. Am. Ceram. Soc.* **1991**, *74*, 1487–1510. [CrossRef]
18. Montazerian, M.; Dutra Zanotto, E. History and trends of bioactive glass-ceramics. *J. Biomed. Mater. Res. Part A* **2016**, *104*, 1231–1249. [CrossRef]
19. Kaur, G.; Pandey, O.P.; Singh, K.; Homa, D.; Scott, B.; Pickrell, G. A review of bioactive glasses: Their structure, properties, fabrication and apatite formation. *J. Biomed. Mater. Res. Part A* **2014**, *102*, 254–274. [CrossRef] [PubMed]
20. Hum, J.; Boccaccini, A.R. Bioactive glasses as carriers for bioactive molecules and therapeutic drugs: A review. *J. Mater. Sci. Mater. Med.* **2012**, *23*, 2317–2333. [CrossRef] [PubMed]
21. Ciraldo, F.E.; Boccardi, E.; Melli, V.; Westhauser, F.; Boccaccini, A.R. Tackling bioactive glass excessive in vitro bioreactivity: Preconditioning approaches for cell culture tests. *Acta Biomater.* **2018**, *75*, 3–10. [CrossRef]
22. Gubler, M.; Brunner, T.J.; Zehnder, M.; Waltimo, T.; Sener, B.; Stark, W.J. Do bioactive glasses convey a disinfecting mechanism beyond a mere increase in pH? *Int. Endod. J.* **2008**, *41*, 670–678. [CrossRef] [PubMed]
23. Peitl, O.; Dutra Zanotto, E.; Hench, L.L. Highly bioactive P_2O_5–Na_2O–CaO–SiO_2 glass-ceramics. *J. Non. Cryst. Solids* **2001**, *292*, 115–126. [CrossRef]
24. Heimke, G.; Griss, P. Ceramic implant materials. *Med. Biol. Eng. Comput.* **1980**, *18*, 503–510. [CrossRef] [PubMed]
25. Crovace, M.C.; Souza, M.T.; Chinaglia, C.R.; Peitl, O.; Zanotto, E.D. Biosilicate®—A multipurpose, highly bioactive glass-ceramic. In vitro, in vivo and clinical trials. *J. Non. Cryst. Solids* **2016**, *432*, 90–110. [CrossRef]
26. Westhauser, F.; Hohenbild, F.; Arango-Ospina, M.; Schmitz, S.I.; Wilkesmann, S.; Hupa, L.; Moghaddam, A.; Boccaccini, A.R. Bioactive Glass (BG) ICIE16 Shows Promising Osteogenic Properties Compared to Crystallized 45S5-BG. *Int. J. Mol. Sci.* **2020**, *21*, 1639. [CrossRef]
27. Fernandes, H.R.; Gaddam, A.; Rebelo, A.; Brazete, D.; Stan, G.E.; Ferreira, J.M.F. Bioactive Glasses and Glass-Ceramics for Healthcare Applications in Bone Regeneration and Tissue Engineering. *Materials* **2018**, *11*, 2530. [CrossRef]
28. Goel, A.; Kapoor, S.; Rajagopal, R.R.; Pascual, M.J.; Kim, H.-W.; Ferreira, J.M.F. Alkali-free bioactive glasses for bone tissue engineering: A preliminary investigation. *Acta Biomater.* **2012**, *8*, 361–372. [CrossRef]
29. Kapoor, S.; Semitela, Â.; Goel, A.; Xiang, Y.; Du, J.; Lourenço, A.H.; Sousa, D.M.; Granja, P.L.; Ferreira, J.M.F. Understanding the composition-structure-bioactivity relationships in diopside ($CaO·MgO·2SiO_2$)-tricalcium phosphate ($3CaO·P_2O_5$) glass system. *Acta Biomater.* **2015**, *15*, 210–226. [CrossRef]
30. Cortez, P.P.; Brito, A.F.; Kapoor, S.; Correia, A.F.; Atayde, L.M.; Dias-Pereira, P.; Maurício, A.C.; Afonso, A.; Goel, A.; Ferreira, J.M.F. The *in Vivo* Performance of an Alkali-free Bioactive Glass for Bone Grafting, FastOs®BG, Assessed with an Ovine. *J. Biomed. Mater. Res. Part B Appl. Biomater.* **2017**, *105*, 30–38. [CrossRef]
31. Bellucci, D.; Sola, A.; Salvatori, R.; Anesi, A.; Chiarini, L.; Cannillo, V. Sol-gel derived bioactive glasses with low tendency to crystallize: Synthesis, post-sintering bioactivity and possible application for the production of porous scaffolds. *Mater. Sci. Eng. C Mater. Biol. Appl.* **2014**, *43*, 573–586. [CrossRef] [PubMed]
32. Ben-Arfa, B.A.E.; Miranda Salvado, I.M.; Ferreira, J.M.F.; Pullar, R.C. A hundred times faster: Novel, rapid sol-gel synthesis of bio-glass nanopowders (Si-Na-Ca-P system, Ca:P = 1.67) without aging. *Int. J. Appl. Glas. Sci.* **2017**, *8*, 337–343. [CrossRef]
33. Schmidt, H. Chemistry of material preparation by the sol-gel process. *J. Non. Cryst. Solids* **1988**, *100*, 51–64. [CrossRef]
34. Popa, A.C.; Stan, G.E.; Husanu, M.A.; Mercioniu, I.; Santos, L.F.; Fernandes, H.R.; Ferreira, J.M.F. Bioglass implant-coating interactions in synthetic physiological fluids with varying degrees of biomimicry. *Int. J. Nanomed.* **2017**, *12*, 683–707. [CrossRef] [PubMed]
35. Dziadek, M.; Zagrajczuk, B.; Jelen, P.; Olejniczak, Z.; Cholewa-Kowalska, K. Structural variations of bioactive glasses obtained by different synthesis routes. *Ceram. Int.* **2016**, *42*, 14700–14709. [CrossRef]
36. Agathopoulos, S.; Tulyaganov, D.U.; Ventura, J.M.G.; Kannan, S.; Karakassides, M.A.; Ferreira, J.M.F. Formation of hydroxyapatite onto glasses of the CaO-MgO-SiO_2 system with B_2O_3, Na_2O, CaF_2 and P_2O_5 additives. *Biomaterials* **2006**, *27*, 1832–1840. [CrossRef] [PubMed]
37. Aguiar, H.; Serra, J.; González, P.; León, B. Structural study of sol–gel silicate glasses by IR and Raman spectroscopies. *J. Non. Cryst. Solids* **2009**, *355*, 475–480. [CrossRef]

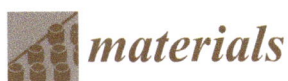

Review

Titanium and Protein Adsorption: An Overview of Mechanisms and Effects of Surface Features

Jacopo Barberi *[ID] and Silvia Spriano [ID]

Department of Applied Science and Technology, Politecnico di Torino, 10129 Turin, Italy; silvia.spriano@polito.it
* Correspondence: jacopo.barberi@polito.it; Tel.: +39-011-0904567

Abstract: Titanium and its alloys, specially Ti6Al4V, are among the most employed materials in orthopedic and dental implants. Cells response and osseointegration of implant devices are strongly dependent on the body–biomaterial interface zone. This interface is mainly defined by proteins: They adsorb immediately after implantation from blood and biological fluids, forming a layer on implant surfaces. Therefore, it is of utmost importance to understand which features of biomaterials surfaces influence formation of the protein layer and how to guide it. In this paper, relevant literature of the last 15 years about protein adsorption on titanium-based materials is reviewed. How the surface characteristics affect protein adsorption is investigated, aiming to provide an as comprehensive a picture as possible of adsorption mechanisms and type of chemical bonding with the surface, as well as of the characterization techniques effectively applied to model and real implant surfaces. Surface free energy, charge, microroughness, and hydroxylation degree have been found to be the main surface parameters to affect the amount of adsorbed proteins. On the other hand, the conformation of adsorbed proteins is mainly dictated by the protein structure, surface topography at the nano-scale, and exposed functional groups. Protein adsorption on titanium surfaces still needs further clarification, in particular concerning adsorption from complex protein solutions. In addition, characterization techniques to investigate and compare the different aspects of protein adsorption on different surfaces (in terms of roughness and chemistry) shall be developed.

Keywords: titanium; protein adsorption; biomaterials; surface modifications; cell interactions

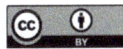

1. Introduction

Almost 1000 tons of titanium-based biomaterials are worldwide used every year as orthopedic and dental implants [1] mainly as commercially pure titanium (cp-Ti) and αβ-alloy Ti6Al4V (Ti64), eventually as extra low interstitial (ELI) [2]. Despite titanium's exceptional biocompatibility implant failure is a current issue. Dental and orthopedic implants have a failure rate ranging from 5 to 10% after up to 15 years [3]. Implant osseointegration is mediated by a complex series of events included in the immune response that are triggered as soon as the tissue are damaged during the surgery. The implant surface is immediately covered by a layer of water molecules and on top of them, a layer of protein is adsorbed within the first few minutes. That, along with cytokines released from the damaged cells and protein-promoted blood coagulation, triggers the foreign body reaction (FBR) of a host body to an implant [4,5]. In order to achieve osseointegration of Ti implants, an equilibrium within the events that occurs during FBR need to be found, in order to avoid chronic inflammation and fibrotic encapsulation. Concerning the inflammatory response, neutrophils and monocytes are recruited at the implant site. Then (after about 48 h) monocytes differentiate into macrophages with a phagocytic function for controlling the immune response. In order to remove larger debris, monocytes and macrophages can fuse together forming foreign body giant cells (FBGCs). Concerning osseointegration, it takes place when mesenchymal stem cells (MSC) differentiate into osteoblasts and osteocytes, leading to new bone formation and it is triggered by an early pro-inflammatory response. When this does not happen, the worst scenario is proliferation of fibroblasts and the formation of a fibrous capsule that engulfs the implant, preventing a correct contact with the bone tissue [4,5]. Formation of the blood clot on the implant surface is of great importance to get the mechanical and biochemical environment for osseointegration. Activation of platelets within the blood clot on the implant surface provides a natural gradient of signal molecules with a high concentration on the surface of the implant and consequent attraction of monocytes, neutrophilis, and mesenchymal cells. This allows the "contact osteogenesis" mechanism with formation of immature bone characterized by irregularly arranged, interwoven collagenous fibers, and, as last, of mature lamellar bone through bone remodeling. Due to this cascade of events, cells do not interact directly with the implant surface, but the interface is strongly mediated and controlled by the adsorbed proteins. Cells exhibit specific binding sites for certain proteins and their activity can be enhanced by those adsorbed onto the material surface. For example, protein such as fibronectin (FN) and vitronectin (VN) are considered adhesive proteins. FN can activate cell $\alpha_5\beta_1$ integrins through the binding domain arginine-glycine-aspartic acid (RGD), which is present in VN as well [6]. Bone morphogenetic (BMP) proteins can promote osseointegration [7] but contemporary increase the inflammatory response to biomaterials [8]. As a consequence, the ability to control the formation of the protein layer, by promoting selective adsorption, is of great interest in the design of novel and more functional biomaterials. Since the '70s of the past century, a great amount of efforts have been put in studying protein adsorption [9]. What happens when a surface gets in contact with a protein containing solution is dictated by a multitude of different factors. According to surface characteristics (roughness, wettability, charge), protein properties (surface charge, hydrophilicity, structure) [9], and even solution parameters (composition, pH, temperature) [10], adsorption of proteins may be driven by hydrophobic interactions, electrostatic attraction, or weak forces, such as Van deer Waals' [11]. Furthermore, the protein layer is a dynamic entity, where adsorbed proteins can be displaced and replaced by the ones still in solution, and according to the so-called Vroman effect, they can change their conformation on the surface, spreading and reorienting themselves, and multilayers of loosely bound proteins can form thanks to protein–protein interactions [12]. Many authors have gathered and reviewed knowledge about driving forces of protein adsorption and their behavior on the surface [12–14]. Nevertheless, despite all these efforts, a fully and comprehensive understanding of adsorption processes and mechanisms is still missing. Even though we found that the protein adsorption on certain biomaterials was reviewed, such as bioactive glasses [15], bioceramics [16], metals of medical interest, steel [17], and magnesium [18], or even nanomaterials for biosensors [19], to our best knowledge, no work of this kind was made for protein adsorption on titanium. This review aims to put together the literature about adsorption of protein on titanium-based materials for osseointegration, trying to depict a comprehensive picture of how surface characteristics affect the way proteins bond to Ti surfaces. After a brief introduction on the main driving forces of protein adsorption, we focused on the principal characteristics of titanium surfaces. The literature was sorted accordingly to how titanium surfaces were treated or modified (kind of surface modification or activation, surface chemical composition, and crystalline structure) in order to explore the specific effect of the different surface features (wettability, roughness, hydroxylation, or charge) on protein adsorption. The same rational was applied to investigate how external parameters can affect the protein–titanium interaction and the correlations among surface features and the competitive adsorption of proteins. This knowledge can lead to an improved design of novel and more effective biomaterials. At last, the characterization techniques applied for studying protein adsorption on titanium-based biomaterials are collected. Due to the great amount of work published on these materials, only adsorption on bulk materials, these being pure Ti, Ti alloys, or titanium oxides (native or modified), is discussed. Adsorption on titania nanoparticles, as well as interaction of proteins with coated or functionalized surfaces were not included unless of interest for the selected topic. Relevant literature of the past 15 years was researched and selected.

2. Driving Forces and Factors Affecting Protein Adsorption

2.1. Driving Forces of Protein Adsorption

Protein adsorption is a complex phenomenon that involves different kinds of protein-substrate interactions and it is influenced by numerous different factors depending on the surfaces features and chemical or biological environment.

It is well acknowledged that protein adsorption can be promoted by several kind of driving forces, these being hydrophobic or electrostatic interactions and van der Waals forces [12,20].

Hydrophobic interactions are fundamental in order to maintain the protein tertiary structure: When a protein is dissolved into a polar solvent, non-polar amino acid residues have the tendency of interact between each other, in the inside of the protein, to limit interaction with solvent. On the reverse, hydrophilic residues are exposed on the protein surface [21]. If a protein approaches a hydrophobic surface, the balance of protein–solvent and intra-protein interactions is disrupted, and hydrophobic residues can interact with the hydrophobic surface. Changes in protein structure lead to entropy gain, with this being a strong driving force for protein adsorption [22]. As a general rule of thumb, proteins adsorbed onto the hydrophobic surfaces undergo greater denaturation than on the hydrophilic ones [10]. Furthermore, dehydration of a surface has to happen for proteins to adsorb. On hydrophobic substrates, this results in reduction of Gibb's free energy and increases protein adsorption [13].

Hydrophobic interactions are the main driving forces of protein adsorption on hydrophobic surface. On the other hand, in case of adsorption on hydrophilic and charged materials, electrostatic and van der Waals interactions take over as primary cause of protein binding to surfaces [20]. When a charged object is immersed into a solution, ions of opposite charges are attracted towards it, forming the so called double layer: the Stern layer, which is composed by ions very close to the surface, and the Gouy-Chapman diffuse layer, which extends towards the solution and exhibits an abundance of ions compensating the surface charge [23]. When proteins approach a surface, the protein diffuse layer overlaps with the one of the substrate and attractive or repulsive forces may arise depending on the zeta potential (ζ). The zeta potential is defined as the electrical potential at the interface dividing the Stern and the Gouy-Chapman layers. Proteins are also sensitive to dipole–dipole interactions, induced or not, commonly referred as van der Waals forces. Usually, van der Waals interactions are attractive at short distances [24]. The contribution of electrostatic interactions and van der Waals forces can be predicted by the DLVO (Derjaguin, Landau, Verwey Overbeek) theory. This theory allows to calculate the total interaction energy between two surfaces, determining if the resulting force is attractive or repulsive in the range of few tens of nanometers [24].

2.2. Surface Effect on Protein Adsorption

As discussed in the previous section, it is clear that the surface properties influence on protein adsorption mechanisms is of great importance. Surface wettability, topography, charge, and chemistry are able to deeply modify surface–protein interactions, as schematized in Figure 1 [12,25].

Wettability of substrates determines the major driving forces for adsorption, and the final result of the whole process may change heavily. It is well accepted that hydrophobic surfaces can adsorb more protein with respect to hydrophilic one [26]. Hydrophobic surfaces can better interact with hydrophobic residues of proteins and water displacement from the surface is more favorable than on hydrophilic surfaces [14]. The pivotal water contact angle (WCA)(θ) dividing hydrophobic from hydrophilic surfaces regarding protein adsorption was set at values near $\theta = 65°$ by different researchers [27,28].

Wettability does not only influence the total amount of proteins, which can be adsorbed onto surfaces, but also their spatial conformation. Different studies investigated the effect of surface wettability on protein conformation upon adsorption, such as FN and bovine serum albumin (BSA), highlighting the fact that proteins adsorbed on more hydrophobic materials present the higher degree of denaturation [29,30].

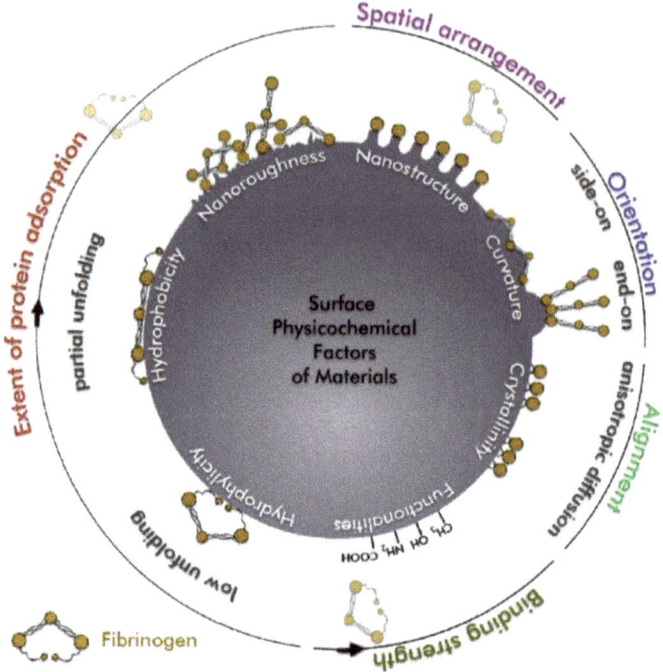

Figure 1. Effects of the physiochemical properties of material surfaces on various aspects of protein adsorption (amount, binding strength, orientation, conformation). Reprinted with permission from ref. [25]. Copyright 2017 WILEY-VCH Verlag GmbH & Co.

Strictly related to surface hydrophilicity/hydrophobicity behavior, there are surface charges. Usually, hydrophobic materials are non-polar, while hydrophilic substrates present a distribution of charges onto their surfaces. Surface charge of solids and particles immersed in solution may vary with the pH of the liquid, and they can be both positive and negative. Thus, according to protein type and substrate, attractive or repulsive interactions may happen [20]. Negatively charged surfaces, such as bioactive glasses in physiological conditions, may hinder adsorption of negative charged proteins [15], and vice versa for positive surfaces [31]. Still, proteins bearing an overall negative charge may adsorb on negatively charged surfaces thanks to the interactions of positive residues that remains on their surfaces, such in the case of BSA [32]. The same can happen with positive charges onto materials, as in the case of block co-polymers [33].

Cells are able to sense micro- and nano- roughness and it affects their adhesion, proliferation, and growth [8]. Similarly, morphological features of surfaces can influence protein adsorption [34]. Increase in surface roughness leads to larger surface area, thus higher protein adsorption. Still, it has been found that in some cases, proteins adsorb on appreciably larger amounts than what might be expected accounting only area increase [35]. Grain size and crystallinity of materials have also been reported to influence the adsorption process on biomaterials [36]

Protein adsorption can be controlled also by changing the chemistry of the surface, for example by functionalization with polymers or polyelectrolyte brush [12,36].

2.3. Protein Characteristics Affecting Adsorption

As well as surface characteristics, protein features like structural stability, charge, and dimension, are of greatly affect the adsorption mechanisms and outcomes.

Structural stability of proteins is related to the easiness to undergo conformational modification. In the late 1990s, Norde introduced the concept of *soft* and *hard* proteins [9] to highlight the different structural behavior of proteins: Soft proteins are less stable and they are more prone to change their conformation after adsorption; on the other hand, hard proteins are more stable and they less prone to be denaturated. Changes in 3D conformation allows optimization of electrostatic interactions on hydrophilic/charged surface, since polar amino acid residues can be close to oppositely charged surfaces. Thus, in general, the soft proteins adsorb in a larger amount than the hard ones [37]. Changes in tertiary and secondary structure of proteins can affect their biological activity. In some cases, denaturation produces a loss of protein activity, as in the case of platelets activation by fibrinogen (FIB) [38]. In another case, denaturation can increase the effect of certain proteins. Denatured FN may expose more integrin-binding sites RGD, increasing cells adhesion [39].

Electrostatic interactions are capable to drive adsorption of proteins on charged surfaces of biomaterials, in a different way according to the overall net charge of proteins and distribution of the electrostatically charged residues within the protein's structure. Proteins' overall net charge is influenced by the presence of polar amino acids in the primary protein structure and by the pH of the solution, depending on the acid/basic behavior of the specific amino acids [40]. The overall net charge of a proteins is positive at pH values below the isoelectric point (IEP), zero at the IEP, and negative above it: It must be remembered that in any case the IEP is due to a balance between the number of positively and negatively charged functional groups which are present at any pH. IEPs of different proteins can vary in a wide range of values, from 4.7 of BSA to about 11 for Lys [41,42]. Still, proteins can adsorb to likely charged surfaces thanks to a non-homogeneous charge distribution within the protein's structure: Positive residues can be selectively exposed on the outside of BSA even at pH 7, allowing its adsorption on a negative surface like titanium [32]. Furthermore, the proteins charges also determine the nature of protein–protein interactions. It is accepted that a higher amount of a protein is adsorbed at the IEP, when electrostatic repulsion between proteins is minimized [12]. Dimension and molecular weight of proteins play an important role too. The smallest proteins can reach the surface before the largest thanks to a higher diffusion coefficient, thus adsorbing in a larger amount at first. In addition, the largest proteins need to displace more water molecules, on hydrophilic surfaces, and higher energy is needed to enter the interface region [43]. On the other side, the largest proteins usually can interact in a stronger manner with the surface, therefore they can displace and substitute the smallest proteins with times. This dynamic behavior of the adsorbed protein layer is known as "the Vroman effect" [12].

2.4. External Parameters Affecting Protein Adsorption

Investigating protein adsorption, it is also fundamental to consider the environment where the process is carried on and the effects of some external parameters. Temperature influences several aspects of the adsorption mechanisms. Increasing temperature allows for higher mobility of proteins in solution, faster adsorption kinetics [44], equilibrium surface concentration [45], and also protein desorption from the surface is easier [29].

A fundamental and determining role is played by the solution where proteins are dissolved. As already mentioned, the pH determines both the charge of protein and surface. Thus, according to its value, the same protein–surface combination may repel or attract one another [46]. Beside pH, other solution parameters have great influence on the adsorption. Presence of ions in the solution has a double effect. The first one regards the ionic strength of the solution, which influences the thickness of the Gouy-Chapman layer and consequently the distance at which the electrostatic interactions take place. Higher ionic concentration and strength result in a thinner diffuse layer both on proteins and surfaces. Thus, an eventual electrostatic repulsion is less relevant on adsorption [47]. As a second effect, ions can also compete with proteins in the adsorption on surfaces. For example, negative phosphate ions in phosphate buffered saline (PBS) solution have been found to depress protein adsorption [48].

Protein concentration in solution is another parameter that can largely impact on adsorption. Several studies describe how an increase of the initial protein concentration results in a higher amount of protein adsorbed onto the surface at the equilibrium [49,50].

The main parameters that affect protein adsorption and the general rules of thumb on the process are collected in Table 1.

Table 1. Main parameters affecting protein adsorption on surfaces.

	Parameters	General Rules of Thumb
Surface	Topography/roughness	Higher surface roughness ≥ higher amount of adsorbed proteins
	Hydrophobicity (non-polar surfaces) Hydrophilicity (polar surfaces, with a net surface charge)-	Higher hydrophobicity ≥ higher amount of adsorbed proteins and denaturation degree; hydrophobic interaction as adsorption mechanism Different mechanisms of adsorption on hydrophilic surfaces: electrostatic, van der Waals, dipole-dipole; adsorbed water must be removed for adsorption
	Chemistry (functional groups, metal ions)	Influence on the surface charge
Protein	Amino acid chain	Affects structural stability
	Hydrophilicity/hydrophobicity	Surface charges and non-polar residues are always present; they can be differently arranged according to the environment; hydrophobic residues interact with hydrophobic surfaces
	Charge	Higher amount of adsorbed proteins at IEP
	Molecular weight	Small proteins adsorb quicker Large proteins replace the smaller ones and make stronger bonds with the hydrophobic surfaces
	Structural stability	Soft proteins change easier configuration and adsorb larger on hydrophilic surfaces; denaturation can enhance or reduce biological activity
Solution	pH	Affects surface charge of both proteins and surfaces
	Ionic strength	Adsorbed ions reduce repulsive effects among proteins; some ions compete with proteins for adsorption
	Protein concentration	Higher protein concentration higher amount of adsorption
	Protein mixture(single, binary or more complex)	Vroman effect
	Temperature	Higher temperature ≥ faster kinetics of adsorption

3. How the Characteristics of Titanium Based Biomaterials Influence Protein Adsorption

3.1. General Consideration on Protein Adsorption on Titanium Based Materials

Titanium peculiar properties have made it one of the most world widespread biomaterials [1]. With respect to other metals, titanium and its alloys possess excellent osseointegration capability, proper mechanical properties, and soft tissue compatibility. They have been extensively described elsewhere, therefore here only the ones of interest for discussing protein adsorption will be briefly reported [8,51,52]. Being a very reactive element, titanium does not exist in its metal form onto its surface, but it is immediately passivated by oxygen and its surface is covered by a thin native oxide layer, which is mainly amorphous TiO_2 about 3–7 nm thick [53]. This layer confers chemical stability, biological inertness and corrosion resistance to the surface. To understand how this biomaterial interacts with the biological environments, it is mandatory to notice that titanium surfaces are highly hydroxylated. OH groups can form by dissociation of water molecules at the five-coordinated Ti sites. Several kinds of hydroxyls can thus form on the surface, differing in their position (terminal or bridging) and in their chemical behavior (acidic or basic). As a consequence, when the surface gets in contact with water, acidic OH groups deprotonate, while basic OH groups protonate themselves, forming both positive and negative charges (Figure 2).

Acidic OH deprotonation: $Ti\text{-}OH + H_2O \leftrightarrow [Ti\text{-}O]^- + H_3O^+$

Basic OH protonation: $Ti\text{-}OH + H_2O \leftrightarrow [Ti\text{-}OH]^+ + OH^-$

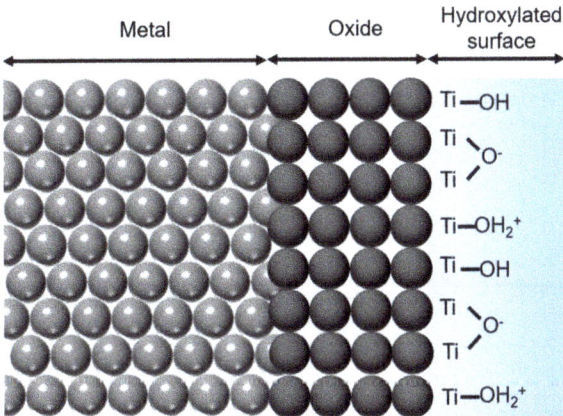

Figure 2. Scheme of hydroxylation of Ti surface and surface charge generation during contact with aqueous solutions.

As consequence of the dissociation constants of both the OH groups, IEP of titanium lies around 5 [54].

Titanium affinity for proteins is well acknowledged. A stable protein layer was found to form in vivo after just three hours [55]. This was observed to prevent precipitation of compound like HA after a week. Ti-based materials can interact with many different proteins, such as serum albumin [56,57], FIB [58], or FN [59]. Many researchers have tried to unveil the mechanisms of interaction between proteins and titanium substrates. By studying the adsorption isotherms of several different proteins (such as human serum albumin (HSA), BSA, lysozyme (LYS), pepsin, myoglobin, and others) at different pH values, Imamura et al. [60] ascribed pseudo-irreversible adsorption of protein to electrostatic interactions between the OH_2^+ groups on the titanium surface and COO^- groups of proteins. Furthermore, negatively charged carboxyl groups can also induce protonation of the OH groups of the surface around the IEP of titanium. Another research group proposed a slightly different interaction mechanism between HSA and titanium [57,61]. They proposed that HSA has a similar effect to a local change of the pH, acting like a reduction of $[H^+]$ and affecting the thickness of the H^+ diffusion layer on the Ti surface. Interactions between albumin and a titanium surface followed the proposed two steps mechanism, which involves a first hydrogen bonding and a subsequent proton transfer.

Hydrogen bonding:

$$\text{Ti}-\text{OH} + {}^-\text{OOC}-\text{R} \rightarrow \text{Ti}-\text{OH}\cdots\text{OOC}-\text{R}$$

Proton transfer:

$$\text{Ti}-\text{OH}\cdots\text{OOC}-\text{R} \rightarrow \text{Ti}=\text{O}^-\cdots\text{HOOC}-\text{R}$$

Even though the interaction mechanisms proposed by Imamura [60] and Camàra [57] are different, they underline the importance of the OH groups on driving protein adsorption. Molecular dynamic simulations observed that an increased density of the OH groups on rutile (1 1 0) means higher affinity for the subdomain IIIb of HSA [62]. Electrostatic interactions with the COO^- and NH_3^+ groups of proteins were greatly enhanced. A key role of the local electrostatic interactions between opposite charges respectively on TiO_2 and organic molecules was also observed for peptides [63]. The charge effect of hydroxyls on the strength of protein adsorption was investigated in another interesting computational studies by Sun et al. [64]. They tuned the hydrophobicity/hydrophilicity of rutile surface by scaling the OH charges of different factors. Lower surface charge, related to higher hydrophobicity, turned out to adsorb lactoferrin and bone morphogenetic protein-2 (BMP-2) in a stronger manner than a hydrophilic surface. Being a soft protein, BMP-2 is also more denaturated. At the same time, protein–surface interactions on hydrophilic TiO_2 surfaces are hindered due to water-surface interactions [65]. Thus, spreading and denaturation of certain adsorbed proteins are limited. OH groups generated onto TiO_2 by vacuum annealing can prevent FIB denaturation by avoiding electron transfer, from the protein to the surface. In this case, hydrophilic TiO_2 surface denatures less proteins than the hydrophobic ones [38]. Less FIB denaturation is related to lower platelet activity and better blood compatibility of biomaterials.

In order to predict the biological behavior of biomaterials, alongside the amount and type of protein adsorbed, it is necessary to be aware of their spatial configuration and orientation with respect to the surface. Proteins can adsorb in a "side-on" or "end-on" orientation, according to the positioning of their main axis [12].

Furthermore, denaturation can occur to different extents with different proteins. As already mentioned, adsorption on titanium substrates lead to denaturation of FIB. Several authors found that FIB can interact with titanium surfaces through αC domains. Since they are positively charged at pH = 7.4, electrostatic attraction between the surface and the protein can occur [58,66]. The strong protein–surface interactions lead to denaturation of FIB [66]. This was confirmed by Zhao et al. [67]. Furthermore, even though binding via αC domains shall result in side-on orientation of the proteins on the surface, FIB was found with preferred end-on orientation [67]. Bimodal adsorption isotherms of immunoglobulin (IgG) suggest that adsorbed proteins may undergo structural rearrangements and orientation modification according to saturation level of the surface [68]. While in some cases no denaturation of BSA was observed upon adsorption on titanium oxide [69], others had observed conformational changes of albumin [56]. Hydrophobicity of titanium may lead to spreading of adsorbed HSA onto its surface [70]. Conformation and adsorption mechanisms are strictly dependent on both surface features and protein composition. Different structures were found for proteins that shall be analogous, such as chicken and human albumin [71]. Adsorption mechanism was also profoundly different: HSA adsorbs as a continuous thin film, while chicken albumin forms adherent flakes on the titanium surface. In addition, relevant peptide sequences, such as RGD domains of FN, may change their spatial configuration after adsorption on rutile or anatase [72]

Surface roughness is a parameter that very often is addressed as pivotal in determining the outcome of protein adsorption, and more in general, cell behavior [73]. It does not only change the effective surface area available for interaction with proteins, but it can also affect the wettability of the materials. It has been acknowledged that roughness in the micro-range enhanced protein adsorption due to increase of specific surface area [74]. Several authors have tried to understand the extent of roughness, in particular in the nano-range, influence on the protein adsorption on titanium-based surfaces. Roughness variations from few to some tens of nm were found not to have a unique effect on all proteins and some results in literature may disagree. BSA adsorption is slightly influenced by roughness between R_a values of 1.57 and 16.44, while in the same range FIB adsorption is increased to a slightly larger extend [75]. Controversially, in a more recent study, Rockwell et al. [76] observed that the increment in the surface area ratio (SAR) due to increased roughness, in the same range as previously reported [75], along sample profile, was not sufficient for explain the increased of normalized adsorption of both FIB and BSA (Figure 3a). Increments on proteins and SAR were up to 50% and 15%, respectively. Instead, the increment in curvature of surface features accounted better for the increment in adsorption (Figure 3b): Higher curvature, meaning smaller features radii, favors end-on FIB adsorption and stabilizes protein secondary structures. Besides, increased roughness, from less than 1 nanometer to about 11, resulted in increased surface free energy (SFE) that promoted better adsorption of FN and VN from fetal bovine serum (FBS) [77]. These results were confirmed also on TiO_2 when other proteins, such as BSA [78] or casein [79], were adsorbed.

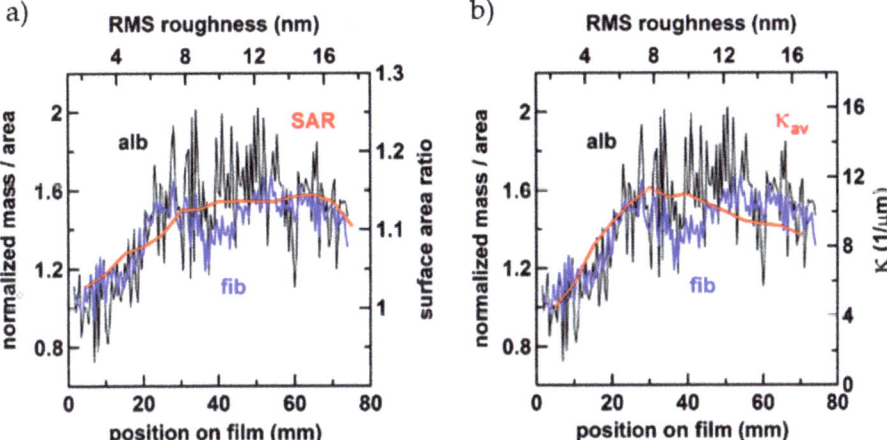

Figure 3. Normalized adsorption profile of bovine serum albumin (BSA) (black) and fibrinogen (FIB) (blue) on Ti with roughness gradient (left y-axes). The overlaid red lines are the SAR profile (**a**) and the curvature profile (**b**) (right y-axes). Adapted with permission from ref. [76]. Copyright 2011 Elsevier B.V.

Roughness of titanium substrates is also capable of influencing the mechanisms of adsorption. While adsorption of BSA, FIB, and streptavidin on flatter substrates occurs mainly as protein monolayers, roughness values about R_{ms} = 29.5 nm can increase protein–protein interactions, resulting in a multilayer type adsorption [80]. Surface features such as protuberances and peaks are not the only topographical characteristics that have influence on proteins adsorption. Surface pores in the meso- and nano-range need to be accounted when the effect of surface roughness on this matter is discussed. Proteins are not able to enter pores smaller than their hydrodynamic radius. In the case of BSA, of which hydrodynamic diameter is about 7.2 nm, mesopores need to be at least about 9 nm for albumin to enter them [81]. Larger mesopores can accommodate more than one BSA molecule, with very little conformational changes, and protein-surface adhesion forces were stronger with respect to smaller pores [82]. Singh et al. [83], due to protein tendency to aggregate into nanopores, concluded that nanometer scale morphology is the main reason for increased protein adsorption, more than the modest increase in wettability of surface with different roughness.

Titanium and its oxide exhibit different adsorption properties with respect to other materials, such as other metals or metal oxides clinically used polymers or dental enamel. In comparison with other metal surfaces such as Au, Pt, and Ir, titanium adsorbs the largest amount of plasma proteins. This is because Ti presents the highest SFE and roughness, as a result of the deposition process of metal thin films [84]. At the opposite, when TiO_2 is compared with other oxides such as ZrO_x, TaO_x, and NbO_x, it showed the least adsorption capability [85] and it is also the flattest and the least energetic surface. ZrO_x interacts the most with albumin being a hydrophobic surface, while the amount of adsorbed BSA correlates well with roughness and polar component of the SFE on the hydrophilic oxides. Similar evidence of different mechanisms of adsorption on hydrophobic or hydrophilic surfaces was found with FIB, investigating fibrinogen adsorption on the same set of oxides [86]. Titanium shows also different retention capability of the adsorbed proteins with respect to the other oxides. Its negative charge makes HSA displacement from its surface faster than on positive charged alumina, at pH 7 [87]. Al_2O_3 adsorbs more BSA than TiO_2 also because of its higher number of OH groups that can form H-bonds with proteins [88]. Adsorption of positively charged proteins such as lactoferrin was enhanced on titanium with respect to stainless steel, ZrO_2, and polymethylmethacrylate (PMMA) thanks to the higher negative surface charge [89]. Still, stronger interactions were found on hydrophobic substrates. In order to better understand why different materials have different behavior during their life as implants, titanium was widely compared to other surfaces of interest in the dental field. Titanium's poor adhesion to gingival tissue may be explained by the fact that, with respect to dentin, it adsorbs less key basal lamina proteins, such as laminin (LAM) α, a protein with a key role in tooth-epithelium adhesion, and nidogen-1 [90]. It was also observed that hydrophobic polymeric materials used in dental field, such as polytetrafluoroethylene (PTFE), polyethylene (PE), and PMMA, adsorb more salivary proteins than Ti, for instance salivary mucins and proline-rich proteins [91,92]. This also reflects in higher adhesion forces between albumin and polymers as PMMA and PTFE with respect to titanium [93]. Interestingly, the interaction force between BSA and Ti is about twofold more than on enamel.

3.2. Effect of Surface Modifications on Titanium: How Topography, Roughness and Surface Chemistry Change Protein Adsorption

3.2.1. Surface Modification by Sand Blasting and Acid Etching (SLA)

Surface roughness and wettability are the main parameters influenced by SLA treatments, thus changes in protein adsorption are mainly ascribed to these materials features. According to our findings in literature, the studies on this kind of surfaces are not in complete agreement. Some of them observed that SLA treatments increases the total amount of adsorbed proteins [94,95], while, in different conditions of adsorption, others observed a neglectable difference [96]. In a remarkable work of Kohavi et al. [94], the authors studied the influence of SLA and acid treatments on Ti64. Proteins adsorption was carried out in vivo during dental implantation surgery. A titanium rod was implanted into the osteotomy and removed after 10 min. Albumin, fibronectin, fibrinogen, and immunoglobulin were quantified by enzyme-linked immunosorbent assay (ELISA). The SLA surfaces adsorbed more than fourfold more of each protein with respect to an untreated surface. Acid etched (AE) titanium surfaces adsorbed only twice more. SLA surfaces were rougher than both AE and flat surfaces (R_a equal to 287.5, 214.5 and 26.8 nm, respectively). Roughness was addressed as the main factor influencing in vivo protein uptake. Prewetting of surfaces also increases protein adsorption. Similar findings on the same surfaces were obtained in vitro [95]. FN resulted the major protein found on a surface in case of adsorption both from a single protein solution and whole plasma. The effect of roughness and increased surface area on protein adsorption was also highlighted by SLA treatment followed by secondary etching [97]. Protein adsorption is only increased to a certain time of etching, since after about 30 min decreasing in specific surface area is experienced. MC3T3 pre-osteoblastic cells viability also correlate well with this observation. Kopf and co-workers [74] put effort in isolate the effect of wettability and roughness. Hydrophilic and hydrophobic SLA surfaces were obtained through proper storage in air or NaCl solutions. On some samples, the storage in NaCl resulted in further nanostructuration of the surface. WCA of hydrophilic and hydrophobic SLA surfaces ranged between less than 10° to 120°, respectively. Simply, SLA-treated surfaces showed no influence of the WCA on adsorption of both FIB and FN. On the contrary, the hydrophilic nanostructured (NS)-SLA samples adsorbed much more than the hydrophobic ones. In both cases, they adsorbed more than the SLA specimens. Thus, it seems that protein adsorption is mainly driven by roughness at the microscale and by a synergistic effect of hydrophilicity and roughness when it comes to nanostrcutures. As an interesting fact, in the same study, it is observed that blood clotting is more improved by hydrophilicity than surface topography. H_2O_2 hydrothermal treatments on SLA-treated dentals screws can promote bioactivity through surface nanostructuration and formation of many OH groups [98]. Better protein adsorption, in particular increased selectivity towards FN, resulted from increased wettability of the implants. Hydroxylation of the surface does not only account for improved wettability and enhanced protein adsorption. SLA-induced OH groups are also responsible for denaturation of proteins, such as statherin [99]. Hydroxyls can bond with proteins through hydrogen bonds, disrupting the equilibrium of forces that maintains the native conformation of proteins. Statherin adsorbed onto polished titanium showed less denaturation.

Some studies focused on how SFE influences the adsorption of proteins. Simple sandblasting of cp-Ti resulted in very different values of surface energy, according to dimension of the blasting particles and even to their composition [100]. On rough surfaces, the authors found a linear correlation between surface energy and amount of adsorbed FN (Figure 4b). Interestingly, the samples treated with SiC particles showed higher SFE, in particular the dispersive component, than the ones processed with alumina particles. As a consequence, FN adsorbed preterably on SiC-blasted samples, regardless of roughness (Figure 4a). The importance of SFE on SLA treatments was also observed very recently by Mussano et al. [101]. Adsorption of different proteins, namely collagen (COL) I, FN, and BSA, was depressed by blasting with alumina if compared with machined surface. SLA treatment restored titanium adsorptive properties, though without enhancement with respect to untreated surface. Blasted surfaces showed lower SFE, while machined and SLA specimens had similar values. This correlates well with the results obtained for alumina blasting particles in ref. [100].

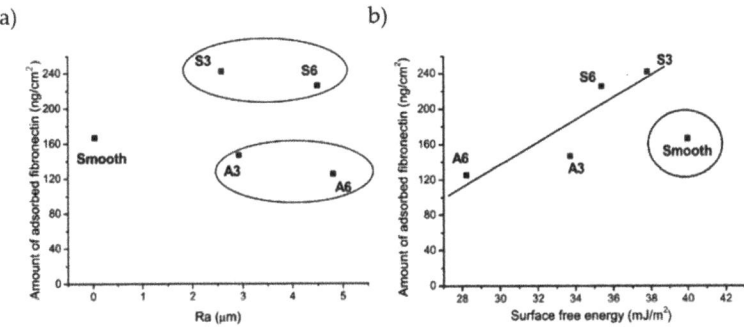

Figure 4. Correlation of FN adsorption with roughness (**a**) and surface free energy (SFE) (**b**) on cp-Ti blasted with different particles: S, SiC particles; A, Al_2O_3 particels; 3, particles of 212–300 μm; 6, 425–600 μm. Adapted with permission from ref. [100]. Copyright 2009 Acta Materialia Inc. Published by Elsevier Ltd.

As previously said, the debate on the effective enhancement of protein adsorption by SLA treatments is an open issue. A recent study observed no difference in adsorption from

FBS on machined or SLA cp-Ti [96]. Still, microrough surfaces elicit murine MC3T3-E1 osteoblastic cell spreading and adhesion. Similar findings were observed also in adsorption kinetics and total amount of adsorbed proteins when FN and BSA are adsorbed from single protein solutions, even when wettability was increased by heat treatment [102]. As an interesting fact, heat treatment promoted selective adsorption of fibrinogen and fibronectin from human serum. Even though hydrophilicity may not increase protein adsorption on SLA surfaces, it can promote the formation of a more homogeneous protein layer [103]. SLA did not seem to enhance adsorption of salivary proteins neither [104].

3.2.2. Surface Modification by Chemical and Hydrothermal Treatments

Acid etching is a very simple kind of chemical treatment employed to enhance biological response of titanium surfaces [51]. Nanopatterning by acid etching was found to affect in different ways adsorption of different proteins [105]. Nanopits, generated by simultaneous acid etching and oxidation with H_2O_2, act as physical traps for proteins that can be accommodated within, such as LYS and growth/differentiation factor 5. Adsorption of larger proteins, such as FN, is hindered due to steric limitations. Acid etching of microgrooved titanium resulted in increased hydrophilicity and consequent enhancement of BSA adsorption and human osteoblast proliferation [106].

Hydrothermal treatments are widespread techniques to obtain surfaces with enhanced cytocompatibility [51]. Immersion in solutions with different chemicals and subsequent heating results in nanostructuration of the surface and modification of its chemistry.

Hydrothermal treatments on Ti64 can also be obtained using simply distilled water [107]. In this way, higher hydrophilicity is obtained without changing surface roughness. Increased wettability led to higher laminin adsorption and consequent improved adhesion of cells through integrins. Hydrogen peroxide is a common reactant for hydrothermal modification of titanium surfaces. Nanoporous structures can be obtained in this way [108]. The increased roughness and SFE of H_2O_2-treated Ti64 results in evident decrease of the WCA, from 49° to 16°, and in a sixfold increase of cytochrome C adsorption. Enhanced serum protein adsorption on this kind of surfaces is also due to the generation of OH groups on titanium surfaces [109]. BSA adsorbs also in a different conformation on H_2O_2-treated Ti64 with respect to the polished surfaces [54]. The higher amount of OH on the treated surface produced adsorption of albumin in a more hydrophilic orientation. FN was proven to adsorb in an island-like manner on this kind of surfaces, by positioning mainly in the surface valleys and forming multilayered globular structures ranging from 55 to 83 nm in diameters [110]. Titanium oxide grown using H_2O_2 treatment adsorbs FN in a more irreversible manner than sputtered TiO_2. On the other side, adsorbed HSA is more easily exchanged by HSA molecules in solution [111].

Bioactive titanium surfaces can be obtained by acid-alkali (AA) treatments, which involve a step of acid etching and a subsequent treatment in alkali solution, mainly NaOH. Both the steps can be performed at temperatures ranging from 30 °C [112] up to 70 °C [113]. These treatments allow to obtain surfaces with nanostructures, enhanced wettability, and different charges with respect to untreated titanium. Nanoscale topography was found responsible for increased protein adsorption of albumin and fibronectin in particular [112]. Treatments in NaOH result in a formation of Ti-O-Na layer that changes the surface electrical charge further increasing adsorption of negatively charged proteins such as albumin. AA treatments are more effective in promoting protein adsorption when compared to other surface treatments, such as alkali-heat (AH) [114] or anodic oxidation treatments (AO) [115] and also SLA modification [116]. Better BSA adsorption capability of AA-Ti than AH-Ti, where samples are heated at 600 °C for 1 h after alkali treatment, relied on the higher number of OH groups and on the positive surface charge of AA-Ti [114]. Hu and Yang observed that the NH_3^+ groups of albumin mainly interact with AA and untreated samples, exposing more COO^- groups while the orientation is different on AH-Ti. Secondary structures of albumin are also affected by the charge of the surfaces and OH groups. Interestingly, they found that BSA preadsorption elicited higher mouse osteoblast proliferation on polished Ti (P-Ti), due to higher content of cell binding α-helices. The same research group observed that AA-Ti adsorbs more osseointegration-relevant proteins, such as FN and bone morphogenetic protein 2 (BMP-2) than AO- and P-Ti [113,115]. They observed that morphology was more relevant than wettability in determining the amount of protein adsorbed: Nanopits on AO-Ti are not able to accommodate large proteins, while grooves on P-Ti and network structure of AA-Ti offers more interaction sites. The latter can act as reservoir for BMP-2 [113]. On the other hand, protein conformation on the surface is dictated by hydroxylation of surfaces. Thus, proteins retained their native structure better on AO-Ti than on AA-Ti. Biological activity of BMP-2 is related to its α-helix content, thus AO-Ti promoted bone formation to a longer extend than AA-Ti, despite adsorbing less. Contrary, adhesive properties of FN are more related to β-sheets, which are consistent with the amount of RGD sequences. In this case, AA-Ti can increase FN effect thanks to the disruption of α-helices and the formation of β-sheets [115]. AA-treatments were also found to increase protein adsorption of SLA modified surfaces by turning the surface from hydrophobic to super-hydrophilic [116]. On hydrophobic samples, air bubbles may be trapped in micropores in a Cassie-Baxter regime, hindering solution-surface interactions thus reducing protein adsorption. Moreover, AA-treatments increase SFE. Alkali-acid treatments were employed also to increase protein adsorption ability of porous titanium scaffolds [117,118]. Various morphology can be easily obtained by changing the treatment parameters such as temperature, time, and solution compositions. Nanoneedles [119], nanopores, or nanoleaves [120] can be obtained on the surfaces. Since nanoneedles showed much higher BSA adsorption than the untreated surfaces, Yu et al. [119] obtained very specific adsorption patterns by texturing nanostructured titanium with laser irradiation (Figure 5).

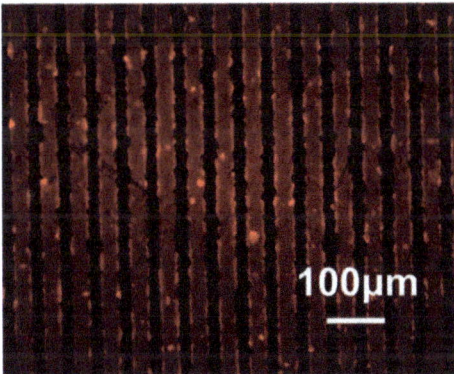

Figure 5. Fluorescent image of BSA adsorbed onto a patterned nanostructured surface: The protein is adsorbed on zones with titanium nanoneedles (red) and not in the zones, which were irradiated with laser. Adapted with permission from ref. [119]. Copyright 2015 WILEY-VCH Verlag GmbH & Co. KGaA, Weinheim.

Morphology has also effect on adsorption selectivity. They present different surface area ratios, SFE, or they can generate physical nanotraps for proteins of certain dimensions [120]. Thus, nanoneedles may overall adsorb less proteins from FBS than nanoleaf or octahedral structures, but still have an equal if not higher number of adhesive proteins such as FN and VN. As result, focal adhesion of human osteoblasts turned out to be larger on this kind of nanostructured surface than on others. Depending on the kind of protein, adsorption may be mainly driven by the contact angle or by roughness. In the case of FIB, adsorption on hydrothermally treated cp-Ti and Ti64 resulted affected more by topography than WCA [121]. Protein adsorption on different morphologies obtained by hydrothermal treatments was also related to their surface potential [122]. High treating temperature,

140 °C, allows to obtain nano-wires on the surface, which exhibit the lowest zeta potential, about −50 mV at pH 7.4, among other nano-structures, such as a nano-network or nano-plate, about −30 and −35 mV at pH 7.4, respectively. Adsorption of BSA and FN was higher on nanowires than on all the other surfaces. Moreover, mouse bone marrow MSCs (BMSCs) had spread better on this kind of surface.

3.2.3. Growth of Titania Nanotubes (TNTs)

A common and easy way to obtain nanotextured titanium surfaces is formation of nanotubes by anodic oxidation [8]. TNTs geometrical features such as diameters, in the range of 15–300 nm, and length are easily tunable with the process parameters. Such surfaces have higher biological response than untreated Ti and can induce cellular differentiation.

At first glance, the enhancement of protein adsorption on TNTs can be ascribed to a much larger surface area than a flat sample [123,124]. At the same time, the oxidized surfaces have higher wettability and SFE, which are factors that contribute to BSA adsorption. The diameters of TNTs further influence the amount of protein adsorbed [125,126]. Increasing diameters from 30 to 100 nm increase adsorption of both FN and COL [125]. Osteoblast viability is higher on 30 nm TNTs when no proteins are adsorbed, while they have the same viability on 30 and 100 nm tubes after adsorption of FN and COL. Computational studies showed that larger diameters correspond to higher interaction energy with collagen, thus increasing protein adsorption [127]. Conformation of the proteins is not affected by TNT's diameters, and collagen lies across several nanotubes. Changes in the 3D structure of other proteins were reported. Smaller diameters correspond to higher α-helix and β-turn content of adsorbed BSA and FIB, while β-sheet showed the inverse behavior. Since the bigger the diameter, the larger flat area on the top of TNTs is, conformation is similar to the proteins adsorbed onto a flat surface. With smaller nanotubes, proteins are more likely to interact with the edge of them, generating differences [126]. A very interesting study by Kulkarni and co-workers [128] defines the synergistic effect of dimensions and charge distribution of TNTs on protein adsorption. The surface charge density is affected by radius of curvature, therefore there is a difference between the outer convex surface and the inner concave surface of TNT. The former presents higher density than the latter. Anyway, the points with higher curvature are the edges at the top of TNTs. Small proteins like histone and albumin can enter TNT with diameter ranging from 15 to 100 nm. Being positively charged, histone can adsorb twofold BSA and also penetrate the space between nanotubes. Albumin cannot do that because of electrostatic repulsion with titanium oxide. Edges at the top of nanotubes are preferential adsorption sites for histone due to higher charge density, as shown in Figure 6

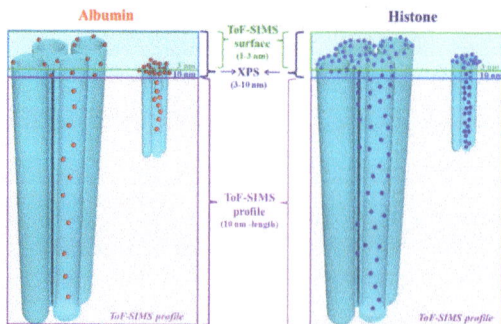

Figure 6. Spatial distribution of albumin and histone adsorbed on titania nanotubes reconstructed by different techniques: Time of flight-secondary ion mass spectroscopy (ToF-SIMS) (1–3 nm depth); X-ray photoelectron spectroscopy (XPS) (3–10 nm depth); Tof-SIMS depth profile (from 10 nm to bottom). Reprinted with permission from ref. [128]. Copyright 2016 Acta Materialia Inc. Published by Elsevier Ltd. Amsterdam, The Netherlands.

Adsorption from platelet rich plasma resulted in lower FIB on TNT surfaces with respect to flat cp-Ti [129]. This is because on more hydrophilic surfaces, such as nanotubes, fibrinogen can be more easily replaced by other proteins, like kininogen, through "the Vroman effect". Adsorption of proteins can be selectively controlled by tuning the diameters of the tube. Smaller TNTs, about 27 nm of diameter, adsorbed more VN from FBS than larger ones, diameters of about 88 nm [130]. Similar effect was obtained for other adhesive proteins such as laminin and fibronectin. Protein adsorption on TNT can be further enhanced by chemical modification of the surface. Hydrogenation of the surface can be achieved by thermal treatments in hydrogenated atmosphere [131]. This is because hydrogenation increase hydrophilicity of TNT and liquid penetration as consequence. Since TNTs substrates can be used as drug-carrier materials, hydrogenation treatment is intriguing because of its effect in changing the release profile of the different proteins.

3.2.4. Other Surface Modification Techniques

SLA, chemical treatments, and growth of TNTs are the most common surface modification techniques for Ti-based biomaterials. Beside those, studies regarding how other kind of surface modifications affect protein adsorption were found.

Electrochemical methods such anodic oxidation allows to grow oxide layers with different nanostrucutres: nanopores [132], nanonetworks [133], or nanorods [134]. By increasing the applied voltage, thickness, micro-roughness, and porosity of the oxide layer increase, resulting in higher BSA adsorption [132]. Higher anodizing voltages resulted, on the other hand, in a rutile layer, which is less biocompatible than anatase. On similar surfaces, no enhancement of adsorbed protein was found when high protein concertation solution as FBS was used [135]. This is a useful reminder that protein adsorption on surfaces is not only dictated by the biomaterials properties but also, and in a significant manner, by the adsorption environment. Subsequent hydrothermal modification of the anodized surfaces highlighted the effect of the surface charge on protein adsorption [136]. Anatase nano-spikes lowered the surface potential of titanium and showed inhomogeneous charge distribution (higher negative charge density on titania tips due to higher curvature). Thus, adsorption of positively charged histone was increased. Au and Ag- nanoparticles (NPs) were successfully embedded into the titanium oxide layer by sequential anodization and soaking in NPs precursor solution and it was found that their presence further increases BSA adsorption [137]. Increased adsorption capability of surfaces with nanonetwork porosity was addressed as result of increased surface area, where pores can easily accommodate BSA and FN [133]. On nanorods, adsorption was found to be mainly driven by the density of the rods. When there are too many or too less structures, adsorption was found to be lower than on untreated titanium. Only intermediate rod density was beneficial for protein adsorption, MC3T3-E1 cell proliferation, and bone formation in vivo [134].

Surface texturing with laser beam is a rather novel way of obtain specific surface pattern in order to increase biological response to biomaterials [138]. It is possible to obtain very complex surface structures, such as micro-pits with nano-ripples at the bottom or at the top, selectively. This results in an accelerated adhesion of MSCs and in a more enhanced osteogenic behavior of the cells [139]. Laser patterning changes surface properties, such as roughness, wettability, chemistry, and charge, to a great extent. Thus, its effect on protein adsorption may vary largely according to the process parameters. Patterning of Ti64 was demonstrated to increase FIB adsorption due to increasing in surface roughness [140]. Furthermore, affinity for FN seemed increased, in particular due to increase in the polar component of the SFE [141]. For the same reason, adsorption of HSA decreased. Lower affinity of textured Ti64 for albumin was also ascribed to a reduction of available binding sites and to chemical modifications and formation of less active titanium oxide forms [142]. Controversy, in a series of studies by Kuczyńska et al. [138,143], an increased adsorption of both BSA and FN was observed. This is the combined result of modified wettability and SFE, morphology, and increased negative charge of the treated surfaces. Conformation of proteins was also affected.

3.3. Effect of Alloying Elements and Surface Ion Doping

Despite being the most widespread materials for orthopedic and dental implants, properties of pure titanium and Ti6Al4V alloy, such as Young's modulus, are not the optimum for instance to avoid stress shield effect. Thus, titanium alloying with several different metals have been developed in order to reduce the elastic modulus or to get other interesting mechanical properties. Nickel is one of the most common alloying elements, TiNi alloys, such as Nitinol (about 50% Ti 50% Ni), possess shape memory and super-elastic properties. Nitinol is largely used in the manufacturing of vascular stent, for example [144].

Alloying elements not only modify the bulk properties of titanium, but also the surface ones. This affect adsorption of proteins. Higher Ni content, from 49.5% to 50.5%, in TiNi alloy results in lower albumin adsorption (from about 90 to 30 ng/cm^2), while FN is quite unaffected. Both resulted in being largely lower than on cp-Ti, twofold and almost 4 times, respectively. Albumin adsorption was found to be proportionally related to the polar component of surface energy, and Ni can reduce it. Fibronectin is more affected by other factors, such as surface charge [145]. Regarding albumin, different results were obtained by Clarke at al. [144] by modifying the composition of the oxide layer on TiNi alloy. They obtained higher adsorption with higher Ni and lower O content in the oxide, regardless of contact angle and roughness. According to Bai studies with binary alloy of Ti with Cr, Al, or Ni oxide layer composition has a larger control on protein adsorption than the bulk ones [146]. In addition, FIB was found to be adsorbed less on Nitinol than on cp-Ti [147]. In both cases, it adsorbs with a "side-on" orientation. FN was found to adsorb in similar manner on cp-Ti also when Zr is introduced into TiNi alloy [148].

Niobium is another very common alloying element for titanium. Nb lowers the Young's modulus of titanium, getting closer to the bone value [149]. β-alloys Ti-Nb-Zr and Ti-Zr showed very little differences in BSA adsorption with cp-Ti and Ti64, but a slight increase can be observed thanks to higher Zr content [150]. The oxide layer drives interactions with proteins also for this kind of alloys. In fact, introduction of boron ions causes a reduction of oxide thickness and hydroxide groups, hindering adsorption of proteins from FBS. This is also detrimental for MG63 human osteosarcoma cells proliferation [151]. Niobium is a beneficial element for proteins also when it is introduced into more complex alloys. The Ti-Zr-Pd-Si-Nb alloy showed enhanced adsorption of BSA and FN with respect to the Nb-free alloy thanks to improved hydrophilicity [152]. The importance of non-polar component in the adsorption of FN was highlighted by Herranz-Diez et al. [153]. They observed that very different Ti-based materials, namely cp-Ti, Ti64, and Ti25Nb21Hf, adsorbed very similar amount of fibronectin, despite various contact angels. Analyzing the components of SFE, they notice different values in the total SFE and polar component, cp-Ti showed the lowest ones. Instead, no variations were found in the dispersive components.

Several metallic ions are well known for being able to stimulate different biological responses, particularly in the field of bioactive glasses. As an example, Ca^{2+} favors osteoblast proliferation and differentiation, Zn^{2+} possess anti-bacterial and anti-inflammatory properties, and Mg^{2+} increase bone cell adhesion and new bone formation [154]. Thus, surface treatments of titanium materials have been developed over past years in order to introduce different ions, in particular within the oxide layer [8]. Presence of ions in the surface results in changes of biomaterials physio-chemical properties and, obviously, this affects protein adsorption. According to several authors, enhancement of protein adsorption is due to increased surface charge of ion-doped titanium materials [31,155] or the bridging effect of divalent ions [155]. Some of the most common methods to produce ion-containing titanium surfaces are hydrothermal treatments [155–158], which allows to obtain at the same time a nanostructured surface and ionic doping. Higher adsorption of albumin was found on treated cp-Ti with Mg^{2+} or Ca^{2+} ions with respect to Na^+. Additionally, increased adsorption was obtained by increasing ions concentration [155]. Magnesium bridging effect towards protein was confirmed in other studies [157] and treated titanium turned out to be bioactive, inducing hydroxyapatite precipitation, and promoting osteoblast attachment and spreading [159]. Anyway, cell adhesion can be depressed by too high Mg concentration in the TiO$_2$ layer due to much higher content of BSA, which reduces cell focal adhesion [160]. Similar results were obtained by lithium ions [31]. Treated surfaces showed super-hydrophilicity, ascribed to increase in surface energy, charge, or OH groups due to Li$^+$. Maximum adsorption of different proteins was found at different lithium concentration, such as FN and BSA. Therefore, it is possible to selectively regulate proteins uptake on the surface and, consequently cellular response. Besides increased protein adsorption, ion presence in a biomaterial is beneficial due to eventual ions release. Co-implantation of Mg and Zn and their release as ions improve adhesion, proliferation, and motility of human gingival fibroblasts [161]. Bridging effect with proteins was confirmed also for trivalent ions such as Fe^{3+} [162], with benefits both in vitro and in vivo. Calcium ions showed further improved protein adsorption, also with respect to other divalent ions such as Mg^{2+} and Sr^{2+} [155,156,163]. Thanks to specific Ca-binding site on some proteins, such as laminin, osteopontin, which is a major non-collagenous bone protein [156], and BSA [163], they adsorb in higher amount on Ca-containing surfaces. Protein adsorption and, more important regarding implants, osteointegration were enhanced also by doping of titanium materials with phosphate ions on TNT [164] or on hydrothermal treated cp-Ti [158]. Growth of TNTs on Ti-Zr-Sn-Mo-Nb alloy resulted into sparse nanotubes due to alloying elements. Spacing between TNTs increased both protein adsorption and rat primary osteoblasts adhesion, proliferation, and activity [165].

All the doping treatments result also in morphological modification of the surface, which may also have a strong effect on protein adsorption. In fewer cases, mainly in the case of doping with monovalent ions such as Na$^+$ [166], researchers found that morphology had a stronger effect than surface chemistry. Monovalent ions do not possess bridging capability towards proteins. Still, many more studies showed how ions presence in titanium-based biomaterials improved biological properties beyond surface nanostructurations [157,163,164].

3.1. Grain Size and Crystalline Phase

Among the factors that influence surface properties such as wettability and surface energy, grain size, and crystalline form of the oxide layer on titanium surface play a major role. It is known that ultrafine-(UG) and nano-grain (NG) metallic surfaces show beneficial behavior with respect to coarse-grain structure. On 301LN stainless steel, grain size of a few nanometers was able to improve BSA adsorption and murine pre-osteoblast cells response [167]. Similar findings, along with improved mechanical properties were obtained on stainless steel 316L [168]. The effect of grain size on protein adsorption has been investigated by several studies, including several types of titanium-based materials such as cp-Ti [169,170], Ti64 [171], and titanium alloy [172,173]. Literature about the effect of nanocrystallization on protein adsorption is not in good agreement. Still, it is important to keep in mind that different results may arise from very different factors, such as surface chemistry, protein concentration in solution, and adsorption conditions. NGs on titanium were mainly obtained by surface mechanical attrition treatment (SMAT) or severe plastic deformation (SPD). The former treatment consists of bombarding the material surface with hardened steel balls [169,172]. The latter is obtained by mechanical stresses such as hydrostatic extrusion [170], sliding friction treatment [171], or high-pressure torsion [173]. All authors assessed that both treatments result in an increased volume of grain boundaries (GBs). They are highly defective sites that contributes to increase the surface energy and the hydrophilicity of titanium-based materials. Usually this resulted in augmented protein adsorption. Bahl et al. [169] applied SMAT to cp-Ti, obtaining nanograins on the surface. Contrary to other studies, nanocrystallization obtained by SMAT decreases BSA adsorption due to changes in electronic and physicochemical properties of the oxide. Still, this is beneficial for attachment and proliferation of human MSCs (hMSCs) and also improved material hemocompatibility thanks to a reduced platelets attachment and corrosion resistance. Corrosion of metallic implants can be enhanced by proteins in solution [174]. Contrary to the adsorption behavior observed by Bahl, Kubacka et al. [170] observed an increase in BSA adsorption on cp-Ti after nanocrystallization through SPD.

They found that adsorption from FBS results in increase of BSA uptake and in reduction of FN. GBs are regions where atoms are prone to be charged, resulting in increase of the acid-base component of the surface energy that is related to adsorption through electrostatic interactions. Thus, authors claimed that in this way non-specific protein adsorption, as BSA, is enhanced. Anyway, higher FN adsorption from FBS, along with VN was obtained on nano-grained Ti64 and Ti-Nb-Mo-Sn-Zr alloys. Huo et al. [171] ascribed enhanced protein adsorption on treated Ti64 to the smaller contact angle of NG surface with respect to coarse-grain and to higher surface energy. Thanks to a greater amount of RGD-containing proteins, these surfaces develop a suitable microenvironment for osteoblasts. β-alloy Ti-Nb-Mo-Sn-Zr subjected to SMAT treatment was found to adsorb twofold more FN and VN than the untreated surfaces [172]. Interestingly, the authors claimed that enhanced cell behavior on these surfaces is also related to proteins being adsorbed in a more active state with respect to coarse-grain surface. RGD groups are better exposed for cell attachment. Similar results were also obtained on Ti-Ni alloy subjected to high-pressure torsion [173]. VN adsorption increased more than BSA. Furthermore, Ni release was found to be hindered after SPD.

Along with grain size, the crystalline phase of titanium surface oxide layer also plays a fundamental role in determining protein–surface interactions. Different titania phases, such as amorphous, rutile, and anatase, and their orientation change surface properties and protein adsorption. TiO_2 phase is easily controlled through heat treatment: By increasing the treating temperature, amorphous titania is transformed into anatase at first and then to rutile, at about 600 °C [175]. The effect of different crystalline phases of titanium on protein adsorption has been investigated largely on TNT substrates [126,175–177]. Native oxide on flat cp-Ti was turned from amorphous to mainly anatase by annealing, showing almost no differences in the adsorption of BSA and FIB [126]. Nevertheless, the crystalline phase has different effects when adsorption from different proteins is investigated. Gong et al. [176] and Li et al. [177] agreed on the fact that anatase showed the lowest adsorption of COL I and FN compared with amorphous titania and rutile, as possible to see in Figure 7. The latter has the highest adsorption capability. On the other hand, adsorption of BSA or FBS were increased by higher annealing temperature [175].

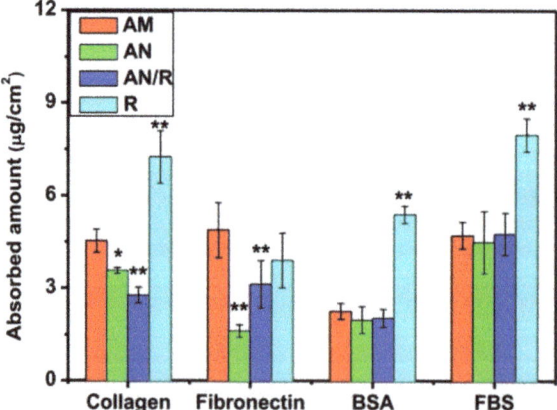

Figure 7. Adsorption of different proteins on Titania Nanotube (TNT) substrates with different crystalline phase: AM, amorphous; AN, pure anatase; AN/R, mainly anatase with rutile presence; R, pure rutile. Statistical difference by ANOVA: **$p < 0.01$ and *$p < 0.05$. Reprinted with permission from ref. [177]. Copyright 2019, King Abdulaziz City for Science and Technology.

Phase transformation highly affect the number of hydroxyl groups on the surface: Anatase has fewer OH groups than amorphous TiO_2 and rutile has the highest number of all [175]. OH groups are fundamental to drive protein–surface interactions, in particular, basic OH groups can promote protein adsorption, and amorphous titania as more of them with respect to anatase [178]. Furthermore, anatase phase is more negatively charged than non-crystalline oxide or rutile, thus less proteins are adsorbed due to electrostatic repulsion [177]. Raffaini and Ganazzoli [179], through molecular modelling, observed that, among titanium oxide polymorphs, anatase provided the highest interaction energy for both BSA and FN. After initial contact, where the adsorption is driven by dipolar and dispersive interactions, both proteins tend to spread on the surface, in order to maximize amino acid residues interacting with the surface. BSA was found to do that on both anatase and rutile, while FN was more compact onto anatase. Higher crystallization obtained by heat treatment was beneficial for protein adsorption also on hydrothermally grown rutile nanoneedles [180]. Beside crystalline phase, also orientation of crystals may affect how proteins arrange on the surface. Molecular dynamic (MD) study allows to investigate protein adsorption by changing crystal's Miller indexes. Myoglobin adsorbs on rutile (1 1 0) or (0 0 1) faces with different orientation [181]. Due to electrostatic repulsion, the HEME group is away from the oxygen rich (1 1 0) rutile face, while it is closer to the (0 0 1) one. Keller et al. [182] proved the effect of anatase orientation on conformation of adsorbed fibrinogen. Low SFE facets, such as the {1 0 0} family, behave as hydrophobic surfaces, favoring protein–protein interactions and formation of FIB networks. (1 0 1) and (1 1 0) crystals have higher hydrophilicity, the latter due to higher surface polarity, and favor adsorption of proteins in a globular-like shape. Globular conformation of FIB may reduce the inflammatory response to a foreign body since it is more similar to its native state.

3.5. Surface Activation

UV-light or plasm activations are very well reported to be a way of improve biological activity of biomaterials surfaces [183,184]. Increase of surface activity is achieved by a three-step mechanism: Removal of hydrocarbon contaminants; induced surface hydrophilicity; change of the surface charge from negative to positive. Medical devices would probably be stored for a very long time before usage, up to 5 years [185], therefore removal of atmospheric contaminants is a priority. This will be discussed deeply later in Section 4.1.

Protein adsorption on cp-Ti, in particular of BSA and FN was found to be strictly correlated to hydrocarbon level [186]. When contaminants are removed by UV, Ti^{4+} sites are exposed, increasing interaction with both protein and cell (Figure 8a).

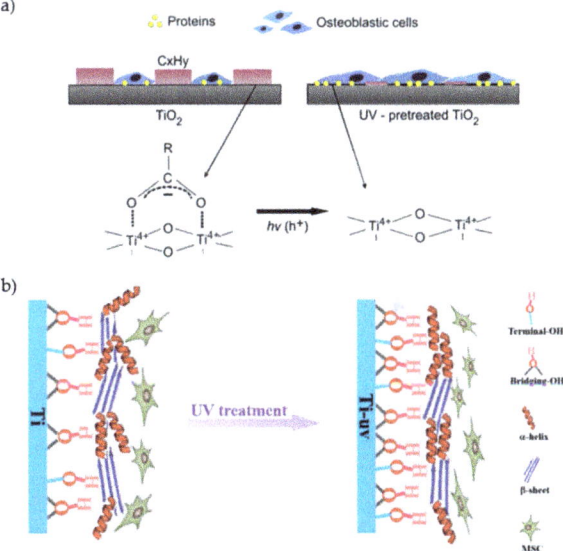

Figure 8. Schematic representation of UV effects on protein adsorption and cell attachment: (a) Removal

of hydrocarbon contamination results in increased protein adsorption and osteoblast adhesion and spreading, adapted from ref. [186]; (**b**) effect of number and type of UV-generated OH groups on protein conformation and subsequent mesenchymal stem cell (MSC) proliferation, adapted with permission from ref. [187]. Copyright 2017 The Royals Society of Chemistry.

Hydrophilicity and positive surface charge of UV-activated surface arise from the same physiochemical modifications of TiO_2 layer, formation of oxygen vacancies, and terminal OH groups. Exposure to UV-light promotes an electron from the valence band to the conduction band. This causes a reduction of Ti^{4+} to Ti^{3+} and, as a consequence, oxygen vacancies are formed [183,188]. Other than increasing positive surface charge, Ti^{3+} are favorable sites for water dissociation, leading to generation of terminal OH groups [187]. Positive surface charge is also promoted by the basic behavior of UV-generated OH groups [189]. On titania nanoparticles, it was proven that basic hydroxyls can form hydrogen bonds with $-NH_3^+$ groups on proteins [178]. Electrostatic nature of protein adsorption enhancement was confirmed by Hori et al. [188]. They observed that more BSA adsorbed onto UV-activated surface from solution at pH 7 but a smaller increase was found at pH 3, compared with untreated Ti. At pH 7, both BSA and Ti are negatively charged. Thus, UV-generated positive charges can attract albumin molecules. At pH 3, BSA is below its IEP, as untreated Ti. Therefore, UV-activation is not as effective. Conformation of proteins is also affected by surface UV-activation, in particular by the terminal OH groups. Yu and coworkers [187] observed an increase of α-helix and a decrease of β-sheet contents in albumin, with respect to adsorption on an untreated surface. They discussed that these conformational changes can be related to increased osteogenic differentiation of MSCs(Figure 8b). Remarkably, while cell adhesion and proliferation on UV treated surfaces are increased, bacteria colonization of surface was hindered [190,191].

Different plasma system can be used in order to obtain activation of the surface: Different kinds of glow discharge plasma, such as atmospheric (APGD) [192], radio frequency (RFGD) [193], vacuum [194]; nonthermal atmospheric pressure plasma (NTAPP) [184]; or argon atmospheric pressure dielectric barrier discharge (APDBD) [195]. As well as UV treatments, plasma can increase protein adsorption thanks to the removal of hydrocarbon contamination [184] but, unlike UV, surface charge become more negative [184,193]. Specifically, employing NTAPP creates -COOH, -OH, and NH_2 groups on the surface [39]. Oxygen-containing groups can generate reactive oxygen species during plasma treatments [184]. NTAPP treatments were found to have analogous effect to UV surface activation in terms of reduction of Ti surface negative charge and adsorption of BSA [196]. To the authors best knowledge, plasma effect was mostly investigated on fibronectin adsorption. Noticeably, FN adsorption was selectively increased in case of single protein solution [39,193] and when mixed to other proteins such as BSA [197] or even from plasma serum [194,198]. FN, as an adhesive protein, is beneficial for cell attachment and spreading *per se*. On plasma-treated Ti, negative plasma-induced charges affect FN conformation, promoting a more bioactive configuration of the protein on the surface. Integrin-binding sites on FN, namely the tripeptide sequence RGD, are more exposed due to conformational changes of the proteins. Thus, interactions with $\alpha_5\beta_1$ integrin on cells are promoted, increasing osteoblast spreading and differentiation [39,193]. Controversy, Santos et al. [199] observed that low-pressure glow discharge plasma did not affect the total amount of adsorbed HSA, IgG, or LAM, nor the adsorption isotherms, when single protein solutions were used. Instead, plasma treatments affected the layer composition of proteins adsorbed from a mixture of the three of them. Adsorption of HSA and LAM were selectively increased and decreased, respectively, while IgG was not changed.

UV photoactivation and plasma treatments are effective ways to promote protein adsorption and surface properties in general. Since surface morphology is not modified, these techniques can provide useful information on adsorption mechanisms, by isolating the effect of surface charges and functional groups. Despite not being addressed as the main adsorption driving force, electrostatic interactions have been proved to play an important role, in particular regarding selective adsorption of proteins and their biological activity.

4. External Parameters Affecting Protein Adsorption on Titanium Surfaces

4.1. Aging and Storage: Contamination of Titanium Surfaces

Biological properties of titanium need to be preserved even through the long-lasting storage of the biomedical devices, up to five years. Implants and dental screw are usually enclosed in a sterile gas-permeable packaging, which keeps the contents sterile but allows contamination of the surfaces by the carbonaceous organic impurities in the atmosphere [185,200]. Very recent molecular dynamic studies performed by Wu et al. [201] demonstrated that carbon contaminants expose C-H bonds, thus greatly reducing surface polarity and dipole–dipole interactions with proteins. Protein adsorption drastically decreases after four-week storage when titanium is placed in sealed container [202]. Proportional correlation between increased WCA and reduced protein adsorption was observed. The same authors observed that inclusion of divalent ions like Ca^{2+} within Ti surface through chemical treatments may hinder depression of bio-properties due to aging [203]. After four weeks, BSA adsorption, and rat BMCs attachment resulted in being higher with respect to untreated surface. Therefore, it is necessary to limit surface contamination of implants during their shelf-life. As described in the previous paragraph, plasma treatments are an effective way to remove carbon contaminants form titanium surface. Despite being very efficient in removal of carbon contaminants, UV and plasma might be time-consuming processes and require delicate equipment. Miki et al. [204] found that simple cleaning of titanium devices with electrolytic reducing ionic water, which has high OH^- concentration, led to similar results in protein adsorption compared with UV. Bone contact is also much higher than the control surfaces. This process can be easily performed in a generic dentistry facility, for example. In the past 10 years, great efforts have been made by researchers to find a suitable storage method. It shall maintain intact the biological properties of a newly manufactured Ti surface and it needs to withstand sterilization. Storage in wet conditions seems to be the most promising way [205,206]. Choi and co-workers observed that soaking in distilled water may retain properties of titanium surface after UV and plasma activation for periods up to eight weeks [206]. UV treatment and wet storage on SLA-modified Ti surface allow to obtain the best results, in terms of protein adsorption and murine osteoblast cells adhesion. Interestingly, storage in water is not only suitable for avoiding carbon contamination, but also it is capable of maintaining the more positive surface charge of the UV-treated titanium [200]. Protein adsorption and cell adhesion can be even increased upon storage by using ion-containing solution [205]. Ca-containing solution can benefit from the protein bridging effects of adsorbed ions and the cellular affinity for these ions. Vacuum storage proved to retain biological activity of alkali-heat treated titanium eve after one year [185]. Wilhelmi et al. [50] confirmed, through time of flight secondary ions mass spectroscopy (Tof-SIMS) analysis, that the maximum adsorption of BSA on cp-Ti is obtained for solution at pH 5.2, and decrease with increasing pH values. This confirm that protein–protein latera interactions play a major role in adsorption mechanisms.

4.2. Influence of the Solution: pH, Temperature and Ions

As discussed in paragraph 2.4, the parameters of the protein solution have a major role in determining various aspect of protein adsorption, such as amount of the protein adsorbed, surface–protein interactions, and adsorption kinetic. The pH value determines charge distribution on both the surface and protein [20]. As a consequence, protein–surface interactions may vary to a great extent by changing pH. This fact also reflects to loosely bound proteins. At pH close to the IEP of a protein, repulsive interactions between BSA molecules are at the lowest, therefore the loosely bound portion of proteins adsorbed is increased [207]. The highest adsorption was observed near the IEP of the BSA, as it is possible to see in Figure 9 [208]. The mechanisms that can explain the pH effect on protein adsorption on Ti was proposed by Imamura et al. [209]. At pH around 4, that is below the IEP of Ti, acidic residues in the proteins, with COO^- groups, are attracted by OH^+ groups on surface. Above pH = 5, the functional groups on the Ti surface turn negatively charged and can interact with $-NH_2^+/-NH=NH_2^+$ groups of the amino acids. They also observed that thickness of the adsorbed protein layer may vary by changing pH. Similar behavior was observed also for titania.

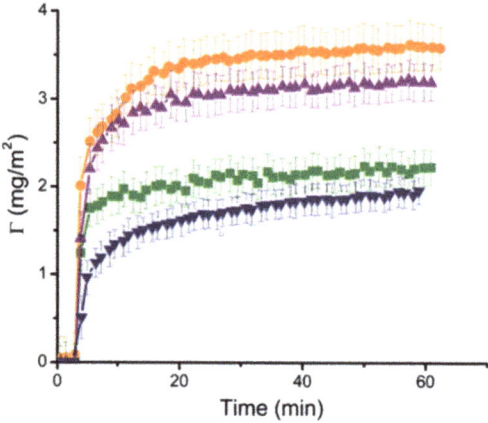

Figure 9. BSA adsorption on TiO$_2$ thin film at different pH values: 3.55 (■), 4.60 (●), 5.60 (▲), and 7.51 (▼). Reprinted with permission from ref. [208]. Copyright 2009 Elsevier B.V.

Still, due to the high adsorption even under adverse electrostatic condition, namely at pH 3.55 and 7.51, the authors claimed that the main driving force for albumin adsorption on titania is hydrophobic interaction. LYS adsorption was also observed to be strongly dependent on pH [210]: When titania is positively charged, at pH lower than 5, almost no adsorption was observed due to electrostatic repulsion, as expected, because at this pH value, LYS is positively charged. In this study, correlation between protein uptake and temperature was also discussed. Increased temperatures lead to higher amount of adsorbed proteins. Combined effect of pH and temperature was studied by Kopac et al. [44]. By fitting adsorption isotherms with Langmuir or Freundlich curves, they observed that the highest adsorption of BSA onto titania can be obtained at 40 °C and pH 4. These data show that adsorption from different solution may results in very different protein layer on the surface of biomaterials.

Ions dissolved within the protein solution compete with protein for interacting with the surface and hinder or elicit protein adsorption. Phosphate ions can easily adsorb on titanium surfaces [56] and they alter BSA adsorption kinetic and conformation on TiO$_2$ [211]. Positive mono- and divalent ions are electrostatically attracted by the negative charges on titanium, subsequently mediating the interaction between the surface and proteins. Monovalent ions, such as K$^+$ and Na$^+$, do not influence to a great extend protein adsorption [59] since once their single positive charge is attracted by the surface, they have no more for proteins to be attracted. On the other hand, divalent ions, Ca^{2+} and Mg^{2+} in particular have a bridging effect toward proteins thanks to spare positive charges after interaction with titanium [212,213]. Kohavi et al. [59] observed that electrostatic interactions may play a major role than surface wettability on protein adsorption. Adsorption of HSA and FN was enhanced by prewetting Ti64 surfaces, with solutions containing divalent ions or not. Wetted surface were hydrophilic, and non-wetted ones were hydrophobic. After being dried, surfaces turned hydrophobic again, and adsorption was still enhanced on the samples that were wetted with Ca^{2+} containing solutions. The interplay between pH and ions dissolved in determining the electrostatic interactions between proteins and surfaces was well described by Hori et al. [188]. Around physiological pH, when both titanium and albumin are negatively charged, divalent ions are effective in increasing protein adsorption. At pH 3, below the IEP of surface and protein both, ions did not alter amount of adsorbed BSA. In the same study, it was also found that anions, as Cl$^-$, can mask UV-generated positive charges and annihilate the beneficial effect of UV treatments. The fact that ions co-adsorption can reduce benefits of positive surface potential on the adsorption of proteins was recently confirmed [214].

After all these considerations, it is possible to state that attention must be paid to the solution parameters, in particular when discussing protein adsorption and comparing results from different studies.

4.3. Protein Concentration in Solution

Human plasma and biological fluids in general contain proteins in a very high concentration. The amount of proteins in human plasma is in the range of 60–80 mg/mL [215]. It is not trivial to reproduce this high concentration in laboratory experiment, mainly due to the high cost of proteins and their availability for purchase. Thus, researchers investigating protein adsorption used to lower protein concentration in solution, from some mg/mL [216] down to small fraction of the biological one [145], for example BSA was employed in concentration ranging from 0.4 to 4 mg/mL while its biological concentration is reported to be as high as 33–52 mg/mL [217]. As pointed out by Hemmersam and co-workers [218], adsorption of proteins from low concentrated solution has a stronger dependence from the substrate than what happens using higher protein concentrations. Using quartz crystal microbalance (QCM) analysis, they found that adsorption of FIB from 0.03 mg/mL solution to Au-, Ti-, or Ta-sensors showed larger differences, both in layer structure and protein amount, than in the case where 1 mg/mL solution was used. In the former case, FIB molecules had time to spread on the surface and to interact with it using both αC and D domains, adhering more strongly. In the latter case, adsorption rate is too fast for this to happen. Strong denaturation of proteins adsorbed from low concentrated solution was observed also for FN on Ti64 [219]. Protein unfolding is also hindered by surface hydrophilicity obtained through UV activation. Reducing the amount of proteins used during an experiment, paying the price of be further away from real physiological conditions, may be necessary to appreciate the influence of the material features on adsorption mechanisms. Beneficial effect on protein adsorption obtained by Argon plasma or UV treatments of pure titanium turns insignificant when adsorption was carried out using 10% FBS solution instead of 2% one [220]. Researchers need to bear in mind that surface effects observed using solution with a very low content of proteins can be reduced, different, or, in the worst case, annihilated in case of the real, biological fluids. This fact applies also for properties and characteristics of the protein adsorbed layers.

5. Protein Co-Adsorption and Competition for the Surface

Human plasma contains about 3020 distinct proteins [221]. As for protein concentration, it is nearly impossible to replicate this enormous complexity on a lab scale. In addition, it would be extremely complex to understand adsorption mechanisms and the specific role of the biomaterial surface in it. Thus, most of researchers conduct their experiments using a single protein solution, as shown previously. Unfortunately, it is not possible to predict the adsorption of proteins from complex mixture just knowing how it happens from the single protein solutions. Researchers tried to expand knowledge of the protein adsorption on titanium-based biomaterials by mostly using binary protein mixture or subsequent adsorption.

Adsorption of BSA on cp-Ti was found to be enhanced when obtained from BSA-LYS containing solutions [222,223]. BSA$^-$LYS$^+$ agglomerates can form in solution and adsorb on the surface, thus increasing the total mass of adsorbed proteins (Figure 10). Relative amounts of adsorbed proteins are influenced both by solution composition and pH, as possible to see in Figure 10a,b. Interestingly, residual enzymatic activity of LYS is not much influenced on protein content in solution [222]. BSA, due to its larger mass, cannot be displaced by LYS in case of sequential adsorption, thus limiting LYS amount on the surface [223].

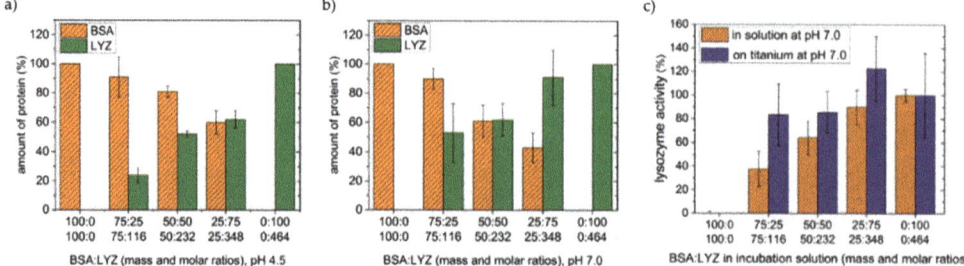

Figure 10. Adsorption on cp-Ti from BSA-LYS mixture: Relative amounts of adsorbed proteins form mixtures with different ratios (BSA: LYS 100:0, 75:25, 50:50, 25:75, 0:100) at different pH, 4.5 (**a**), 7.0 (**b**) (amount is expressed as percentage of adsorbed protein from a pure solution); LYS enzymatic activity, relative to pure LYS solution, in mixture with BSA and after adsorption from same mixture (**c**). Adapted with permission from ref. [222]. Copyright 2016 Elsevier B.V.

Physiochemical characteristics of surfaces have a strong role in determining protein competition for the surface. Hydrophilic titanium surfaces, such as SLA-treated substrates, have been found to promote FN adsorption during competition with albumin, even when a biological BSA:FN ratio of about 100:1 is maintained in the solution [224]. The first protein to adsorb on the surface can inhibit sequential adsorption of other proteins [225], but higher affinity with the surface can result in protein displacement and substitution [225,226]. Felgueiras et al. [226] showed that FN and COL I can block sequential albumin adsorption on Ti64 due to their larger mass, and that they are able to displace albumin when adsorbed as second proteins. Interaction between FN and COL I are dependent on the kind of the surface. As in the case of LYS, albumin can form complexes with COL I in solution resulting in higher number of proteins adsorbed with respect to the single protein solutions. Contrary to these results, BSA was found to be able to displace larger proteins such as FIB or FN on TiO$_2$ surfaces [227] due to higher affinity for the surface. On a pre-existing BSA layer, FIB and FN forms a layer on the albumin instead of displacing it.

Being quite simple, binary protein solutions are still not very much representative of actual biological fluids. Some researchers moved further on in complexity of systems by investigating through proteomic analysis the exact composition of protein layers adsorbed on several titanium surfaces from real and whole biological fluids such as plasma [221,228,229] or saliva [230–232]. Among the thousands of proteins present in human plasma, the most adsorbed was FN, followed by albumin, alipoprotein, and fibrinogen [221]. From saliva, which contains about 750 different proteins, less than half of them were found on titanium [232], mainly amylase and lysozyme [230]. The effect of surface modification on the protein pellicle composition was also evaluated. In case of adsorption from saliva, very low specificity was observed for different titanium surfaces, smooth, SLA-treated, and SLA-treated+stored in ionic solution [231]. On the contrary, differences were observed between smooth and SLA surfaces by using human serum [229]. One hundred and eighty-one and 162 proteins were identified on smooth and blasted/acid-etched surfaces, respectively. Proteins adsorbed onto smooth Ti are involved in a higher number of biological pathways, such as clotting, cytokines-mediated inflammation response, integrin signaling, and glycolysis, the latter being absent on SLA-treated titanium. SLA treatments were also found to affect the proteome on Ti-Zr alloy, from both plasma and saliva [233]. Adsorption from saliva resulted in 389 common adsorbed proteins, 40 adsorbed uniquely on the machined samples, and 14 on the SLA treated ones. The proteome from blood plasma was much more similar with only three unique proteins, on both machined and SLA surfaces, and 145 common proteins. Even though UV activation of the surface has been reported to improve adsorption of proteins [188], proteomic analyses found that light treatment on cp-Ti, hydrothermally coated with nano-structured TiO$_2$, depress proteins adsorption from plasma [228]. Much lower content of FIB, immunoglobulins, and other proteins were found on pre-activated surfaces. Authors addressed this decrease to a mutual combination of surface properties: Roughness, charge, intrinsic, and photo-induced wettability. Reduction of inflammation-promoting proteins such as immunoglobulins and FIB may be beneficial for osseointegration. Even if adsorption from complex biological fluids can be more significant than adsorption from a single protein solution for understanding the fate of biomaterials, this might not be still enough. Jager et al. [234] studied the composition of the protein layer formed onto explanted hip implants. They found that proteome formed onto a titanium implants is different with respect of the one that forms from plasma. Among the 2802 unique proteins founded on the implant, cell-free hemoglobin was the most abundant, almost two-fold albumin. Most of them were of intracellular origin and, interestingly, fibronectin was absent.

Adsorption from single protein solution can be useful for a preliminary understanding of how the different surface features may interact with biological fluids after being implanted. Anyhow, it is evident that this is not sufficient and it is quite necessary to test protein-biomaterials interactions using complex solutions.

6. Methods for Investigating Protein Adsorption on Titanium-Based Materials

During the past years, researchers have developed and optimized a huge number of experimental techniques in order to overcome the challenges of investigating adsorption of proteins on surfaces with very different features. Characterization techniques for proteins adsorption, and biomolecules adsorption in general, are extensively reviewed elsewhere [235,236]. Here, a brief overview is reported of the techniques used in literature specifically for characterizing adsorption on titanium-based biomaterials. Different aspects of proteins adsorption need to be targeted by characterization techniques, for instance protein quantification, conformation of the adsorbed proteins, protein–surface interactions, and protein type recognition. Experimental techniques will be described according to the information that they can provide about the protein adsorption phenomenon, their advantages, and drawbacks in the characterization of biomaterials, as summarized in Table 2.

One of the first issue when studying protein adsorption is to quantify the molecules adsorbed onto the surface. Two main strategies are at the disposal of researchers to perform a direct quantification of the adsorbed protein: Unlabeled proteins and labeled proteins. In the latter case, proteins can be labeled with iodine isotope ^{125}I [144,145] or with fluorophores, as rhodamines [74,100]. The use of fluorescent markers allows also to image the protein layer. Quantification of proteins can be achieved with label-free techniques. Bicinchoninic acid assay (BCA) is one of the most employed analytical assay for the quantification of proteins [98,101], alongside the Bradford method [224]. With these techniques, adsorbed protein can be determined by removing the proteins form the material surface or by measuring the remaining concentration in the uptake solution. Underestimation of the adsorbed proteins may occur if proteins are not completely detached from the surface. Protein concentration in solution can be evaluated thanks to the Lambert-Beer law, using a wavelength of 280 nm [81,117] Other techniques may be adapted from biochemistry in order to quantify and recognize adsorbed proteins. In some studies, the use of gold-labeled [131] or fluorescent-marked antibodies [107] is reported, which allows to target specific proteins and quantify or even image them. With these methods, it is also possible to search specific proteins within mixture. ELISA is another suitable and widespread method to evaluate the amount of very specific proteins adsorbed ono the surface [104,128,129,152]. Determination of the specific composition of the protein layer formed onto a surface can be performed using different methods: Gel electrophoresis is commonly used in various forms, such as Western blot or sodium dodecyl sulphate–polyacrylamide gel electrophoresis (SDS-PAGE) [130,162,199,230], to separate and recognize different proteins; liquid chromatography electrospray ionization tandem mass spectrometry (LC-ESI-MS/MS) is another largely used method to identify proteins within a complex layer [90,221,231]. Conventional techniques for surface chemical analysis in material science are also valuable for evaluating presence of protein on a surface. XPS [75,123] and Tof-SIMS [50,128,223] can detect elements or functional groups characteristic of proteins and also identify specific proteins. Furthermore, XPS can also be employed for investigating protein–surface interactions [114,148]. X-ray wavelength dispersion spectroscopy (WSD) was also reported as effective for detect adsorbed proteins in a large concentration range, from ng/cm^2 to µg/cm^2 [76,147]. Imaging and qualitative detection of proteins onto a surface can be also performed by atomic forces microscopy (AFM) [58,110,143]. It is possible to image single proteins or agglomerates on the surface [58] or, thanks to appropriate tip modifications, it is also possible to measure the interaction forces between the proteins and surfaces [82]. Distribution of proteins onto a surface can be imaged thanks to the use of confocal laser scanning microscopy (CLSM) coupled with use of fluorescent-labeled proteins [95,100]. Qualitative evaluation of protein adsorption can be performed directly visualizing the adsorbed layer by transmission electron microscopy (TEM) [180]. Zeta potential measurements is usually applied for nanoparticles or particles in suspension [196], but it is also possible to obtain titration curves on bulky samples [54]. IEP shift and curve shapes can provide information on the surface coverage and protein conformation. Real-time monitoring of adsorption process can be obtained by QCM. With this technique, proteins adsorbed onto the surface can be weighted [112]. Different QCM set ups allow to collet further information: QCM with dissipation (QCM-D) allows to measure the dissipation of energy in the adsorbed layer, thus providing information about the flexibility and the water content of the adsorbed layer [67,126,227]; QCM can be coupled with electrochemical and impedance measurements (EQCI) [66]. Mechanisms of protein adsorption are very complex to be characterized. The family of spectroscopic techniques comprehend several powerful methods, which allows to investigate protein secondary structure, layer thickness, and chemical environment of certain amino acidic residues. Protein conformation, in terms of α-helix, β-sheet, and random coils content, can be determined by Fourier transform infrared (FTIR) spectroscopy, in particular in Attenuated Total Reflection (ATR), thanks to deconvolution of Amide I band [113,216]. Amide I and II band intensity can also provide quantitative information about adsorbed proteins [88,123]. Raman spectroscopy is a technique mostly applied for studying adsorption on nanoparticles [36,237], which was also reported to be used, with 2D-correlation analysis, for adsorption on bulk materials [71]. The evolution of the adsorbing layer can be monitored in situ by spectroscopic ellipsometry by measuring the thickness of the layer, according to the variation of the ellipsometric angles Δ and Ψ [86,208,209]. Some amino acids are intrinsically fluorescent, tryptophan and tyrosine in particular, and their emission is sensitive to the chemical environment around them. By choosing a suitable Δλ, synchronous fluorescent spectroscopy (SFS) can be applied to monitor the conformation of proteins around such residues [113–115]. The electrochemical behavior at the protein–surface interface can provide information about the evolution of the layer and protein–surface interactions. This information can be obtained by electrochemical impedance spectroscopy (EIS) performed in protein-containing solutions [57,61,169,212]. Information about the denaturation of proteins after adsorption can be obtained by exploiting circular dichroism (CD) analysis [187].

Table 2. Characterization techniques commonly used for protein investigation on titanium-based surface. The output about protein adsorption, the kind of substrates that can be analyzed, the possibility of in situ (without protein detachment) and real-time measurement, and main advantages and drawbacks are reported.

	Technique	Output	Substrate	In Situ/Real Time	Advantages	Drawbacks	References
Labeled proteins	^{125}I-labeling	Quantification	Any	Yes/no	Direct quantification	Change of protein properties, handling issues	[144,145]
	Fluorescent labeling	Quantification and imaging	Any	Yes/no	Direct quantification, competitive adsorption evaluation	Change of protein properties, expensive reagents	[74,80,100,116]
UV-vis spectroscopy	BCA	Quantification	Any	No/no	Low cost, large range of concentrations	Protein detachment needed	[98,101,114,115]
	Bradford assay	Quantification	Any	No/no	Low time consume	Protein detachment needed, sensible to surfactant	[88,155,224]
	Spectrophotometry ($\lambda = 280$ nm)	Quantification	Any	No/no	No reactant needed	Protein detachment needed, inaccurate with complex samples	[81,117]
	Labeled antibodies	Quantification, protein recognition and imaging	Any	Yes/no	Targeting of specific proteins	Time consuming, specific reagents	[94,107,131,173]
	ELISA	Quantification and protein recognition	Any	Yes/no	High specificity	Time consuming, specific reagents	[104,128,129,152]
	Western blot	Quantification and protein recognition	Any	No/no	No toxic chemicals	Sample preparation, poor band separation	[102,130]
Gel electrophoresis	SDS-PAGE	Quantification and protein recognition	Any	No/no	High sensitivity, small samples needed	Poor band resolution, toxic chemicals	[109,230]
	LC-EIS-MS/MS	Proteomic analysis	Any	No/no	High specificity and sensitivity	High costs	[229,233,234]

Table 2. *Cont.*

Technique	Output	Substrate	In Situ/Real Time	Advantages	Drawbacks	References
XPS	Quantification, protein-surface interaction	Any	Yes/no	High sensitivity, simultaneous evaluation of surface chemistry, depth profiling	No absolute quantification, complex data analysis	[110,114,133,212]
Tof-SIMS	Quantification, protein recognition	Any	Yes/no	High sensitivity, possible orientation and conformation analysis, depth profiling	No absolute quantification, complex data analysis	[50,128,223]
WSD	Quantification	Any	Yes/no	Sensitive to a wide range of protein surface concentration	Thorough calibration needed	[76,147]
AFM	Imaging, adhesion forces, conformation	Flat substrates	Yes/no	High resolution, customizable tip	Low throughput, time consuming	[58,82,110,143]
CLSM	Imaging, relative quantification	Any	Yes/no	High resolution, 3D distribution into surface features	Expensive reagents	[95,100]
TEM	Imaging, thickness measurement	Any	Yes/no	Direct visualization of protein layer	Complex sample preparation	[180]
Zeta potential	Adsorption evaluation, protein conformation	Powder or planar samples	Yes/no	Simple measurement	No protein recognition, preliminary information needed	[54,78,228]
QCM	Quantification, viscoelastic properties of layer, changes in conformation	Sputtered sensors	Yes/Yes	High sensitivity, real time measurement, possibility to change the uptake solution	Co-adsorbed solvent weighted. Mass calculation affected by energy dissipation	[67,112,226,227,238]
FTIR (ATR)	Secondary structure, relative quantification	Planar samples	Yes/no	Very specific protein band	Not highly sensitive, data deconvolution needed	[113,114,216]

Table 2. Cont.

Technique	Output	Substrate	In Situ/Real Time	Advantages	Drawbacks	References
Raman spectroscopy	Secondary structure, relative quantification	Any	Yes/no	Very specific protein band	Not highly sensitive, complex data interpretation	[71]
SE	Layer thickness measurement	Flat surfaces	Yes/yes	High sensitivity, low cost, fast measurement	Difficult optical modeling of rough and structured surfaces	[86,208,209]
SFS	Protein conformation	Any	Yes/no	Sensitive, high selectivity towards specific amino acids	Possible instrument artifacts	[113–115]
EIS	Layer evolution, protein-surface interactions	Planar samples	Yes/yes	High sensitivity, possible to study adsorption in different condition	Complex modelling and data interpretation	[57,61,169,212]
CD	Protein conformation	Planar samples	Yes/no	Specific bands for secondary structures	Band deconvolution needed	[187]

7. Key Concepts

Protein adsorption is a fundamental step in the interaction of implantable biomaterials, such as titanium and titanium alloys, with the biological environment. The positive or negative outcome of tissue integration of an implant depends on the interplay between the body and the implant surface. How cells and bacteria adhere, proliferate, and compete is strongly dictated by the protein layer that forms on the device surface within the first minutes after implantation. The understanding of these phenomena is necessary to develop always better implants and to reduce possible adverse reactions. Thus, in past years, great efforts have been put to gain knowledge about the aspects that regulate proteins adsorption on titanium. A large variety of different surface–protein combinations have been investigated, including different type of titanium, titanium oxide, and titanium alloys, several kinds of surface treatments aimed to improve Ti osseointegration and a wide range of proteins in a simpler or more complex environment. Due to the enormous variability and complexity of the protein adsorption processes, a unique and fully agreed explanation of adsorption on titanium was not found in literature, some aspects being clearer than others. Impact of surface properties, such as roughness, morphology, chemistry, surface energy, wettability, and charge, need further investigation. The main effects of titanium surface features are summarized in Table 3.

Increased surface roughness in the micro scale seems to be capable of increasing the adsorption due to a greater number of active sites and features such as pores, nanotubes, or pits can accommodate proteins. On the other hand, no clear effect was found for nano-roughness. In this case, topography effect is mediated by other properties, such as charge or wettability. Electrostatic attraction may increase protein adsorption, while repulsion seems not enough to completely avoid protein binding with the surface. The role of wettability in adsorption is the most controverse. As a rule of thumb, proteins prefer to adsorb on hydrophobic surfaces, since water is more easily displaced from the surface and hydrophobic interactions between ammino acid residue and surface can be strong. In fact, this has been reported in some cases for adsorption on titanium surfaces. On the other hand, hydrophilic surfaces usually present more OH groups, higher surface charge, and SFE. These factors can promote surface–protein interactions, making adsorption favorable also on wettable surfaces. Furthermore, wettability can enhance solution-surface contact by turning it from a Cassie-Baxter to a Wenzel regime. These factors are able to promote protein adsorption against the generally accepted rule of thumb. The ongoing research on development of new and more bioactive surfaces had introduced more factors that can influence protein adsorption: The presence of ions within the oxide layer or of metals as alloying elements, the control over grain size, and surface activation treatments. All these features strongly change surface properties, namely wettability, hydroxylation, charge, SFE, roughness, making it less trivial to discriminate what features influence proteins adsorption and how. Conformation and orientation of adsorbed proteins are also heavily affected by surface properties in a non-unique way. Aspect ratio of surface features can change how proteins accommodate on the surface, higher hydroxylation may promote denaturation and spreading of certain proteins, while in other cases, OH groups increase wettability consequently reducing protein–surface interactions.

Besides, the poor standardization and use of testing protocols among researchers led to different conclusions about protein adsorption. The wide variety of protein concentrations, solution composition, and experimental methods make it very difficult to compare different works and to state if a system is an effective representation of the real adsorption process as occurring in vivo, within the human body. The complexity level of the system used can completely change how proteins interact with a surface, and scaling up from a simple single protein solution seems not to be an effective way to understand how materials behave when put in contact with biological fluids.

Table 3. Effect of titanium surface properties on protein adsorption (amount of adsorbed proteins, protein conformation on surface, and mechanism of protein–surface interaction) and impact of each feature on adsorption. ≈: no clear impact; ↑: mild impact; ↑↑: high impact; n.r.: effect not reported.

Surface Characteristic	Impact on Protein Adsorption	Conformation	Mechanism	Examples
Microroughness	↑	n.r.	Higher interaction area, physical adsorption	SLA surfaces adsorb fourfold more of albumin, fibronectin, fibrinogen and immunoglobulin vs. untreated surface because of roughness. Laser patterning increases adsorption of FIB.
Nanoroughness	≈	↑	Dependent on other characteristics. Aspect ratio of nanofeatures can influence protein conformation.	BSA aggregates into nanopores larger than its hydrodynamic radius with a strong interaction with the surface, while FN is too large. BSA/FIB adsorb as multilayer with stronger protein–protein interaction on nano-rough surfaces
Hydroxylation	↑↑	↑	According to the specific adsorbed proteins, OH can promote or hinder interaction with the surface	BSA adsorbs through hydrogen bonding and proton transfer with interaction with OH surface groups. FIB adsorbs through positive charged αC domains. Rutile adsorbs more COL, FN and BSA than anatase or amorphous titania due to higher OH density
SFE	↑↑	n.r.	High surface energy, in particular the polar component, increases adsorption	Ti adsorbs larger amount of plasma proteins vs. other metals with lower SFE, but TiO$_2$ adsorbs less proteins and in a weaker manner than other oxides with higher SFE. Ti adsorbs less basal lamina and salivary proteins than polymers for dentistry. Sandblasting with SiC induces higher SFE and preferential adsorption of FN. Laser patterning induces higher adsorption of FN by increasing the polar component of SFE. Nanograined surfaces have higher volumes of grain boundaries, which increase the SFE and adsorption of FN and VN
Charge	↑↑	↑	Can promote or limit protein adsorption, depending on charge of both surface and proteins	BSA is adsorbed in a lower amount on negatively charged surfaces while it is the opposite for histone that is positively charged. UV-generated positive surface can adsorb more BSA at pH 7, when the protein is negatively charged.
Chemistry (alloying metals, ions)	↑	n.r.	Increase protein adsorption, divalent ions in particular	TiNi alloys results in lower BSA (dependent on Ni content), FIB, and FN adsorption vs. cp-Ti. Ion-doped Ti has increased surface charge and protein adsorption because of bridging effect of divalent ions or specific chemical bonds (Ag)

161

Today, knowledge about protein adsorption on actual implant surface is also limited by the fact that it is not trivial to find characterization techniques that can provide information about adsorption mechanisms on real surfaces. In the literature, a lot of techniques have been used to investigate protein adsorption on titanium materials (see Table 2), but some of them may not be appliable on a bulky and surface treated titanium sample because they need specific characteristics, such as surface flatness, planar specimen or surfaces need to be grown on the instrument sensors. These kinds of model surfaces may not be representative of the surface of a real implant.

8. Conclusions

In conclusion, in the past 15 years, great efforts have been put into building deeper knowledge of how proteins and titanium-based biomaterials interact. Many different aspects of the complex adsorption phenomenon have been investigated by using a wide range of different surfaces, tailoring specific characteristics and exploiting adsorption environments ranging from a simple single protein solution to actual human biological fluids or even in human body. However, no generally accepted adsorption mechanisms have been found, with researchers sometimes being in disagreement about how surface properties or surface treatments affect protein adsorption. This can be ascribed to the absence of standardized and commonly used experimental protocols: protein concentration, adsorption condition and eventual rising methodology, all may alter the formation and evolution of the protein layer on materials surfaces. It is desirable that, in future, protein adsorption will be investigated through more common and shared methodology, obtaining comparable results. Furthermore, the researchers shall both study simple model systems and mimic, as close as possible, the physiological condition, as in case of protein concentration. This may be not trivial, but it allows comprehension of both very detailed aspects of the adsorption mechanisms and how actual implant surfaces will behave when employed as biomaterials. In parallel, further efforts have to be spent into development or optimization of the characterization techniques that can be applied on a wide range of materials in terms of sample shape and surface characteristics, mainly surface roughness. This is necessary for a correct evaluation of adsorption properties of biomaterials that may be actually employed as implants. Being extremely sensitive to surface features, protein–surface interactions may not be reproduced in an effective way on model surfaces.

In any case, according to the literature reviewed here, surface modifications that enhance adsorption of proteins, in particular adhesive ones such as fibronectin and vitronectin, are generally the same, which are able to increase cell proliferation and to promote osteoblast differentiation and in vivo bone integration. Deeper and better comprehension of protein adsorption will allow also a more efficient design of biomaterial surfaces, chasing the perfect implant.

Twenty years have passed since Imamura and co-workers described protein adsorption on solid surfaces as "a common but very complicated phenomenon" [239], and in this time, thousands of papers addressing this issue have been published. Nevertheless, protein adsorption is such a complex matter that a fully and comprehensive explanation of it is still missing. Research groups need to put further efforts to enlighten hidden aspects of protein adsorption and to put an end to the "quest for a universal mechanism" [240].

Author Contributions: J.B. wrote the first draft and participated the revision; S.S. participated in the drafting and revised its final version. All authors have read and agreed to the published version of the manuscript.

Funding: This research received no external funding.

Institutional Review Board Statement: Not applicable.

Informed Consent Statement: Not applicable.

Data Availability Statement: Not applicable.

Conflicts of Interest: The authors declare no conflict of interest.

References

1. Wilson, J. Metallic biomaterials: State of the art and new challenges. In *Fundamental Biomaterials: Metals*; Balakrishnan, P., Sreekala, M.S., Sabu, T., Eds.; Elsevier: Amsterdam, The Netherlands, 2018; pp. 1–33. ISBN 978-0-08-102206-1.
2. Oldani, C.; Dominguez, A. Titanium as a Biomaterial for Implants. In *Recent Advances in Arthroplasty*; InTech: Rijeka, Croatia, 2011.
3. Buser, D.; Janner, S.F.M.; Wittneben, J.G.; Brägger, U.; Ramseier, C.A.; Salvi, G.E. 10-Year Survival and Success Rates of 511 Titanium Implants with a Sandblasted and Acid-Etched Surface: A Retrospective Study in 303 Partially Edentulous Patients. *Clin. Implant Dent. Relat. Res.* **2012**, *14*, 839–851. [CrossRef]
4. Trindade, R.; Albrektsson, T.; Tengvall, P.; Wennerberg, A. Foreign Body Reaction to Biomaterials: On Mechanisms for Buildup and Breakdown of Osseointegration. *Clin. Implant Dent. Relat. Res.* **2016**, *18*, 192–203. [CrossRef]
5. Anderson, J.M.; Jiang, S. Implications of the Acute and Chronic Inflammatory Response and the Foreign Body Reaction to the Immune Response of Implanted Biomaterials. In *The Immune Response to Implanted Materials and Devices*; Corradetti, B., Ed.; Springer: Cham, Switzerland, 2016; ISBN 9783319454337.
6. Pegueroles, M.; Aguirre, A.; Engel, E.; Pavon, G.; Gil, F.J.; Planell, J.A.; Migonney, V.; Aparicio, C. Effect of blasting treatment and Fn coating on MG63 adhesion and differentiation on titanium: A gene expression study using real-time RT-PCR. *J. Mater. Sci. Mater. Med.* **2011**, *22*, 617–627. [CrossRef] [PubMed]
7. Sun, Y.S.; Chang, J.H.; Huang, H.H. Enhancing the biological response of titanium surface through the immobilization of bone morphogenetic protein-2 using the natural cross-linker genipin. *Surf. Coat. Technol.* **2016**, *303*, 289–297. [CrossRef]
8. Spriano, S.; Yamaguchi, S.; Baino, F.; Ferraris, S. A critical review of multifunctional titanium surfaces: New frontiers for improving osseointegration and host response, avoiding bacteria contamination. *Acta Biomater.* **2018**, *79*, 1–22. [CrossRef] [PubMed]
9. Norde, W. My voyage of discovery to proteins in flatland...and beyond. *Colloids Surf. B Biointerfaces* **2008**, *61*, 1–9. [CrossRef]
10. Yano, Y.F. Kinetics of protein unfolding at interfaces. *J. Phys. Condens. Matter* **2012**, *24*, 503101. [CrossRef] [PubMed]
11. Gray, J.J. The interaction of proteins with solid surfaces. *Curr. Opin. Struct. Biol.* **2004**, *14*, 110–115. [CrossRef]
12. Rabe, M.; Verdes, D.; Seeger, S. Understanding protein adsorption phenomena at solid surfaces. *Adv. Colloid Interface Sci.* **2011**, *162*, 87–106. [CrossRef]
13. Norde, W. Driving forces for protein adsorption at solid surfaces. *Macromol. Symp.* **1996**, *103*, 5–18. [CrossRef]
14. Vogler, E.A. Protein adsorption in three dimensions. *Biomaterials* **2012**, *33*, 1201–1237. [CrossRef]
15. Zheng, K.; Kapp, M.; Boccaccini, A.R. Protein interactions with bioactive glass surfaces: A review. *Appl. Mater. Today* **2019**, *15*, 350–371. [CrossRef]
16. Lee, W.H.; Loo, C.Y.; Rohanizadeh, R. A review of chemical surface modification of bioceramics: Effects on protein adsorption and cellular response. *Colloids Surf. B Biointerfaces* **2014**, *122*, 823–834. [CrossRef]
17. Hedberg, Y.; Wang, X.; Hedberg, J.; Lundin, M.; Blomberg, E.; Odnevall Wallinder, I. Surface-protein interactions on different stainless steel grades: Effects of protein adsorption, surface changes and metal release. *J. Mater. Sci. Mater. Med.* **2013**, *24*, 1015–1033. [CrossRef]
18. Höhn, S.; Virtanen, S.; Boccaccini, A.R. Protein adsorption on magnesium and its alloys: A review. *Appl. Surf. Sci.* **2019**, *464*, 212–219. [CrossRef]
19. Bhakta, S.A.; Evans, E.; Benavidez, T.E.; Garcia, C.D. Protein adsorption onto nanomaterials for the development of biosensors and analytical devices: A review. *Anal. Chim. Acta* **2015**, *872*, 7–25. [CrossRef] [PubMed]
20. Tsapikouni, T.S.; Missirlis, Y.F. Protein–material interactions: From micro-to-nano scale. *Mater. Sci. Eng. B* **2008**, *152*, 2–7. [CrossRef]
21. Godbey, W.T. Proteins. In *An Introduction to Biotechnology*; Elsevier: Amsterdam, The Netherlands, 2014; pp. 9–33. ISBN 9781907568282.
22. Czeslik, C. Factors Ruling Protein Adsorption. *Z. Phys. Chem.* **2004**, *218*, 771–801. [CrossRef]
23. Metwally, S.; Stachewicz, U. Surface potential and charges impact on cell responses on biomaterials interfaces for medical applications. *Mater. Sci. Eng. C* **2019**, *104*, 109883. [CrossRef] [PubMed]
24. Adair, J.H.; Suvaci, E.; Sindel, J. Surface and Colloid Chemistry. In *Encyclopedia of Materials: Science and Technology*; Elsevier: Amsterdam, The Netherlands, 2001; Volume 3, pp. 1–10.
25. Firkowska-Boden, I.; Zhang, X.; Jandt, K.D. Controlling Protein Adsorption through Nanostructured Polymeric Surfaces. *Adv. Healthc. Mater.* **2018**, *7*, 1–19. [CrossRef]
26. Felgueiras, H.P.; Antunes, J.C.; Martins, M.C.L.; Barbosa, M.A. *Fundamentals of Protein and Cell Interactions in Biomaterials*; Elsevier: Amsterdam, The Netherlands, 2018; ISBN 9780081008522.
27. Vogler, E.A. Structure and reactivity of water at biomaterial surfaces. *Adv. Colloid Interface Sci.* **1998**, *74*, 69–117. [CrossRef]
28. Xu, L.C.; Siedlecki, C.A. Effects of surface wettability and contact time on protein adhesion to biomaterial surfaces. *Biomaterials* **2007**, *28*, 3273–3283. [CrossRef] [PubMed]
29. Michael, K.E.; Vernekar, V.N.; Keselowsky, B.G.; Meredith, J.C.; Latour, R.A.; García, A.J. Adsorption-induced conformational changes in fibronectin due to interactions with well-defined surface chemistries. *Langmuir* **2003**, *19*, 8033–8040. [CrossRef]

30. Roach, P.; Farrar, D.; Perry, C.C. Interpretation of protein adsorption: Surface-induced conformational changes. *J. Am. Chem. Soc.* **2005**, *127*, 8168–8173. [CrossRef]
31. Isoshima, K.; Ueno, T.; Arai, Y.; Saito, H.; Chen, P.; Tsutsumi, Y.; Hanawa, T.; Wakabayashi, N. The change of surface charge by lithium ion coating enhances protein adsorption on titanium. *J. Mech. Behav. Biomed. Mater.* **2019**, *100*, 103393. [CrossRef]
32. Kubiak-Ossowska, K.; Jachimska, B.; Al Qaraghuli, M.; Mulheran, P.A. Protein interactions with negatively charged inorganic surfaces. *Curr. Opin. Colloid Interface Sci.* **2019**, *41*, 104–117. [CrossRef]
33. Xie, H.G.; Li, X.X.; Lv, G.J.; Xie, W.Y.; Zhu, J.; Luxbacher, T.; Ma, R.; Ma, X.J. Effect of surface wettability and charge on protein adsorption onto implantable alginate-chitosan-alginate microcapsule surfaces. *J. Biomed. Mater. Res. Part A* **2010**, *92*, 1357–1365. [CrossRef]
34. Bousnaki, M.; Koidis, P. Advances on Biomedical Titanium Surface Interactions. *J. Biomim. Biomater. Tissue Eng.* **2014**, *19*, 43–64. [CrossRef]
35. Rechendorff, K.; Hovgaard, M.B.; Foss, M.; Zhdanov, V.P.; Besenbacher, F. Enhancement of protein adsorption induced by surface roughness. *Langmuir* **2006**, *22*, 10885–10888. [CrossRef]
36. Fernández-Montes Moraleda, B.; Román, J.S.; Rodríguez-Lorenzo, L.M. Influence of surface features of hydroxyapatite on the adsorption of proteins relevant to bone regeneration. *J. Biomed. Mater. Res. Part A* **2013**, *101A*, 2332–2339. [CrossRef]
37. Yu, L.; Zhang, L.; Sun, Y. Protein behavior at surfaces: Orientation, conformational transitions and transport. *J. Chromatogr. A* **2015**, *1382*, 118–134. [CrossRef]
38. Zhao, A.; Wang, Z.; Zhou, S.; Xue, G.; Wang, Y.; Ye, C.; Huang, N. Titanium oxide films with vacuum thermal treatment for enhanced hemocompatibility. *Surf. Eng.* **2015**, *31*, 898–903. [CrossRef]
39. Lee, E.-J.; Kwon, J.-S.; Om, J.-Y.; Moon, S.-K.; Uhm, S.-H.; Choi, E.H.; Kim, K.-N. The enhanced integrin-mediated cell attachment and osteogenic gene expression on atmospheric pressure plasma jet treated micro-structured titanium surfaces. *Curr. Appl. Phys.* **2014**, *14*, S167–S171. [CrossRef]
40. Blanco, A.; Blanco, G. Proteins. In *Medical Biochemistry*; Elsevier: Amsterdam, The Netherlands, 2017; pp. 21–71. ISBN 978-0-12-803550-4.
41. Bharti, B. *Adsorption, Aggregation and Structure Formation in Systems of Charged Particles*; Springer Theses; Springer International Publishing: Cham, Switzerland, 2014; ISBN 978-3-319-07736-9.
42. Li, R.; Wu, Z.; Wangb, Y.; Ding, L.; Wang, Y. Role of pH-induced structural change in protein aggregation in foam fractionation of bovine serum albumin. *Biotechnol. Rep.* **2016**, *9*, 46–52. [CrossRef] [PubMed]
43. Barnthip, N.; Parhi, P.; Golas, A.; Vogler, E.A. Volumetric interpretation of protein adsorption: Kinetics of protein-adsorption competition from binary solution. *Biomaterials* **2009**, *30*, 6495–6513. [CrossRef] [PubMed]
44. Kopac, T.; Bozgeyik, K.; Yener, J. Effect of pH and temperature on the adsorption of bovine serum albumin onto titanium dioxide. *Colloids Surf. A Physicochem. Eng. Asp.* **2008**, *322*, 19–28. [CrossRef]
45. Valero Vidal, C.; Olmo Juan, A.; Igual Muñoz, A. Adsorption of bovine serum albumin on CoCrMo surface: Effect of temperature and protein concentration. *Colloids Surf. B Biointerfaces* **2010**, *80*, 1–11. [CrossRef] [PubMed]
46. Kubiak-Ossowska, K.; Cwieka, M.; Kaczynska, A.; Jachimska, B.; Mulheran, P.A. Lysozyme adsorption at a silica surface using simulation and experiment: Effects of pH on protein layer structure. *Phys. Chem. Chem. Phys.* **2015**, *17*, 24070–24077. [CrossRef] [PubMed]
47. Tercinier, L.; Ye, A.; Singh, A.; Anema, S.G.; Singh, H. Effects of Ionic Strength, pH and Milk Serum Composition on Adsorption of Milk Proteins on to Hydroxyapatite Particles. *Food Biophys.* **2014**, *9*, 341–348. [CrossRef]
48. Wei, T.; Kaewtathip, S.; Shing, K. Buffer Effect on Protein Adsorption at Liquid/Solid Interface. *J. Phys. Chem. C* **2009**, *113*, 2053–2062. [CrossRef]
49. Gondim, D.R.; Cecilia, J.A.; Santos, S.O.; Rodrigues, T.N.B.; Aguiar, J.E.; Vilarrasa-García, E.; Rodríguez-Castellón, E.; Azevedo, D.C.S.; Silva, I.J. Influence of buffer solutions in the adsorption of human serum proteins onto layered double hydroxide. *Int. J. Biol. Macromol.* **2018**, *106*, 396–409. [CrossRef]
50. Wilhelmi, M.; Müller, C.; Ziegler, C.; Kopnarski, M. BSA adsorption on titanium: ToF-SIMS investigation of the surface coverage as a function of protein concentration and pH-value. *Anal. Bioanal. Chem.* **2011**, *400*, 697–701. [CrossRef]
51. Hanawa, T. Titanium-tissue interface reaction and its control with surface treatment. *Front. Bioeng. Biotechnol.* **2019**, *7*. [CrossRef] [PubMed]
52. Brunette, D.M.; Tengvall, P.; Textor, M.; Thomsen, P. (Eds.) *Titanium in Medicine*, 1st ed; Engineering Materials; Springer: Berlin/Heidelberg, Germany, 2001; ISBN 978-3-642-63119-1.
53. Textor, M.; Sittig, C.; Frauchiger, V.; Tosatti, S.; Brunette, D. Properties and Biological Significance of Natural Oxide Films on Titanium and Its Alloys. In *Titanium in Medicine*; Brunette, D.M., Tengvall, P., Textor, M., Thomsen, P., Eds.; Springer: Berlin/Heidelberg, Germany, 2001.
54. Ferraris, S.; Cazzola, M.; Peretti, V.; Stella, B.; Spriano, S. Zeta potential measurements on solid surfaces for in Vitro biomaterials testing: Surface charge, reactivity upon contact with fluids and protein absorption. *Front. Bioeng. Biotechnol.* **2018**, *6*, 1–7. [CrossRef] [PubMed]
55. Watanabe, K.; Okawa, S.; Kanatani, M.; Homma, K. Surface analysis of commercially pure titanium implant retrieved from rat bone. part 1: Initial biological response of sandblasted surface. *Dent. Mater. J.* **2009**, *28*, 178–184. [CrossRef] [PubMed]

56. Ionita, D.; Popescu, R.; Tite, T.; Demetrescu, I. The Behaviour of Pure Titanium in Albumin Solution. *Mol. Cryst. Liq. Cryst.* **2008**, *486*, 166–174. [CrossRef]
57. Cámara, O.R.; Avalle, L.B.; Oliva, F.Y. Protein adsorption on titanium dioxide: Effects on double layer and semiconductor space charge region studied by EIS. *Electrochim. Acta* **2010**, *55*, 4519–4528. [CrossRef]
58. Van De Keere, I.; Willaert, R.; Hubin, A.; Vereecken, J. Interaction of human plasma fibrinogen with commercially pure titanium as studied with atomic force microscopy and X-ray photoelectron spectroscopy. *Langmuir* **2008**, *24*, 1844–1852. [CrossRef]
59. Kohavi, D.; Badihi Hauslich, L.; Rosen, G.; Steinberg, D.; Sela, M.N. Wettability versus electrostatic forces in fibronectin and albumin adsorption to titanium surfaces. *Clin. Oral Implant. Res.* **2013**, *24*, 1002–1008. [CrossRef]
60. Imamura, K.; Shimomura, M.; Nagai, S.; Akamatsu, M.; Nakanishi, K. Adsorption characteristics of various proteins to a titanium surface. *J. Biosci. Bioeng.* **2008**, *106*, 273–278. [CrossRef]
61. Oliva, F.Y.; Cámara, O.R.; Avalle, L.B. Adsorption of human serum albumin on electrochemical titanium dioxide electrodes: Protein–oxide surface interaction effects studied by electrochemical techniques. *J. Electroanal. Chem.* **2009**, *633*, 19–34. [CrossRef]
62. Kang, Y.; Li, X.; Tu, Y.; Wang, Q.; Ågren, H. On the Mechanism of Protein Adsorption onto Hydroxylated and Nonhydroxylated TiO 2 Surfaces. *J. Phys. Chem. C* **2010**, *114*, 14496–14502. [CrossRef]
63. Mao, C.M.; Sampath, J.; Sprenger, K.G.; Drobny, G.; Pfaendtner, J. Molecular Driving Forces in Peptide Adsorption to Metal Oxide Surfaces. *Langmuir* **2019**, *35*, 5911–5920. [CrossRef]
64. Sun, T.; Han, G.; Lindgren, M.; Shen, Z.; Laaksonen, A. Adhesion of lactoferrin and bone morphogenetic protein-2 to a rutile surface: Dependence on the surface hydrophobicity. *Biomater. Sci.* **2014**, *2*, 1090–1099. [CrossRef] [PubMed]
65. Utesch, T.; Daminelli, G.; Mroginski, M.A. Molecular dynamics simulations of the adsorption of bone morphogenetic protein-2 on surfaces with medical relevance. *Langmuir* **2011**, *27*, 13144–13153. [CrossRef] [PubMed]
66. Yang, Q.; Zhang, Y.; Liu, M.; Ye, M.; Zhang, Y.; Yao, S. Study of fibrinogen adsorption on hydroxyapatite and TiO2 surfaces by electrochemical piezoelectric quartz crystal impedance and FTIR–ATR spectroscopy. *Anal. Chim. Acta* **2007**, *597*, 58–66. [CrossRef]
67. Zhao, A.; Wang, Z.; Zhu, X.; Maitz, M.F.; Huang, N. Real-Time Characterization of Fibrinogen Interaction with Modified Titanium Dioxide Film by Quartz Crystal Microbalance with Dissipation. *Chin. J. Chem. Phys.* **2014**, *27*, 355–360. [CrossRef]
68. Moulton, S.E.; Barisci, J.N.; Bath, A.; Stella, R.; Wallace, G.G. Investigation of Ig.G adsorption and the effect on electrochemical responses at titanium dioxide electrode. *Langmuir* **2005**, *21*, 316–322. [CrossRef] [PubMed]
69. Bouhekka, A.; Bürgi, T. In situ ATR-IR spectroscopy study of adsorbed protein: Visible light denaturation of bovine serum albumin on TiO 2. *Appl. Surf. Sci.* **2012**, *261*, 369–374. [CrossRef]
70. Van De Keere, I.; Willaert, R.; Tourwé, E.; Hubin, A.; Vereecken, J. The interaction of human serum albumin with titanium studied by means of atomic force microscopy. *Surf. Interface Anal.* **2008**, *40*, 157–161. [CrossRef]
71. Wesełucha-Birczyńska, A.; Stodolak-Zych, E.; Piś, W.; Długoń, E.; Benko, A.; Błażewicz, M. A model of adsorption of albumin on the implant surface titanium and titanium modified carbon coatings (MWCNT-EPD). 2D correlation analysis. *J. Mol. Struct.* **2016**, *1124*, 61–70. [CrossRef]
72. Zhang, H.P.; Lu, X.; Fang, L.M.; Weng, J.; Huang, N.; Leng, Y. Molecular dynamics simulation of RGD peptide adsorption on titanium oxide surfaces. *J. Mater. Sci. Mater. Med.* **2008**, *19*, 3437–3441. [CrossRef]
73. Deligianni, D.D.; Katsala, N.; Ladas, S.; Sotiropoulou, D.; Amedee, J.; Missirlis, Y.F. Effect of surface roughness of the titanium alloy Ti-6Al-4V on human bone marrow cell response and on protein adsorption. *Biomaterials* **2001**, *22*, 1241–1251. [CrossRef]
74. Kopf, B.S.; Ruch, S.; Berner, S.; Spencer, N.D.; Maniura-Weber, K. The role of nanostructures and hydrophilicity in osseointegration: In-vitro protein-adsorption and blood-interaction studies. *J. Biomed. Mater. Res. Part A* **2015**, *103*, 2661–2672. [CrossRef] [PubMed]
75. Cai, K.; Bossert, J.; Jandt, K.D. Does the nanometre scale topography of titanium influence protein adsorption and cell proliferation? *Colloids Surf. B Biointerfaces* **2006**, *49*, 136–144. [CrossRef] [PubMed]
76. Rockwell, G.P.; Lohstreter, L.B.; Dahn, J.R. Fibrinogen and albumin adsorption on titanium nanoroughness gradients. *Colloids Surfaces B Biointerfaces* **2012**, *91*, 90–96. [CrossRef]
77. Lu, J.; Yao, C.; Yang, L.; Webster, T.J. Decreased Platelet Adhesion and Enhanced Endothelial Cell Functions on Nano and Submicron-Rough Titanium Stents. *Tissue Eng. Part A* **2012**, *18*, 1389–1398. [CrossRef]
78. Kopac, T.; Bozgeyik, K. Effect of surface area enhancement on the adsorption of bovine serum albumin onto titanium dioxide. *Colloids Surf. B Biointerfaces* **2010**, *76*, 265–271. [CrossRef]
79. Liu, L.; Bhatia, R.; Webster, T. Atomic layer deposition of nano-TiO2 thin films with enhanced biocompatibility and antimicrobial activity for orthopedic implants. *Int. J. Nanomed.* **2017**, *12*, 8711–8723. [CrossRef]
80. Scopelliti, P.E.; Borgonovo, A.; Indrieri, M.; Giorgetti, L.; Bongiorno, G.; Carbone, R.; Podestà, A.; Milani, P. The Effect of Surface Nanometre-Scale Morphology on Protein Adsorption. *PLoS ONE* **2010**, *5*, e11862. [CrossRef] [PubMed]
81. Liu, C.; Guo, Y.; Hong, Q.; Rao, C.; Zhang, H.; Dong, Y.; Huang, L.; Lu, X.; Bao, N. Bovine Serum Albumin Adsorption in Mesoporous Titanium Dioxide: Pore Size and Pore Chemistry Effect. *Langmuir* **2016**, *32*, 3995–4003. [CrossRef] [PubMed]
82. An, R.; Zhuang, W.; Yang, Z.; Lu, X.; Zhu, J.; Wang, Y.; Dong, Y.; Wu, N. Protein adsorptive behavior on mesoporous titanium dioxide determined by geometrical topography. *Chem. Eng. Sci.* **2014**, *117*, 146–155. [CrossRef]
83. Singh, A.V.; Vyas, V.; Patil, R.; Sharma, V.; Scopelliti, P.E.; Bongiorno, G.; Podestà, A.; Lenardi, C.; Gade, W.N.; Milani, P. Quantitative Characterization of the Influence of the Nanoscale Morphology of Nanostructured Surfaces on Bacterial Adhesion and Biofilm Formation. *PLoS ONE* **2011**, *6*, e25029. [CrossRef] [PubMed]

84. Selvakumaran, J.; Keddie, J.L.; Ewins, D.J.; Hughes, M.P. Protein adsorption on materials for recording sites on implantable microelectrodes. *J. Mater. Sci. Mater. Med.* **2008**, *19*, 143–151. [CrossRef] [PubMed]
85. Silva-Bermudez, P.; Rodil, S.E.; Muhl, S. Albumin adsorption on oxide thin films studied by spectroscopic ellipsometry. *Appl. Surf. Sci.* **2011**, *258*, 1711–1718. [CrossRef]
86. Silva-Bermudez, P.; Muhl, S.; Rodil, S.E. A comparative study of fibrinogen adsorption onto metal oxide thin films. *Appl. Surf. Sci.* **2013**, *282*, 351–362. [CrossRef]
87. Arvidsson, S.; Askendal, A.; Tengvall, P. Blood plasma contact activation on silicon, titanium and aluminium. *Biomaterials* **2007**, *28*, 1346–1354. [CrossRef]
88. Song, L.; Yang, K.; Jiang, W.; Du, P.; Xing, B. Adsorption of bovine serum albumin on nano and bulk oxide particles in deionized water. *Colloids Surf. B Biointerfaces* **2012**, *94*, 341–346. [CrossRef]
89. Yoshida, E.; Hayakawa, T. Adsorption Analysis of Lactoferrin to Titanium, Stainless Steel, Zirconia, and Polymethyl Methacrylate Using the Quartz Crystal Microbalance Method. *BioMed Res. Int.* **2016**, *2016*, 1–7. [CrossRef]
90. Abdallah, M.-N.; Abughanam, G.; Tran, S.D.; Sheikh, Z.; Mezour, M.A.; Basiri, T.; Xiao, Y.; Cerruti, M.; Siqueira, W.L.; Tamimi, F. Comparative adsorption profiles of basal lamina proteome and gingival cells onto dental and titanium surfaces. *Acta Biomater.* **2018**, *73*, 547–558. [CrossRef]
91. Schweikl, H.; Hiller, K.-A.; Carl, U.; Schweiger, R.; Eidt, A.; Ruhl, S.; Müller, R.; Schmalz, G. Salivary protein adsorption and Streptococccus gordonii adhesion to dental material surfaces. *Dent. Mater.* **2013**, *29*, 1080–1089. [CrossRef]
92. Miyake, A.; Komasa, S.; Hashimoto, Y.; Komasa, Y.; Okazaki, J. Adsorption of Saliva Related Protein on Denture Materials: An X-Ray Photoelectron Spectroscopy and Quartz Crystal Microbalance Study. *Adv. Mater. Sci. Eng.* **2016**, *2016*, 1–9. [CrossRef]
93. Müller, C.; Lüders, A.; Hoth-Hannig, W.; Hannig, M.; Ziegler, C. Initial bioadhesion on dental materials as a function of contact time, pH, surface wettability, and isoelectric point. *Langmuir* **2010**, *26*, 4136–4141. [CrossRef]
94. Kohavi, D.; Badihi, L.; Rosen, G.; Steinberg, D.; Sela, M.N. An in vivo method for measuring the adsorption of plasma proteins to titanium in humans. *Biofouling* **2013**, *29*, 1215–1224. [CrossRef]
95. Sela, M.N.; Badihi, L.; Rosen, G.; Steinberg, D.; Kohavi, D. Adsorption of human plasma proteins to modified titanium surfaces. *Clin. Oral Implant. Res.* **2007**, *18*, 630–638. [CrossRef] [PubMed]
96. Parisi, L.; Toffoli, A.; Cutrera, M.; Bianchi, M.G.; Lumetti, S.; Bussolati, O.; Macaluso, G.M. Plasma Proteins at the Interface of Dental Implants Modulate Osteoblasts Focal Adhesions Expression and Cytoskeleton Organization. *Nanomaterials* **2019**, *9*, 1407. [CrossRef] [PubMed]
97. Huang, Y.; Zha, G.; Luo, Q.; Zhang, J.; Zhang, F.; Li, X.; Zhao, S.; Zhu, W.; Li, X. The construction of hierarchical structure on Ti substrate with superior osteogenic activity and intrinsic antibacterial capability. *Sci. Rep.* **2015**, *4*, 6172. [CrossRef]
98. Ferraris, S.; Bobbio, A.; Miola, M.; Spriano, S. Micro- and nano-textured, hydrophilic and bioactive titanium dental implants. *Surf. Coat. Technol.* **2015**, *276*, 374–383. [CrossRef]
99. Lu, X.; Xiong, S.; Chen, Y.; Zhao, F.; Hu, Y.; Guo, Y.; Wu, B.; Huang, P.; Yang, B. Effects of statherin on the biological properties of titanium metals subjected to different surface modification. *Colloids Surf. B Biointerfaces* **2020**, *188*, 110783. [CrossRef]
100. Pegueroles, M.; Aparicio, C.; Bosio, M.; Engel, E.; Gil, F.J.; Planell, J.A.; Altankov, G. Spatial organization of osteoblast fibronectin matrix on titanium surfaces: Effects of roughness, chemical heterogeneity and surface energy. *Acta Biomater.* **2010**, *6*, 291–301. [CrossRef] [PubMed]
101. Mussano, F.; Genova, T.; Laurenti, M.; Gaglioti, D.; Scarpellino, G.; Rivolo, P.; Faga, M.G.; Fiorio, P.A.; Munaron, L.; Mandracci, P.; et al. Beta1-integrin and TRPV4 are involved in osteoblast adhesion to different titanium surface topographies. *Appl. Surf. Sci.* **2020**, *507*, 145112. [CrossRef]
102. Toffoli, A.; Parisi, L.; Bianchi, M.G.; Lumetti, S.; Bussolati, O.; Macaluso, G.M. Thermal treatment to increase titanium wettability induces selective proteins adsorption from blood serum thus affecting osteoblasts adhesion. *Mater. Sci. Eng. C* **2020**, *107*, 110250. [CrossRef] [PubMed]
103. Tugulu, S.; Löwe, K.; Scharnweber, D.; Schlottig, F. Preparation of superhydrophilic microrough titanium implant surfaces by alkali treatment. *J. Mater. Sci. Mater. Med.* **2010**, *21*, 2751–2763. [CrossRef]
104. Martínez-Hernández, M.; García-Pérez, V.I.; Almaguer-Flores, A. Potential of salivary proteins to reduce oral bacterial colonization on titanium implant surfaces. *Mater. Lett.* **2019**, *252*, 120–122. [CrossRef]
105. Richert, L.; Variola, F.; Rosei, F.; Wuest, J.D.; Nanci, A. Adsorption of proteins on nanoporous Ti surfaces. *Surf. Sci.* **2010**, *604*, 1445–1451. [CrossRef]
106. Lee, M.H.; Oh, N.; Lee, S.W.; Leesungbok, R.; Kim, S.E.; Yun, Y.P.; Kang, J.H. Factors influencing osteoblast maturation on microgrooved titanium substrata. *Biomaterials* **2010**, *31*, 3804–3815. [CrossRef]
107. Sakamoto, Y.; Ayukawa, Y.; Furuhashi, A.; Kamo, M.; Ikeda, J.; Atsuta, I.; Haraguchi, T.; Koyano, K. Effect of hydrothermal treatment with distilled water on titanium alloy for epithelial cellular attachment. *Materials* **2019**, *12*, 2748. [CrossRef]
108. Yoneyama, Y.; Matsuno, T.; Hashimoto, Y.; Satoh, T. In vitro evaluation of H2O2 hydrothermal treatment of aged titanium surface to enhance biofunctional activity. *Dent. Mater. J.* **2013**, *32*, 115–121. [CrossRef]
109. Yang, J.; Wang, J.; Yuan, T.; Zhu, X.D.; Xiang, Z.; Fan, Y.J.; Zhang, X.D. The enhanced effect of surface microstructured porous titanium on adhesion and osteoblastic differentiation of mesenchymal stem cells. *J. Mater. Sci. Mater. Med.* **2013**, *24*, 2235–2246. [CrossRef]

110. Sousa, S.R.; Brás, M.M.; Moradas-Ferreira, P.; Barbosa, M.A. Dynamics of Fibronectin Adsorption on TiO 2 Surfaces. *Langmuir* **2007**, *23*, 7046–7054. [CrossRef] [PubMed]
111. Sousa, S.R.; Lamghari, M.; Sampaio, P.; Moradas-Ferreira, P.; Barbosa, M.A. Osteoblast adhesion and morphology on TiO2 depends on the competitive preadsorption of albumin and fibronectin. *J. Biomed. Matter. Res. A.* **2008**, *84*, 281–290. [CrossRef]
112. Zeng, Y.; Yang, Y.; Chen, L.; Yin, D.; Zhang, H.; Tashiro, Y.; Inui, S.; Kusumoto, T.; Nishizaki, H.; Sekino, T.; et al. Optimized Surface Characteristics and Enhanced in Vivo Osseointegration of Alkali-Treated Titanium with Nanonetwork Structures. *Int. J. Mol. Sci.* **2019**, *20*, 1127. [CrossRef] [PubMed]
113. Xiao, M.; Biao, M.; Chen, Y.; Xie, M.; Yang, B. Regulating the osteogenic function of rhBMP 2 by different titanium surface properties. *J. Biomed. Mater. Res. Part A* **2016**, *104*, 1882–1893. [CrossRef]
114. Hu, X.N.; Yang, B.C. Conformation change of bovine serum albumin induced by bioactive titanium metals and its effects on cell behaviors. *J. Biomed. Mater. Res. Part A* **2014**, *102*, 1053–1062. [CrossRef]
115. Biao, M.N.; Chen, Y.M.; Xiong, S.B.; Wu, B.Y.; Yang, B.C. Synergistic effects of fibronectin and bone morphogenetic protein on the bioactivity of titanium metal. *J. Biomed. Mater. Res. Part A* **2017**, *105*, 2485–2498. [CrossRef] [PubMed]
116. Jia, S.; Zhang, Y.; Ma, T.; Chen, H.; Lin, Y. Enhanced hydrophilicity and protein adsorption of titanium surface by sodium bicarbonate solution. *J. Nanomater.* **2015**, *2015*. [CrossRef]
117. Chen, Y.; Feng, B.; Zhu, Y.; Weng, J.; Wang, J.; Lu, X. Preparation and characterization of a novel porous titanium scaffold with 3D hierarchical porous structures. *J. Mater. Sci. Mater. Med.* **2011**, *22*, 839–844. [CrossRef] [PubMed]
118. Yao, Y.; Liu, S.; Swain, M.V.; Zhang, X.; Zhao, K.; Jian, Y. Effects of acid-alkali treatment on bioactivity and osteoinduction of porous titanium: An in vitro study. *Mater. Sci. Eng. C* **2019**, *94*, 200–210. [CrossRef]
119. Yu, P.; Zhu, X.; Wang, X.; Wang, S.; Li, W.; Tan, G.; Zhang, Y.; Ning, C. Periodic Nanoneedle and Buffer Zones Constructed on a Titanium Surface Promote Osteogenic Differentiation and Bone Calcification In Vivo. *Adv. Healthc. Mater.* **2016**, *5*, 364–372. [CrossRef]
120. Rani, V.V.D.; Manzoor, K.; Menon, D.; Selvamurugan, N.; Nair, S.V. The design of novel nanostructures on titanium by solution chemistry for an improved osteoblast response. *Nanotechnology* **2009**, *20*, 195101. [CrossRef]
121. Manivasagam, V.K.; Popat, K.C. In Vitro Investigation of Hemocompatibility of Hydrothermally Treated Titanium and Titanium Alloy Surfaces. *ACS Omega* **2020**, *5*, 8108–8120. [CrossRef]
122. Qian, L.; Yu, P.; Zeng, J.; Shi, Z.; Wang, Q.; Tan, G.; Ning, C. Large-scale functionalization of biomedical porous titanium scaffolds surface with TiO2 nanostructures. *Sci. China Mater.* **2018**, *61*, 557–564. [CrossRef]
123. Shi, J.; Feng, B.; Lu, X.; Weng, J. Adsorption of bovine serum albumin onto titanium dioxide nanotube arrays. *Int. J. Mater. Res.* **2012**, *103*, 889–896. [CrossRef]
124. Zhao, D.P.; Tang, J.C.; Nie, H.M.; Zhang, Y.; Chen, Y.K.; Zhang, X.; Li, H.X.; Yan, M. Macro-micron-nano-featured surface topography of Ti-6Al-4V alloy for biomedical applications. *Rare Met.* **2018**, *37*, 1055–1063. [CrossRef]
125. Yang, W.; Xi, X.; Shen, X.; Liu, P.; Hu, Y.; Cai, K. Titania nanotubes dimensions-dependent protein adsorption and its effect on the growth of osteoblasts. *J. Biomed. Mater. Res. Part A* **2014**, *102*, 3598–3608. [CrossRef]
126. Jia, E.; Zhao, X.; Lin, Y.; Su, Z. Protein adsorption on titanium substrates and its effects on platelet adhesion. *Appl. Surf. Sci.* **2020**, *529*, 146986. [CrossRef]
127. Yang, W.; Xi, X.; Ran, Q.; Liu, P.; Hu, Y.; Cai, K. Influence of the titania nanotubes dimensions on adsorption of collagen: An experimental and computational study. *Mater. Sci. Eng. C* **2014**, *34*, 410–416. [CrossRef]
128. Kulkarni, M.; Mazare, A.; Park, J.; Gongadze, E.; Killian, M.S.; Kralj, S.; von der Mark, K.; Iglič, A.; Schmuki, P. Protein interactions with layers of TiO2 nanotube and nanopore arrays: Morphology and surface charge influence. *Acta Biomater.* **2016**, *45*, 357–366. [CrossRef] [PubMed]
129. Sabino, R.M.; Kauk, K.; Movafaghi, S.; Kota, A.; Popat, K.C. Interaction of blood plasma proteins with superhemophobic titania nanotube surfaces. *Nanomed. Nanotechnol. Biol. Med.* **2019**, *21*, 102046. [CrossRef]
130. Wu, S.; Zhang, D.; Bai, J.; Zheng, H.; Deng, J.; Gou, Z.; Gao, C. Adsorption of serum proteins on titania nanotubes and its role on regulating adhesion and migration of mesenchymal stem cells. *J. Biomed. Mater. Res. Part A* **2020**, *108*, 2305–2318. [CrossRef]
131. Lu, R.; Wang, C.; Wang, X.; Wang, Y.; Wang, N.; Chou, J.; Li, T.; Zhang, Z.; Ling, Y.; Chen, S. Effects of hydrogenated TiO2 nanotube arrays on protein adsorption and compatibility with osteoblast-like cells. *Int. J. Nanomed.* **2018**, *13*, 2037–2049. [CrossRef]
132. Teng, F.; Li, J.; Wu, Y.; Chen, H.; Zhang, Q.; Wang, H.; Ou, G. Fabrication and bioactivity evaluation of porous anodised TiO2 films in vitro. *Biosci. Trends* **2014**, *8*, 260–265. [CrossRef]
133. Yang, W.-E.; Huang, H.-H. Multiform TiO2 nano-network enhances biological response to titanium surface for dental implant applications. *Appl. Surf. Sci.* **2019**, *471*, 1041–1052. [CrossRef]
134. Ning, C.; Wang, S.; Zhu, Y.; Zhong, M.; Lin, X.; Zhang, Y.; Tan, G.; Li, M.; Yin, Z.; Yu, P.; et al. Ti nanorod arrays with a medium density significantly promote osteogenesis and osteointegration. *Sci. Rep.* **2016**, *6*, 19047. [CrossRef] [PubMed]
135. Bayrak, Ö.; Ghahramanzadeh Asl, H.; Ak, A. Protein adsorption, cell viability and corrosion properties of Ti6Al4V alloy treated by plasma oxidation and anodic oxidation. *Int. J. Miner. Metall. Mater.* **2020**, *27*, 1269–1280. [CrossRef]
136. Lin, D.J.; Fuh, L.J.; Chen, W.C. Nano-morphology, crystallinity and surface potential of anatase on micro-arc oxidized titanium affect its protein adsorption, cell proliferation and cell differentiation. *Mater. Sci. Eng. C* **2020**, *107*, 110204. [CrossRef] [PubMed]
137. Fadlallah, S.A.; Amin, M.A.; Alosaimi, G.S. Construction of Nanophase Novel Coatings-Based Titanium for the Enhancement of Protein Adsorption. *Acta Metall. Sin. Eng. Let.* **2016**, *29*, 243–252. [CrossRef]

138. Kuczyńska, D.; Kwaśniak, P.; Pisarek, M.; Borowicz, P.; Garbacz, H. Influence of surface pattern on the biological properties of Ti grade 2. *Mater. Charact.* **2018**, *135*, 337–347. [CrossRef]
139. Dumas, V.; Guignandon, A.; Vico, L.; Mauclair, C.; Zapata, X.; Linossier, M.T.; Bouleftour, W.; Granier, J.; Peyroche, S.; Dumas, J.C.; et al. Femtosecond laser nano/micro patterning of titanium influences mesenchymal stem cell adhesion and commitment. *Biomed. Mater.* **2015**, *10*, 055002. [CrossRef]
140. Mukherjee, S.; Dhara, S.; Saha, P. Enhancing the biocompatibility of Ti6Al4V implants by laser surface microtexturing: An in vitro study. *Int. J. Adv. Manuf. Technol.* **2015**, *76*, 5–15. [CrossRef]
141. Hao, L.; Lawrence, J. Wettability modification and the subsequent manipulation of protein adsorption on a Ti6Al4V alloy by means of CO2 laser surface treatment. *J. Mater. Sci. Mater. Med.* **2007**, *18*, 807–817. [CrossRef] [PubMed]
142. Parmar, V.; Kumar, A.; Mani Sankar, M.; Datta, S.; Vijaya Prakash, G.; Mohanty, S.; Kalyanasundaram, D. Oxidation facilitated antimicrobial ability of laser micro-textured titanium alloy against gram-positive Staphylococcus aureus for biomedical applications. *J. Laser Appl.* **2018**, *30*, 032001. [CrossRef]
143. Kuczyńska, D.; Kwaśniak, P.; Marczak, J.; Bonarski, J.; Smolik, J.; Garbacz, H. Laser surface treatment and the resultant hierarchical topography of Ti grade 2 for biomedical application. *Appl. Surf. Sci.* **2016**, *390*, 560–569. [CrossRef]
144. Clarke, B.; Kingshott, P.; Hou, X.; Rochev, Y.; Gorelov, A.; Carroll, W. Effect of nitinol wire surface properties on albumin adsorption. *Acta Biomater.* **2007**, *3*, 103–111. [CrossRef] [PubMed]
145. Michiardi, A.; Aparicio, C.; Ratner, B.D.; Planell, J.A.; Gil, J. The influence of surface energy on competitive protein adsorption on oxidized NiTi surfaces. *Biomaterials* **2007**, *28*, 586–594. [CrossRef] [PubMed]
146. Bai, Z.; Filiaggi, M.J.; Sanderson, R.J.; Lohstreter, L.B.; McArthur, M.A.; Dahn, J.R. Surface characteristics and protein adsorption on combinatorial binary Ti-M (Cr, Al, Ni) and Al-M (Ta, Zr) library films. *J. Biomed. Mater. Res. Part A* **2010**, *92*, 521–532. [CrossRef]
147. Bai, Z.; Filiaggi, M.J.; Dahn, J.R. Fibrinogen adsorption onto 316L stainless steel, Nitinol and titanium. *Surf. Sci.* **2009**, *603*, 839–846. [CrossRef]
148. Lefaix, H.; Galtayries, A.; Prima, F.; Marcus, P. Nano-size protein at the surface of a Ti–Zr–Ni quasi-crystalline alloy: Fibronectin adsorption on metallic nano-composites. *Colloids Surf. A Physicochem. Eng. Asp.* **2013**, *439*, 207–214. [CrossRef]
149. Chen, L.; Wei, K.; Qu, Y.; Li, T.; Chang, B.; Liao, B.; Xue, W. Characterization of plasma electrolytic oxidation film on biomedical high niobium-containing β-titanium alloy. *Surf. Coat. Technol.* **2018**, *352*, 295–301. [CrossRef]
150. Cordeiro, J.M.; Beline, T.; Ribeiro, A.L.R.; Rangel, E.C.; da Cruz, N.C.; Landers, R.; Faverani, L.P.; Vaz, L.G.; Fais, L.M.G.; Vicente, F.B.; et al. Development of binary and ternary titanium alloys for dental implants. *Dent. Mater.* **2017**, *33*, 1244–1257. [CrossRef]
151. Majumdar, P.; Singh, S.B.; Dhara, S.; Chakraborty, M. Influence of boron addition to Ti–13Zr–13Nb alloy on MG63 osteoblast cell viability and protein adsorption. *Mater. Sci. Eng. C* **2015**, *46*, 62–68. [CrossRef] [PubMed]
152. Blanquer, A.; Musilkova, J.; Barrios, L.; Ibáñez, E.; Vandrovcova, M.; Pellicer, E.; Sort, J.; Bacakova, L.; Nogués, C. Cytocompatibility assessment of Ti-Zr-Pd-Si-(Nb) alloys with low Young's modulus, increased hardness, and enhanced osteoblast differentiation for biomedical applications. *J. Biomed. Mater. Res. Part B Appl. Biomater.* **2018**, *106*, 834–842. [CrossRef]
153. Herranz-Diez, C.; Gil, F.; Guillem-Marti, J.; Manero, J. Mechanical and physicochemical characterization along with biological interactions of a new Ti25Nb21Hf alloy for bone tissue engineering. *J. Biomater. Appl.* **2015**, *30*, 171–181. [CrossRef]
154. Hoppe, A.; Güldal, N.S.; Boccaccini, A.R. A review of the biological response to ionic dissolution products from bioactive glasses and glass-ceramics. *Biomaterials* **2011**, *32*, 2757–2774. [CrossRef]
155. Ren, N.; Li, J.; Qiu, J.; Sang, Y.; Jiang, H.; Boughton, R.I.; Huang, L.; Huang, W.; Liu, H. Nanostructured titanate with different metal ions on the surface of metallic titanium: A facile approach for regulation of rBMSCs fate on titanium implants. *Small* **2014**, *10*, 3169–3180. [CrossRef]
156. Haraguchi, T.; Ayukawa, Y.; Shibata, Y.; Takeshita, T.; Atsuta, I.; Ogino, Y.; Yasunami, N.; Yamashita, Y.; Koyano, K. Effect of Calcium Chloride Hydrothermal Treatment of Titanium on Protein, Cellular, and Bacterial Adhesion Properties. *J. Clin. Med.* **2020**, *9*, 2627. [CrossRef]
157. Shi, X.; Nakagawa, M.; Kawachi, G.; Xu, L.; Ishikawa, K. Surface modification of titanium by hydrothermal treatment in Mg-containing solution and early osteoblast responses. *J. Mater. Sci. Mater. Med.* **2012**, *23*, 1281–1290. [CrossRef]
158. Jiang, N.; Guo, Z.; Sun, D.; Li, Y.; Yang, Y.; Chen, C.; Zhang, L.; Zhu, S. Promoting osseointegration of Ti implants through micro/nanoscaled hierarchical Ti phosphate/Ti oxide hybrid coating. *ACS Nano* **2018**, *12*, 7883–7891. [CrossRef] [PubMed]
159. Lingli, X.; Xingling, S.; Chun, O.; Wen, L. In vitro Apatite Formation, Protein Adsorption and Initial Osteoblast Responses on Titanium Surface Enriched with Magnesium. *Rare Met. Mater. Eng.* **2017**, *46*, 1512–1517. [CrossRef]
160. Shi, X.; Tsuru, K.; Xu, L.; Kawachi, G.; Ishikawa, K. Effects of solution pH on the structure and biocompatibility of Mg-containing TiO2 layer fabricated on titanium by hydrothermal treatment. *Appl. Surf. Sci.* **2013**, *270*, 445–451. [CrossRef]
161. Wang, L.; Luo, Q.; Zhang, X.; Qiu, J.; Qian, S.; Liu, X. Co-implantation of magnesium and zinc ions into titanium regulates the behaviors of human gingival fibroblasts. *Bioact. Mater.* **2021**, *6*, 64–74. [CrossRef]
162. Yuan, Z.; Liu, P.; Liang, Y.; Tao, B.; He, Y.; Hao, Y.; Yang, W.; Hu, Y.; Cai, K. Investigation of osteogenic responses of Fe-incorporated micro/nano-hierarchical structures on titanium surfaces. *J. Mater. Chem. B* **2018**, *6*, 1359–1372. [CrossRef] [PubMed]
163. Anbazhagan, E.; Rajendran, A.; Natarajan, D.; Kiran, M.S.; Pattanayak, D.K. Divalent ion encapsulated nano titania on Ti metal as a bioactive surface with enhanced protein adsorption. *Colloids Surf. B Biointerfaces* **2016**, *143*, 213–223. [CrossRef]

164. Soares, P.; Dias-Netipanyj, M.F.; Elifio-Esposito, S.; Leszczak, V.; Popat, K. Effects of calcium and phosphorus incorporation on the properties and bioactivity of TiO 2 nanotubes. *J. Biomater. Appl.* **2018**, *33*, 410–421. [CrossRef]
165. Mei, S.; Zhao, L.; Wang, W.; Ma, Q.; Zhang, Y. Biomimetic titanium alloy with sparsely distributed nanotubes could enhance osteoblast functions. *Adv. Eng. Mater.* **2012**, *14*, 166–174. [CrossRef]
166. Cai, K.Y. Surface modification of titanium films with sodium ion implantation: Surface properties and protein adsorption. *Acta Metall. Sin. Eng. Lett.* **2007**, *20*, 148–156. [CrossRef]
167. Misra, R.D.K.; Nune, C.; Pesacreta, T.C.; Somani, M.C.; Karjalainen, L.P. Interplay between grain structure and protein adsorption on functional response of osteoblasts: Ultrafine-grained versus coarse-grained substrates. *J. Biomed. Mater. Res. Part A* **2013**, *101A*, 1–12. [CrossRef]
168. Yin, F.; Xu, R.; Hu, S.; Zhao, K.; Yang, S.; Kuang, S.; Li, Q.; Han, Q. Enhanced Mechanical and Biological Performance of an Extremely Fine Nanograined 316L Stainless Steel Cell-Substrate Interface Fabricated by Ultrasonic Shot Peening. *ACS Biomater. Sci. Eng.* **2018**, *4*, 1609–1621. [CrossRef] [PubMed]
169. Bahl, S.; Aleti, B.T.; Suwas, S.; Chatterjee, K. Surface nanostructuring of titanium imparts multifunctional properties for orthopedic and cardiovascular applications. *Mater. Des.* **2018**, *144*, 169–181. [CrossRef]
170. Kubacka, D.; Yamamoto, A.; Wieciński, P.; Garbacz, H. Biological behavior of titanium processed by severe plastic deformation. *Appl. Surf. Sci.* **2019**, *472*, 54–63. [CrossRef]
171. Huo, W.T.; Zhao, L.Z.; Zhang, W.; Lu, J.W.; Zhao, Y.Q.; Zhang, Y.S. In vitro corrosion behavior and biocompatibility of nanostructured Ti6Al4V. *Mater. Sci. Eng. C* **2018**, *92*, 268–279. [CrossRef] [PubMed]
172. Huang, R.; Zhang, L.; Huang, L.; Zhu, J. Enhanced in-vitro osteoblastic functions on β-type titanium alloy using surface mechanical attrition treatment. *Mater. Sci. Eng. C* **2019**, *97*, 688–697. [CrossRef] [PubMed]
173. Awang Shri, D.N.; Tsuchiya, K.; Yamamoto, A. Effect of high-pressure torsion deformation on surface properties and biocompatibility of Ti-50.9 mol. %Ni alloys. *Biointerphases* **2014**, *9*, 029007. [CrossRef] [PubMed]
174. Talha, M.; Ma, Y.; Kumar, P.; Lin, Y.; Singh, A. Role of protein adsorption in the bio corrosion of metallic implants—A review. *Colloids Surfaces B Biointerfaces* **2019**, *176*, 494–506. [CrossRef]
175. Dias-Netipanyj, M.F.; Cowden, K.; Sopchenski, L.; Cogo, S.C.; Elifio-Esposito, S.; Popat, K.C.; Soares, P. Effect of crystalline phases of titania nanotube arrays on adipose derived stem cell adhesion and proliferation. *Mater. Sci. Eng. C* **2019**, *103*, 109850. [CrossRef] [PubMed]
176. Gong, Z.; Hu, Y.; Gao, F.; Quan, L.; Liu, T.; Gong, T.; Pan, C. Effects of diameters and crystals of titanium dioxide nanotube arrays on blood compatibility and endothelial cell behaviors. *Colloids Surf. B Biointerfaces* **2019**, *184*, 110521. [CrossRef]
177. Li, Y.; Dong, Y.; Zhang, Y.; Yang, Y.; Hu, R.; Mu, P.; Liu, X.; Lin, C.; Huang, Q. Synergistic effect of crystalline phase on protein adsorption and cell behaviors on TiO2 nanotubes. *Appl. Nanosci.* **2020**, *10*, 3245–3257. [CrossRef]
178. Hong, Y.; Yu, M.; Lin, J.; Cheng, K.; Weng, W.; Wang, H. Surface hydroxyl groups direct cellular response on amorphous and anatase TiO2 nanodots. *Colloids Surf. B Biointerfaces* **2014**, *123*, 68–74. [CrossRef]
179. Raffaini, G.; Ganazzoli, F. Molecular modelling of protein adsorption on the surface of titanium dioxide polymorphs. *Philos. Trans. R. Soc. A Math. Phys. Eng. Sci.* **2012**, *370*, 1444–1462. [CrossRef]
180. Liu, Y.; Cheng, K.; Weng, W.; Yu, M.; Lin, J.; Wang, H.; Du, P.; Han, G. Influence of rod-surface structure on biological interactions between TiO2 nanorod films and proteins/cells. *Thin Solid Films* **2013**, *544*, 285–290. [CrossRef]
181. Yang, C.; Peng, C.; Zhao, D.; Liao, C.; Zhou, J.; Lu, X. Molecular simulations of myoglobin adsorbed on rutile (110) and (001) surfaces. *Fluid Phase Equilib.* **2014**, *362*, 349–354. [CrossRef]
182. Keller, T.F.; Reichert, J.; Thanh, T.P.; Adjiski, R.; Spiess, L.; Berzina-Cimdina, L.; Jandt, K.D.; Bossert, J. Facets of protein assembly on nanostructured titanium oxide surfaces. *Acta Biomater.* **2013**, *9*, 5810–5820. [CrossRef] [PubMed]
183. Sugita, Y.; Saruta, J.; Taniyama, T.; Kitajima, H.; Hirota, M.; Ikeda, T.; Ogawa, T. UV-pre-treated and protein-adsorbed titanium implants exhibit enhanced osteoconductivity. *Int. J. Mol. Sci.* **2020**, *21*, 4194. [CrossRef]
184. Jeong, W.S.; Kwon, J.S.; Choi, E.H.; Kim, K.M. The Effects of Non-Thermal Atmospheric Pressure Plasma treated Titanium Surface on Behaviors of Oral Soft Tissue Cells. *Sci. Rep.* **2018**, *8*, 1–13. [CrossRef]
185. Kamo, M.; Kyomoto, M.; Miyaji, F. Time course of surface characteristics of alkali- and heat-treated titanium dental implants during vacuum storage. *J. Biomed. Mater. Res. Part B Appl. Biomater.* **2016**, *105*, 1453–1460. [CrossRef]
186. Aita, H.; Hori, N.; Takeuchi, M.; Suzuki, T.; Yamada, M.; Anpo, M.; Ogawa, T. The effect of ultraviolet functionalization of titanium on integration with bone. *Biomaterials* **2009**, *30*, 1015–1025. [CrossRef]
187. Yu, M.; Gong, J.; Zhou, Y.; Dong, L.; Lin, Y.; Ma, L.; Weng, W.; Cheng, K.; Wang, H. Surface hydroxyl groups regulate the osteogenic differentiation of mesenchymal stem cells on titanium and tantalum metals. *J. Mater. Chem. B* **2017**, *5*, 3955–3963. [CrossRef]
188. Hori, N.; Ueno, T.; Minamikawa, H.; Iwasa, F.; Yoshino, F.; Kimoto, K.; Il Lee, M.C.; Ogawa, T. Electrostatic control of protein adsorption on UV-photofunctionalized titanium. *Acta Biomater.* **2010**, *6*, 4175–4180. [CrossRef]
189. Wu, J.; Zhou, L.; Ding, X.; Gao, Y.; Liu, X. Biological Effect of Ultraviolet Photocatalysis on Nanoscale Titanium with a Focus on Physicochemical Mechanism. *Langmuir* **2015**, *31*, 10037–10046. [CrossRef] [PubMed]
190. Zhang, H.; Komasa, S.; Mashimo, C.; Sekino, T.; Okazaki, J. Effect of ultraviolet treatment on bacterial attachment and osteogenic activity to alkali-treated titanium with nanonetwork structures. *Int. J. Nanomed.* **2017**, *12*, 4633–4646. [CrossRef] [PubMed]

191. Dini, C.; Nagay, B.E.; Cordeiro, J.M.; da Cruz, N.C.; Rangel, E.C.; Ricomini-Filho, A.P.; de Avila, E.D.; Barão, V.A.R. UV-photofunctionalization of a biomimetic coating for dental implants application. *Mater. Sci. Eng. C* **2020**, *110*, 110657. [CrossRef]
192. Han, I.; Vagaska, B.; Seo, H.J.; Kang, J.K.; Kwon, B.-J.; Lee, M.H.; Park, J.-C. Promoted cell and material interaction on atmospheric pressure plasma treated titanium. *Appl. Surf. Sci.* **2012**, *258*, 4718–4723. [CrossRef]
193. Rapuano, B.E.; MacDonald, D.E. Surface oxide net charge of a titanium alloy: Modulation of fibronectin-activated attachment and spreading of osteogenic cells. *Colloids Surf. B Biointerfaces* **2011**, *82*, 95–103. [CrossRef]
194. Yamamoto, H.; Shibata, Y.; Miyazaki, T. Anode Glow Discharge Plasma Treatment of Titanium Plates Facilitates Adsorption of Extracellular Matrix Proteins. *J. Dent. Res.* **2005**, *84*, 668–671. [CrossRef] [PubMed]
195. Canullo, L.; Genova, T.; Wang, H.-L.; Carossa, S.; Mussano, F. Plasma of Argon Increases Cell Attachment and Bacterial Decontamination on Different Implant Surfaces. *Int. J. Oral Maxillofac. Implant.* **2017**, *32*, 1315–1323. [CrossRef]
196. Choi, S.-H.; Jeong, W.-S.; Cha, J.-Y.; Lee, J.-H.; Yu, H.-S.; Choi, E.-H.; Kim, K.-M.; Hwang, C.-J. Time-dependent effects of ultraviolet and nonthermal atmospheric pressure plasma on the biological activity of titanium. *Sci. Rep.* **2016**, *6*, 33421. [CrossRef] [PubMed]
197. Han, I.; Vagaska, B.; Joo Park, B.; Lee, M.H.; Jin Lee, S.; Park, J.C. Selective fibronectin adsorption against albumin and enhanced stem cell attachment on helium atmospheric pressure glow discharge treated titanium. *J. Appl. Phys.* **2011**, *109*, 124701. [CrossRef]
198. Zhu, W.; Teel, G.; O'Brien, C.M.; Zhuang, T.; Keidar, M.; Zhang, L.G. Enhanced human bone marrow mesenchymal stem cell functions on cathodic arc plasma-treated titanium. *Int. J. Nanomed.* **2015**, *10*, 7385–7396.
199. Santos, O.; Svendsen, I.E.; Lindh, L.; Arnebrant, T. Adsorption of HSA, IgG and laminin-1 on model titania surfaces—Effects of glow discharge treatment on competitively adsorbed film composition. *Biofouling* **2011**, *27*, 1003–1015. [CrossRef] [PubMed]
200. Choi, S.-H.; Jeong, W.-S.; Cha, J.-Y.; Lee, J.-H.; Lee, K.-J.; Yu, H.-S.; Choi, E.-H.; Kim, K.-M.; Hwang, C.-J. Overcoming the biological aging of titanium using a wet storage method after ultraviolet treatment. *Sci. Rep.* **2017**, *7*, 3833. [CrossRef]
201. Wu, X.; Hao, P.; He, F.; Yao, Z.; Zhang, X. Molecular dynamics simulations of BSA absorptions on pure and formate-contaminated rutile (1 1 0) surface. *Appl. Surf. Sci.* **2020**, *533*, 147574. [CrossRef]
202. Hori, N.; Att, W.; Ueno, T.; Sato, N.; Yamada, M.; Saruwatari, L.; Suzuki, T.; Ogawa, T. Age-dependent degradation of the protein adsorption capacity of titanium. *J. Dent. Res.* **2009**, *88*, 663–667. [CrossRef]
203. Att, W.; Hori, N.; Takeuchi, M.; Ouyang, J.; Yang, Y.; Anpo, M.; Ogawa, T. Time-dependent degradation of titanium osteoconductivity: An implication of biological aging of implant materials. *Biomaterials* **2009**, *30*, 5352–5363. [CrossRef] [PubMed]
204. Miki, T.; Matsuno, T.; Hashimoto, Y.; Miyake, A.; Satomi, T. In Vitro and In Vivo Evaluation of Titanium Surface Modification for Biological Aging by Electrolytic Reducing Ionic Water. *Appl. Sci.* **2019**, *9*, 713. [CrossRef]
205. Lu, H.; Zhou, L.; Wan, L.; Li, S.; Rong, M.; Guo, Z. Effects of storage methods on time-related changes of titanium surface properties and cellular response. *Biomed. Mater.* **2012**, *7*, 055002. [CrossRef] [PubMed]
206. Choi, S.-H.; Ryu, J.-H.; Kwon, J.-S.; Kim, J.-E.; Cha, J.-Y.; Lee, K.-J.; Yu, H.-S.; Choi, E.-H.; Kim, K.-M.; Hwang, C.-J. Effect of wet storage on the bioactivity of ultraviolet light- and non-thermal atmospheric pressure plasma-treated titanium and zirconia implant surfaces. *Mater. Sci. Eng. C* **2019**, *105*, 110049. [CrossRef]
207. Kratz, F.; Müller, C.; Körber, N.; Umanskaya, N.; Hannig, M.; Ziegler, C. Characterization of protein films on dental materials: Bicinchoninic acid assay (BCA) studies on loosely and firmly adsorbed protein layers. *Phys. Status Solidi Appl. Mater. Sci.* **2013**, *210*, 964–967. [CrossRef]
208. Wehmeyer, J.L.; Synowicki, R.; Bizios, R.; García, C.D. Dynamic adsorption of albumin on nanostructured TiO2 thin films. *Mater. Sci. Eng. C* **2010**, *30*, 277–282. [CrossRef]
209. Imamura, K.; Oshita, M.; Iwai, M.; Kuroda, T.; Watanabe, I.; Sakiyama, T.; Nakanishi, K. Influences of properties of protein and adsorption surface on removal kinetics of protein adsorbed on metal surface by H2O2-electrolysis treatment. *J. Colloid Interface Sci.* **2010**, *345*, 474–480. [CrossRef]
210. Forov, Y.; Paulus, M.; Dogan, S.; Salmen, P.; Weis, C.; Gahlmann, T.; Behrendt, A.; Albers, C.; Elbers, M.; Schnettger, W.; et al. Adsorption Behavior of Lysozyme at Titanium Oxide-Water Interfaces. *Langmuir* **2018**, *34*, 5403–5408. [CrossRef] [PubMed]
211. Xu, Z.; Grassian, V.H. Bovine serum albumin adsorption on TiO2 nanoparticle surfaces: Effects of ph and coadsorption of phosphate on protein-surface interactions and protein structure. *J. Phys. Chem. C* **2017**, *121*, 21763–21771. [CrossRef]
212. Burgos-Asperilla, L.; García-Alonso, M.C.; Escudero, M.L.; Alonso, C. Study of the interaction of inorganic and organic compounds of cell culture medium with a Ti surface. *Acta Biomater.* **2010**, *6*, 652–661. [CrossRef]
213. Sultan, A.M.; Hughes, Z.E.; Walsh, T.R. Effect of calcium ions on peptide adsorption at the aqueous rutile titania (110) interface. *Biointerphases* **2018**, *13*, 06D403. [CrossRef] [PubMed]
214. Hashimoto, M.; Kitaoka, S.; Furuya, M.; Kanetaka, H.; Hoshikaya, K.; Yamashita, H.; Abe, M. Enhancement of cell differentiation on a surface potential-controlled nitrogen-doped TiO_2 surface. *J. Ceram. Soc. Jpn.* **2019**, *127*, 636–641. [CrossRef]
215. Leeman, M.; Choi, J.; Hansson, S.; Storm, M.U.; Nilsson, L. Proteins and antibodies in serum, plasma, and whole blood—Size characterization using asymmetrical flow field-flow fractionation (AF4). *Anal. Bioanal. Chem.* **2018**, *410*, 4867–4873. [CrossRef]
216. Boix, M.; Eslava, S.; Costa Machado, G.; Gosselin, E.; Ni, N.; Saiz, E.; De Coninck, J. ATR-FTIR measurements of albumin and fibrinogen adsorption: Inert versus calcium phosphate ceramics. *J. Biomed. Mater. Res. Part A* **2015**, *103*, 3493–3502. [CrossRef] [PubMed]
217. Hoppe, J.D.; Scriba, P.C.; Klüter, H. 5 Human Albumin. In *Transfusion Medicine and Hemotherapy: Offizielles Organ der Deutschen Gesellschaft fur Transfusionsmedizin und Immunhamatologie*; Karger Publishers: Basel, Switzerland, 2009; Volume 36, pp. 399–407.

218. Hemmersam, A.G.; Foss, M.; Chevallier, J.; Besenbacher, F. Adsorption of fibrinogen on tantalum oxide, titanium oxide and gold studied by the QCM-D technique. *Colloids Surf. B Biointerfaces* **2005**, *43*, 208–215. [CrossRef]
219. Vadillo-Rodríguez, V.; Pacha-Olivenza, M.A.; Gönzalez-Martín, M.L.; Bruque, J.M.; Gallardo-Moreno, A.M.; Gónzalez-Martín, M.L.; Bruque, J.M.; Gallardo-Moreno, A.M. Adsorption behavior of human plasma fibronectin on hydrophobic and hydrophilic Ti6Al4V substrata and its influence on bacterial adhesion and detachment. *J. Biomed. Mater. Res. Part A* **2013**, *101A*, 1397–1404. [CrossRef] [PubMed]
220. Canullo, L.; Genova, T.; Tallarico, M.; Gautier, G.; Mussano, F.; Botticelli, D. Plasma of Argon Affects the Earliest Biological Response of Different Implant Surfaces. *J. Dent. Res.* **2016**, *95*, 566–573. [CrossRef]
221. Dodo, C.G.; Senna, P.M.; Custodio, W.; Paes Leme, A.F.; Del Bel Cury, A.A. Proteome analysis of the plasma protein layer adsorbed to a rough titanium surface. *Biofouling* **2013**, *29*, 549–557. [CrossRef] [PubMed]
222. Rösch, C.; Kratz, F.; Hering, T.; Trautmann, S.; Umanskaya, N.; Tippkötter, N.; Müller-Renno, C.; Ulber, R.; Hannig, M.; Ziegler, C. Albumin-lysozyme interactions: Cooperative adsorption on titanium and enzymatic activity. *Colloids Surf. B Biointerfaces* **2017**, *149*, 115–121. [CrossRef]
223. Wald, J.; Müller, C.; Wahl, M.; Hoth-Hannig, W.; Hannig, M.; Kopnarski, M.; Ziegler, C. ToF-SIMS investigations of adsorbed proteins on dental titanium. *Phys. Status Solidi* **2010**, *207*, 831–836. [CrossRef]
224. Parisi, L.; Ghezzi, B.; Bianchi, M.G.; Toffoli, A.; Rossi, F.; Bussolati, O.; Macaluso, G.M. Titanium dental implants hydrophilicity promotes preferential serum fibronectin over albumin competitive adsorption modulating early cell response. *Mater. Sci. Eng. C* **2020**, *117*, 111307. [CrossRef]
225. Felgueiras, H.; Migonney, V.; Sommerfeld, S.; Murthy, N.; Kohn, J. Competitive Adsorption of Albumin, Fibronectin and Collagen Type I on Different Biomaterial Surfaces: A QCM-D Study. In *XIII Mediterranean Conference on Medical and Biological Engineering and Computing 2013*; IFMBE Proceedings; Roa Romero, L.M., Ed.; Springer International Publishing: Cham, Switzerland, 2014; Volume 41, pp. 1597–1600.
226. Felgueiras, H.P.; Murthy, N.S.; Sommerfeld, S.D.; Brás, M.M.; Migonney, V.; Kohn, J. Competitive Adsorption of Plasma Proteins Using a Quartz Crystal Microbalance. *ACS Appl. Mater. Interfaces* **2016**, *8*, 13207–13217. [CrossRef]
227. Pegueroles, M.; Tonda-Turo, C.; Planell, J.A.; Gil, F.-J.; Aparicio, C. Adsorption of Fibronectin, Fibrinogen, and Albumin on TiO2: Time-Resolved Kinetics, Structural Changes, and Competition Study. *Biointerphases* **2012**, *7*, 48. [CrossRef]
228. Lorenzetti, M.; Bernardini, G.; Luxbacher, T.; Santucci, A.; Kobe, S.; Novak, S. Surface properties of nanocrystalline TiO2 coatings in relation to the in vitro plasma protein adsorption. *Biomed. Mater.* **2015**, *10*, 045012. [CrossRef] [PubMed]
229. Romero-Gavilán, F.; Gomes, N.C.; Ródenas, J.; Sánchez, A.; Azkargorta, M.; Iloro, I.; Elortza, F.; García Arnáez, I.; Gurruchaga, M.; Goñi, I.; et al. Proteome analysis of human serum proteins adsorbed onto different titanium surfaces used in dental implants. *Biofouling* **2017**, *33*, 98–111. [CrossRef]
230. Svendsen, I.E.; Lindh, L. The composition of enamel salivary films is different from the ones formed on dental materials. *Biofouling* **2009**, *25*, 255–261. [CrossRef] [PubMed]
231. Zuanazzi, D.; Xiao, Y.; Siqueira, W.L. Evaluating protein binding specificity of titanium surfaces through mass spectrometry–based proteomics. *Clin. Oral Investig.* **2020**. [CrossRef]
232. Wei, C.-X.; Burrow, M.F.; Botelho, M.G.; Lam, H.; Leung, W.K. In Vitro Salivary Protein Adsorption Profile on Titanium and Ceramic Surfaces and the Corresponding Putative Immunological Implications. *Int. J. Mol. Sci.* **2020**, *21*, 3083. [CrossRef] [PubMed]
233. Souza, J.G.S.; Bertolini, M.; Costa, R.C.; Lima, C.V.; Barão, V.A.R. Proteomic profile of the saliva and plasma protein layer adsorbed on Ti–Zr alloy: The effect of sandblasted and acid-etched surface treatment. *Biofouling* **2020**, *36*, 428–441. [CrossRef] [PubMed]
234. Jäger, M.; Jennissen, H.P.; Haversath, M.; Busch, A.; Grupp, T.; Sowislok, A.; Herten, M. Intrasurgical Protein Layer on Titanium Arthroplasty Explants: From the Big Twelve to the Implant Proteome. *PROTEOMICS Clin. Appl.* **2019**, *13*, 1800168. [CrossRef]
235. Martins, M.C.L.; Sousa, S.R.; Antunes, J.C.; Barbosa, M.A. Protein adsorption characterization. *Methods Mol. Biol.* **2012**, *811*, 141–161.
236. Migliorini, E.; Weidenhaupt, M.; Picart, C. Practical guide to characterize biomolecule adsorption on solid surfaces (Review). *Biointerphases* **2018**, *13*, 06D303. [CrossRef]
237. Ledesma, A.E.; Chemes, D.M.; de los Angeles Frías, M.; Torres, M.D.P.G. Spectroscopic characterization and docking studies of ZnO nanoparticle modified with BSA. *Appl. Surf. Sci.* **2017**, *412*, 177–188. [CrossRef]
238. Hemmersam, A.G.; Rechendorff, K.; Foss, M.; Sutherland, D.S.; Besenbacher, F. Fibronectin adsorption on gold, Ti-, and Ta-oxide investigated by QCM-D and RSA modelling. *J. Colloid Interface Sci.* **2008**, *320*, 110–116. [CrossRef] [PubMed]
239. Nakanishi, K.; Sakiyama, T.; Imamura, K. On the adsorption of proteins on solid surfaces, a common but very complicated phenomenon. *J. Biosci. Bioeng.* **2001**, *91*, 233–244. [CrossRef]
240. Adamczyk, Z. Protein adsorption: A quest for a universal mechanism. *Curr. Opin. Colloid Interface Sci.* **2019**, *41*, 50–65. [CrossRef]

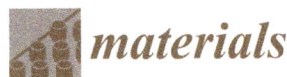

Review

Evaluation of Bone Gain and Complication Rates after Guided Bone Regeneration with Titanium Foils: A Systematic Review

Elisabet Roca-Millan [1], Enric Jané-Salas [2], Albert Estrugo-Devesa [2] and José López-López [2,*]

1. Faculty of Medicine and Health Sciences (School of Dentistry), University of Barcelona, 08907 Barcelona, Spain; erocamil@gmail.com
2. Oral Health and Masticatory System Group-IDIBELL, Faculty of Medicine and Health Sciences (School of Dentistry), Odontological Hospital University of Barcelona, University of Barcelona, 08907 Barcelona, Spain; enjasa19734@gmail.com (E.J.-S.); albertestrugodevesa@gmail.com (A.E.-D.)
* Correspondence: jl.lopez@ub.edu or 18575jll@gmail.com

Received: 29 October 2020; Accepted: 23 November 2020; Published: 25 November 2020

Abstract: Guided bone regeneration techniques are increasingly used to enable the subsequent placement of dental implants. This systematic review aims to analyze the success rate of these techniques in terms of bone gain and complications rate using titanium membranes as a barrier element. Electronic and hand searches were conducted in PubMed/Medline, Scielo, Scopus and Cochrane Library databases for case reports, case series, cohort studies and clinical trials in humans published up to and including 19 September 2020. Thirteen articles were included in the qualitative analysis. Bone gain both horizontally and vertically was comparable to that obtained with other types of membranes more commonly used. The postoperative complication rate was higher that of native collagen membranes and non-resorbable titanium-reinforced membranes, and similar that of crosslinked collagen membranes and titanium meshes. The survival rate of the implants was similar to that of implants placed in native bone. Due to the limited scientific literature published on this issue, more randomized clinical trials comparing occlusive titanium barriers and other types of membranes are necessary to reach more valid conclusions.

Keywords: titanium membrane; titanium foil; occlusive titanium barrier; bone augmentation; guided bone regeneration

---

1. Introduction

The four classical principles of guided bone regeneration (GBR) are primary closure, angiogenesis, space maintenance and blood clot stability [1] (Figure 1).

Based on these concepts, different techniques and a wide variety of biomaterials have been developed with the aim of achieving greater predictability, lower risk of complications, lower morbidity and shorter operative time in this type of treatment, which is becoming more and more common [2,3]. Research on new biomaterials for bone regeneration is advancing rapidly; even recently they have been manufactured by combining biopolymers and natural nanoparticles [4,5]. Ideally, the proposed method should provide a solution to the four precepts [2,3].

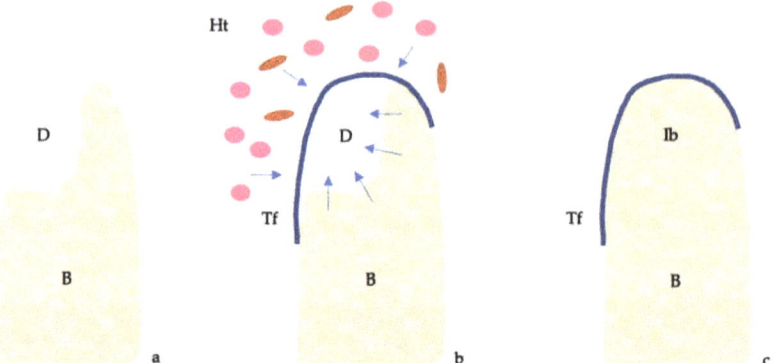

Figure 1. Guided bone regeneration (GBR) mechanism. (**a**) Bone defect. (**b**) The titanium barrier prevents the penetration of epithelial cells and fibroblasts and allows access to the defect of osteogenic and stem cells originating from the native bone. (**c**) Regeneration of the bone defect. Abbreviations: B, bone; D, defect; Ht, healing tissue; Ib, immature bone; Tf, titanium foil.

On the other hand, the properties that an ideal biomaterial should fulfill are osteogenesis, osteoconduction and osteoinduction. Therefore, autologous bone is considered the gold standard [2]. However, the great resorption, the unlimited availability, the morbidity and the longer surgical time represent inconveniences in its use. That is why a combination of several biomaterials is generally used in GBR procedures [2,3,6].

Since clot formation is the first and essential step in bone healing [7,8], in the last years, there have been numerous studies that focus on the use of blood concentrates (platelet-rich plasma (PRP), platelet-rich fibrin (PRF) and platelet-rich growth factor (PRGF)) in these surgical procedures [9–11].

However, due to the presence of erythrocytes, blood has a greater capacity to generate thrombin and activate platelets than these concentrates [12]. Likewise, the lower porosity and density of the fibrin layer present in the complete clot facilitate cell migration [13]. However, to benefit from its properties, it would be necessary to at least maintain the space and stabilize the clot [14–16].

To comply with these two principles, there are different types of membranes or barrier elements, such as titanium-reinforced polytetrafluoroethylene membranes, perforated titanium meshes and titanium foils [17]. The main drawback of the first two is the high exposure rate, associated with a high failure rate [3,6,18]. However, titanium barriers tolerate prolonged exposure to the oral environment, with good hygiene and the use of antiseptics to avoid bacterial colonization being essential [19–21].

Several studies published in recent years defend the use of these barrier elements in the regeneration of large maxillary atrophies [20–24], in post-extraction socket reconstruction [19,25,26], in the regeneration of periodontal defects [27] and even simultaneously with implant placement [28].

The concept of using these barriers is to take advantage of the properties of the blood clot, which is why, in some studies, they are used without biomaterial filling [21,24]; although, in other publications, these membranes have been used in combination with PRF [19], allograft [20,22,23,29], xenograft [25,26,30], mixed autograft and allograft [31] or even tricalcium β-phosphate [28].

Given that titanium barriers comply with the two aforementioned precepts and have tolerance to prolonged exposure, the objective of this systematic review is to study the success rate of GBR through the use of this type of membranes in terms of the amount of new bone formed and the complications associated with this surgical technique.

2. Materials and Methods

This systematic review was conducted according to the guidelines of the Preferred Reporting Items of Systematic Reviews and Meta-Analyses (PRISMA) statement [32]. Before starting the review, a detailed protocol of the methodology was developed. The protocol was not registered.

2.1. Focused Questions

1. Is the use of occlusive titanium barriers alone or in combination with biomaterial a predictable treatment in terms of amount of new bone formed? (primary question)
2. What is the complication rate regarding membrane exposure and infection? (primary question)
3. What is the survival and success rate of implants placed after this regenerative procedure? (secondary question)

2.2. PICO Question

P: Patients with partial or total edentulism.
I: Guided bone regeneration using occlusive titanium barriers alone or in combination with biomaterials.
C: Guided bone regeneration using other type of membranes.
O: Amount of new bone formed and rate of membrane exposure and infection.

2.3. Eligibility Criteria

Inclusion criteria: Case reports, case series, cohort studies and clinical trials written in English or Spanish that analyze the use of titanium foils in GBR procedures were considered for inclusion.

Exclusion criteria: animal studies. No limitations were used for publication date, sample size, follow-up period, type of bone defect treated or filler biomaterial.

2.4. Search Strategy

An electronic search was performed by two reviewers (E.R-M and E.J-S) for articles published up to and including September 2020. The databases consulted were MEDLINE/PubMed, Scielo, Scopus and Cochrane Library. An additional hand search was conducted to identify potential articles of interest in the references of the studies found. Both searches were performed on 19 September 2020.

The following term combination was used in the electronic search: ("titanium membrane [All Fields]" OR "occlusive titanium barrier [All Fields]" OR "titanium foil [All Fields]") AND ("bone regeneration [All Fields]" OR "bone formation [All Fields]" OR "bone augmentation [All Fields]" OR "guided bone regeneration [All Fields]" OR "guided tissue regeneration [All Fields]").

2.5. Study Selection

After screening titles and discarding duplicates, those studies whose abstract met the inclusion criteria were selected. The full text of these articles was read to verify that they met the eligibility criteria. Disagreements during the study selection were solved by consulting a third author (J.L-L).

2.6. Data Extraction and Method of Analysis

The data were extracted by two authors (E.R-M and A.E-D) and entered into a data collection form (Microsoft Excel version 16.35). In case of disagreement, a third author (E.J-S or J.L-L) was consulted, to get a consensus. The following data were collected: author(s), year of publication, type of study, number of titanium foils, type of defect, filling material, time of membrane removal, amount of bone gain, percentage membrane exposure, percentage of infection, number of patients, number of implants placed, survival and success rates of the implants, and follow-up period. Corresponding authors were contacted and asked if they could provide missing data. To summarize the data, the mean rates of exposure, infection, implant survival and implant infection were calculated.

2.7. Quality Assessment and Risk of Bias

The Strength of Recommendation Taxonomy (SORT) criteria were used to assess the quality of the evidence provided in the included studies [33]. This classification groups the articles into three levels: Level 1 (good-quality patient-oriented evidence), Level 2 (limited-quality patient-oriented evidence) and Level 3 (other evidence). Version 2 of the Cochrane Collaboration's tool for assessing risk of bias in randomized trials (RoB 2) [34] was implemented to evaluate the risk of bias of the randomized clinical trials and the Cochrane tool for assessing risk of bias in non-randomized studies of interventions (ROBINS-1) [35] was implemented to assess the risk of bias of the included retrospective cohort study.

3. Results

3.1. Study Selection

Through the electronic and manual searches, a total of 118 records were identified. After reading the titles and, if necessary, the abstracts and identifying duplicate articles, a total of 101 papers were discarded. Of these 17 studies assessed for eligibility, one was discarded after reading the full text because the titanium foil was placed in order to stabilize the jaw and prevent its fracture [36]. Three other articles were discarded, as they appear to be the same study as another two of the included papers but in earlier stages [20,21,23]. A total of 13 articles were included in the qualitative analysis [19,22,24–31,37–39] (Figure 2). A quantitative analysis could not be performed due to the lack of information provided and the great heterogeneity of the studies, in terms of sample size, type of defect to be regenerated, time of membrane removal and filling material used.

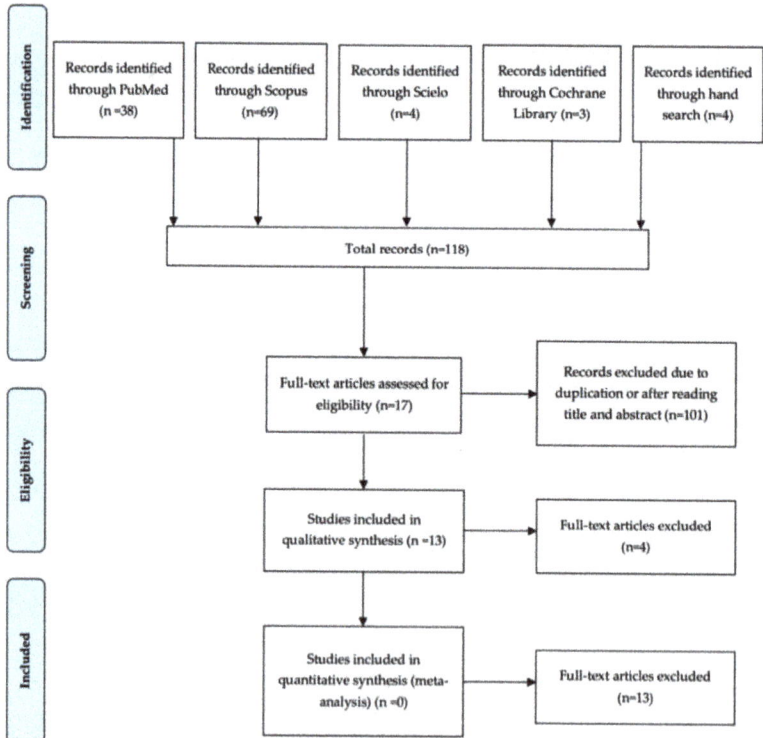

Figure 2. Preferred Reporting Items of Systematic Reviews and Meta-Analyses (PRISMA) flow diagram of selection process.

3.2. Study Methods and Characteristics

Two of the included articles were case reports [28,30], seven were case series [19,22,25,26,29,31,39], three were split-mouth randomized clinical trials [27,37,38] and only one was a retrospective cohort study [24]. The studies were published between 1999 and 2020 (Figure 3 and Table 1).

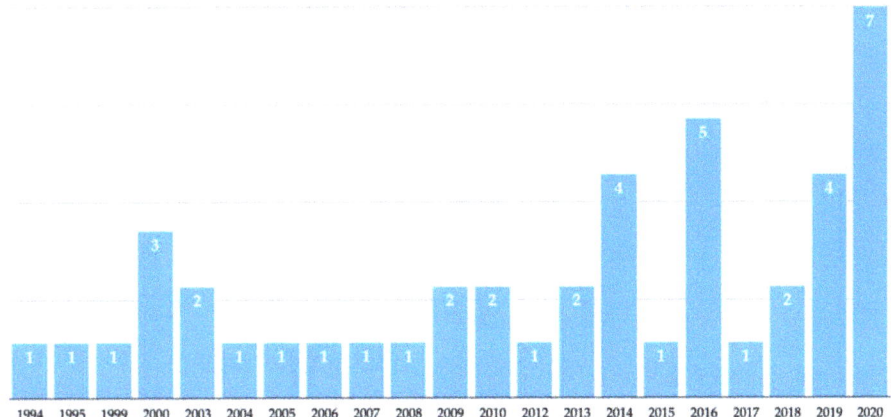

Figure 3. Results by year of the electronic search in PubMed.

The total population was 200 patients (72 women, 54 men, and 74 not specified), in which 260 titanium foils were placed. In two of the studies, the membrane was custom-fit manufactured from a previous computerized tomography [22,24]. The follow-up period was between two months and nine years. In six of the included studies [19,22,24,26,28,30], implants were placed in the regenerated area, with 88 implants placed in 39 patients. The time of membrane removal was between 21 days and 17 months; although, in some studies, it is not specified [19,28,31].

A wide variety of bone defects were treated: horizontal [25,28–30,39], horizontal and vertical [22,24,26,28,39], periodontal intrabony defects [27,37], post-extraction sockets [19,38], peri-implant defects [31,39] and sinus-floor augmentation [39].

The filling material was different depending on the study: blood clot [24,27,37,38], xenograft [25,26,30], allograft [22,29], β-Tricalcium phosphate [28], PRF or PRF + tricalcium phosphate + hydroxyapatite [19], autograft [38], autograft or/and hydroxyapatite [39] and autograft + xenograft [31].

3.3. Quality Assessment and Risk of Bias

According to the Strength of Recommendation Taxonomy (SORT) criteria, four of the studies included obtained a Level 2 of evidence [24,27,37,38] while the others obtained a Level 3 [19,22,25,26,28–31,39], so it should be noted that the quality of the included studies is limited and greater value should be given to the results obtained in Level 2 articles. Table 2 presents the risk of bias of the randomized clinical trials (RCT) [27,37,38] and the cohort study [24] assessed by using RoB 2 and ROBINS-1, respectively, with an overall judgment of low–moderate risk of bias. The present review itself fulfils 22 items in the PRISMA statement [32].

Table 1. Summary of the included studies.

Author	Type of Study	Level of Evidence	N (Titanium Foils)	Type of Defect	Filling Material	Membrane Removal (Months)	Bone Gain (mm)	Membrane Exposure (%)	Infection (%)
Kfir et al., 2007 [19]	Case series	Level 3	15	Post-extraction socket	PRF or PRF + TCP + HAP	NS	NS	47%	0%
Bassi et al., 2016 [22]	Case series	Level 3	13	HV	Allograft	6.35 ± 2.15	5.9 ± 2.1 V; 8.9 ± 3.5 H	38.5%	0%
Maeda et al., 2020 [25]	Case series	Level 3	15	H	Xenograft	21 days	8.02 ± 2.43 (P1); 8.71 ± 2.26 (P2); 9.00 ± 2.52 (P3)	100% (intentionally exposed)	0%
Pernet et al., 2019 [26]	Case series	Level 3	6	HV	Xenograft	4	7.3 ± 2.2 (P1) 4.2 ± 1.2 (P2) V; 2.3 ± 1.0 H	100% (intentionally exposed)	0%
Engelke et al., 2014 [28]	Case report	Level 3	2	1HV; 1H	β-Tricalcium phosphate	3; NS	NS	0%	0%
Molly et al., 2006 [24]	Retrospective study	Level 2	11	HV	Blood clot	9–17	NS	45.5%	NS
Toygar et al., 2009 [27]	RCT	Level 2	16	Periodontal Intrabony Defect	Blood clot	1–1.5	NS	43.75%	NS
Gaggl et al., 1999 [31]	Case series	Level 3	42	Peri-implant Defect	Autograft + xenograft	NS	4.5 ± 0.2	21.43%	11.90%
Beltrán et al., 2013 [30]	Case report	Level 3	1	H	Xenograft	7	4 mm	0%	0%
Beltrán et al., 2014 [29]	Case series	Level 3	5	H	Allograft	6	2.3 (P1); 2.7 (P2); 2.9 (P3)	0%	0%
Khanna et al., 2016 [37]	RCT	Level 2	12	Periodontal Intrabony Defect	Blood clot	5–6 weeks	54.69% defect fill	33.33%	0%
Pinho et al., 2006 [38]	RCT	Level 2	10	Post-extraction socket	Blood clot (CS); autograft (TS)	Maximum 6 months	8.80 ± 2.93 (C); 8.40 ± 3.35 (T)	50%	0%
Watzinger et al., 2000 [39]	Case series	Level 3	112	Different type defects	Autograft and/or hydroxyapatite	4.6	NS	30%	NS

Abbreviations: C, control; CS, control socket; H, horizontal; HAP, hydroxyapatite; HV, horizontal and vertical; NS, not specified; P, point; PRF, platelet-rich fibrin; RCT, randomized clinical trial; T, test; TCP, tricalcium phosphate; TS, test socket; V, vertical.

Table 2. Risk of bias across randomized clinical trials and the cohort study.

Bias Domain ROBINS-1	Molly et al. [24]	Bias Domain RoB 2	Khanna et al. [37]	Pinho et al. [38]	Toygar et al. [27]
Confounding	Low	Randomization process	Unclear	Unclear	Unclear
Selection of participants	High				
Classification of interventions	Low				
Deviations from intended interventions	Low	Deviations from intended interventions	Low	Low	Low
Missing data	Low	Missing data	Low	Low	Unclear
Measurement of outcomes	Low	Measurement of outcomes	Unclear	Low	Low
Selection of reported result	Unclear	Selection of reported result	Low	Low	Low
Overall bias	Unclear				

3.4. Bone Gain

Of the 13 studies included, four did not specify or evaluate the amount of new bone formed [19,24,27,28]. In two of them, a sufficient amount of bone was gained in all cases [19,28]. Another, which studied the regeneration of periodontal intrabony defects, did not evaluate this parameter [27]. The other one did not specify the values obtained but clarified that, in most cases, a sufficient bone augmentation was obtained for implant placement [24].

In the other nine studies, in which a wide variety of bone defects were treated, considerable bone gain was obtained after using titanium foils, regardless of the type of defect. Vertical bone gain, excluding the post-extraction sockets, was between 4.5 mm (autograft + xenograft) [31] and 7.3 mm (xenograft) [26]. Horizontal bone gain was between 2.3 mm (allograft) [29] and 9 mm (xenograft) [25]. In the study that quantified the regeneration of periodontal intrabony defects, a filling of 54.69% was obtained [37].

3.5. Complications

In two of the studies, titanium barriers were intentionally left exposed [25,26]. Three other articles reported not having had any exposure prior to membrane removal [26,27,29]. In the rest of the studies, the exposures ranged between 21.43% and 50% [19,22,24,27,31,37–39]. The mean percentage of accidental exposure was 23.81%. Only one article reported having cases of graft infection, with a percentage of 11.9% [31].

It must be taken in account that one of these articles reported an exposure of the 43.75% of the membranes; however, this percentage is higher, since the study discarded those patients who had had an exposure greater than a quarter of the membrane in the first four to six weeks [27].

As another complication, in one of the studies two patients were excluded due to displacement of the titanium barrier [37].

3.6. Implant Survival and Success Rates

In six of the included studies [19,22,24,26,28,30], implants were placed in the regenerated area, with 88 implants placed in 39 patients. The mean survival rate was 96.5% (82.6–100%), and the mean success rate was 91.3% (82.6–100%). It must be considered that only two studies evaluated the success rate [22,26]. The follow-up period for these implants was between one and nine years (Table 3). The study with the lowest survival rate was the one with the longest follow-up period [24].

Table 3. Implants survival and success rates.

Author	N Patients	N Implants	Survival Rate	Success Rate	Follow-Up
Kfir et al., 2007 [19]	8	9	-	-	-
Bassi et al., 2016 [22]	13	23	100%	82.6%	1 year
Perret et al., 2019 [26]	6	6	100%	100%	2 years
Engelke et al., 2014 [28]	2	3	100%	-	2 years
Molly et al., 2006 [24]	9	46	82.6%	-	6–9 years
Beltrán et al., 2013 [30]	1	1	100%	-	-
Total	39	88	96.5%	91.3%	1–9 years

4. Discussion

According to the results obtained in the present systematic review, the horizontal bone gain was between 2.3 and 9 mm [22,25,26,29,30], and the vertical between 4.5 and 7.3 mm [22,26,31]. These last values without taking into account the randomized clinical trial in which alveolar ridge preservation of well-conserved post-extraction sockets was performed, in which the mean vertical gain was greater than 8 mm [38].

In a recent RCT comparing vertical bone gain by using d-PTFE titanium-reinforced membranes or titanium meshes, a gain of 4.2 ± 1.0 mm (range 2.7–5.8) and 4.1 ± 1.0 mm (range 2.6–6.3) was obtained, respectively [40]. Likewise, a meta-analysis obtained similar results, with a mean vertical bone gain of 4.42 mm by using non-resorbable membranes (d-PTFE and e-PTFE), of 4.26 mm by using titanium meshes covered by resorbable membranes and of 5.2 mm by using titanium meshes alone [41].

Based on these data, it appears that the use of titanium foils is predictable in terms of the amount of bone gain, regardless of the filling material, and the gain may be even higher than with the use of other commonly used non-resorbable membranes or meshes.

With regard to horizontal bone gain, the values obtained in the different studies analyzed are very heterogeneous and do not seem to be related to the filling material used either. Other studies in which horizontal regeneration procedures were performed with collagen membranes and particulate grafts obtained average bone gains of 2.27 ± 1.68 mm [42], 5.68 ± 1.42 mm [43] and 5.03 ± 2.15 mm [44]. Thus, it seems that, in terms of horizontal bone gain, titanium barriers are comparable to collagen membranes, the most widely used in horizontal ridge augmentation procedures.

Based on the included articles, there is no evidence to believe that a filling material is better than another or even blood clot, in combination with occlusive titanium barriers. Furthermore, this type of membrane could be useful in the regeneration of defects of different types, from contained defects such as a post-extraction socket to a combined vertical and horizontal defect such as a posterior mandibular atrophy.

Regarding complications, it appears that titanium foils are prone to exposure, as is the case of titanium meshes and non-resorbable membranes with titanium reinforcement. The mean exposure rate in the present work was 23.81% (range 0–50%) [19,22,24,27–31,37–39], and the mean infection rate was 1.19% (range 0–11.9%) [19,22,25,26,28–31,37,38]. If these results are compared with those of other studies, it can be observed that the rate of postoperative complications of titanium foils is slightly higher than that of GBR procedures with other types of membranes. In an RCT in which the rate of complications in vertical ridge augmentation was evaluated through the use of titanium meshes covered with collagen membranes and the use of non-resorbable membranes with titanium reinforcement, a postoperative complication rate (exposure and infection) of 21.1% and 15% was obtained, respectively [40]. A meta-analysis obtained an intra- and postoperative complications rate of 21% for titanium meshes covered with resorbable membranes, of 6.9% for non-resorbable membranes and of 20% for titanium meshes [41].

In different studies on the use of native collagen membranes in horizontal bone regeneration, a percentage of complications of 3.2% [43] and 0% [44] was recorded. In a recent meta-analysis, an exposure rate of 28.62% for crosslinked membranes and of 20.74 for non-crosslinked membranes was obtained [42].

The postoperative complication rate of titanium barriers was higher than that of native collagen membranes and non-resorbable titanium-reinforced membranes, and similar to that of crosslinked collagen membranes and titanium meshes.

It must be taken into account that the complication rate obtained in this systematic review is surely lower than the real one in the included studies, since, in some articles, patients were excluded due to membrane displacement [37] or very premature exposure [27], not taking into account these cases in the complication rate reported. Furthermore, in two of the studies, some exposed membranes are associated with graft failure, but it is not specified whether it is due to graft infection [24,39].

On the one hand, some of the included articles defend that the exposure of the titanium foil does not influence the success of the GBR [19,22,37,38], even if one of them sustains that the very early exposure favors the increase in width of the attached gingiva, unlike what happens with a later exposure [22]. On the other hand, two studies support that early exposure (before 14 days) has a worse prognosis than late exposure, with very poor bone gain [24,39].

From the results obtained, it appears that the survival rate of implants placed in regenerated bone is similar to that of implants placed in native bone [45].

This review is based on the scant scientific literature published on the matter so far, and, for the moment, it is the only existing systematic review, so the results obtained cannot be compared and cannot be given much value. Other limitations are the heterogeneity of the included studies, the small sample size of some of them and the lack of information regarding bone gain or membrane removal. For these reasons, a quantitative analysis could not be performed.

5. Conclusions

Based on the data presented above, titanium membranes in GBR should be considered as an incipient technique, versatile in terms of the type of bone defect to regenerate, in which there is still no evidence of the need of filling material and which is the most appropriate, that can better tolerate exposure than titanium meshes and titanium-reinforced non-resorbable membranes and that can be tailored to the patient's bone defect.

More randomized clinical trials comparing occlusive titanium barriers and other types of membranes are necessary to obtain more robust data that allow us to reach solid conclusions regarding the predictability and complications rate associated with the use of titanium foils, and how to manage complications when they occur.

Author Contributions: Conceptualization, E.R.-M. and A.E.-D.; methodology, E.R.-M. and A.E.-D.; validation, E.R.-M., E.J.-S. and J.L.-L.; formal analysis, E.R.-M. and A.E.-D.; investigation, E.R.-M. and A.E.-D.; resources, J.L.-L.; data Curation, E.R.-M. and J.L.-L.; writing—original draft preparation, E.R.-M. and A.E.-D.; writing—review and editing, E.J.-S. and J.L.-L.; visualization, E.R.-M. and J.L.-L.; supervision, E.J.-S. and J.L.-L.; project administration, A.E.-D. and J.L.-L. All authors have read and agreed to the published version of the manuscript.

Funding: This research received no external funding.

Conflicts of Interest: The authors declare no conflict of interest.

References

1. Wang, H.-L.; Boyapati, L. "PASS" principles for predictable bone regeneration. *Implant Dent.* **2006**, *15*, 8–17. [CrossRef] [PubMed]
2. McAllister, B.S.; Hahgighat, K. Bone augmentation techniques. *J. Periodontol.* **2007**, *78*, 277–296. [CrossRef] [PubMed]
3. Benic, G.I.; Hämmerle, C.H.F. Horizontal bone augmentation by means of guided bone regeneration. *Periodontology 2000* **2014**, *66*, 13–40. [CrossRef]
4. Bertolino, V.; Cavallaro, G.; Milioto, S.; Lazzara, G. Polysaccharides/Halloysite nanotubes for smart bionanocomposite materials. *Carbohydr. Polym.* **2020**, *245*, 116502. [CrossRef] [PubMed]
5. Cavallaro, C.; Lazzara, G.; Fakhrullin, R. Mesoporous inorganic nanoscale particles for drug adsorption and controlled release. *Ther. Deliv.* **2018**, *9*, 287–301. [CrossRef]
6. Soldatos, N.K.; Stylianou, P.; Koidou, V.P.; Angelov, N.; Yukna, R.; Romanos, G.E. Limitations and options using resorbable versus nonresorbable membranes for successful guided bone regeneration. *Quintessence Int.* **2017**, *48*, 131–147.
7. Cardaropoli, G.; Araújo, M.; Lindhe, J. Dynamics of bone tissue formation in tooth extraction sites. An experimental study in dogs. *J. Clin. Periodontol.* **2003**, *30*, 809–819. [CrossRef]
8. Araújo, M.G.; Lindhe, J. Dimensional ridge alterations following tooth extraction. An experimental study in dog. *J. Clin. Periodontol.* **2005**, *32*, 212–218. [CrossRef]
9. Srinivas, B.; Das, P.; Rana, M.M.; Qureshi, A.Q.; Vaidya, K.C.; Raziuddin, S.J.A. Wound healing and bone regeneration in postextraction sockets with and without platelet-rich fibrin. *Ann. Maxillofac. Surg.* **2018**, *8*, 28–34.
10. Li, J.; Chen, M.; Wei, X.; Hao, Y.; Wang, J. Evaluation of 3D-printed polycaprolactone scaffolds coated with freeze-dried platelet-rich plasma for bone regeneration. *Materials* **2017**, *10*, 831. [CrossRef]
11. Batas, L.; Tsalikis, L.; Stavropoulos, A. PRGF as adjunct to DBB in maxillary sinus floor augmentation: Histological results of a pilot Split-mouth study. *Int. J. Implant Dent.* **2019**, *5*, 14. [CrossRef] [PubMed]
12. Gersh, K.C.; Nagaswami, C.; Weisel, J.W. Fibrin network structure and clot mechanical properties are altered by incorporation of erythrocytes. *Thromb. Haemost.* **2009**, *102*, 1169–1175. [CrossRef] [PubMed]

13. Thor, A.; Rasmusson, L.; Wennerberg, A.; Thomsen, P.; Hirsch, J.-M.; Nilsson, B.; Hong, J. The role of whole blood in thrombin generation in contact with various titanium surfaces. *Biomaterials* **2007**, *28*, 966–974. [CrossRef] [PubMed]
14. Polimeni, G.; Koo, K.-T.; Qahash, M.; Xiropaidis, A.V.; Albandar, J.M.; Wikesjö, M.E. Prognostic factors for alveolar regeneration: Effect of a space-providing biomaterial on guided tissue regeneration. *J. Clin. Periodontol.* **2004**, *31*, 725–729. [CrossRef]
15. Jovanovic, S.S.; Nevins, M. Bone formation utilizing titanium-reinforced barrier membranes. *Int. J. Periodontics Restor. Dent.* **1995**, *15*, 56–69. [CrossRef]
16. Simion, M.; Trisi, P.; Piattelli, A. Vertical risge augmentation using a membrane technique associated with osseointegrated implants. *Int. J. Periodontics Restor. Dent.* **1994**, *14*, 496–511.
17. Elgali, I.; Omar, O.; Dahlin, C.; Thomsen, P. Guided bone regeneration: Materials and biological mechanisms revisited. *Eur. J. Oral Sci.* **2017**, *125*, 315–337. [CrossRef]
18. Caballé-Serrano, J.; Munar-Frau, A.; Ortiz-Puigpelat, O.; Soto-Penaloza, D.; Peñarrocha, M.; Herández-Alfaro, F. On the search of the ideal barrier membrane for guided bone regeneration. *J. Clin. Exp. Dent.* **2018**, *10*, e477–e483. [CrossRef]
19. Kfir, E.; Kfir, V.; Kaluski, E. Immediate bone augmentation after infected tooth extraction using titanium membranes. *J. Oral Implantol.* **2007**, *33*, 133–138. [CrossRef]
20. Bassi, M.A.; Andrisani, C.; Lico, S.; Ormanier, Z.; Ottria, L.; Gargari, M. Guided bone regeneration via a performed titanium foil: Clinical, histological and histomorphometric outcome of a case series. *Oral Implantol.* **2016**, *9*, 164–174.
21. Van Steenberghe, D.; Johansson, C.; Quirynen, M.; Molly, L.; Albrektsson, T.; Naert, I. Bone augmentation by means of a stiff occlusive titanium barrier. *Clin. Oral Implants Res.* **2003**, *14*, 63–71. [CrossRef] [PubMed]
22. Bassi, M.A.; Andrisani, C.; López, M.A.; Gaudio, R.M.; Lombardo, L.; Lauritano, D. Guided bone regeneration in distal mandibular atrophy by means of a performed titanium foil: A case series. *J. Biol. Regul. Homeost. Agents* **2016**, *30*, 61–68.
23. Bassi, M.A.; Andrisani, C.; López, M.A.; Gaudio, R.M.; Lombardo, L.; Carinci, F. Guided bone regeneration by means of a preformed titanium foil: A case of severe atrophy of edentulous posterior mandible. *J. Biol. Homeost. Agents* **2016**, *30*, 35–41.
24. Molly, L.; Quirynen, M.; Michiels, K.; van Steenberghe, D. Comparison between jaw bone augmentation by means of a stiff occlusive titanium membrane or an autologous hip graft: A retrospective clinical assessment. *Clin. Oral Implants Res.* **2006**, *17*, 481–487. [CrossRef]
25. Mauricio, E.J.M.; Faveri, M.; de Silva, H.D.P. Alveolar ridge regeneration of damaged extraction sockets using bovine-derived bone graft in association with a titanium foil: Prospective case series. *J. Int. Acad. Periodontol.* **2020**, *22*, 109–116.
26. Perret, F.; Romano, F.; Ferrarotti, F.; Aimetti, M. Occlusive titanium barrier for immediate bone augmentation of severely resorbed alveolar sockets with secondary soft tissue healing: A 2-year case series. *Int. J. Periodontics Restor. Dent.* **2019**, *39*, 97–105. [CrossRef]
27. Toygar, H.U.; Guzeldemir, E.; Cilasun, U.; Akkor, D.; Arpak, N. Long-term clinical evaluation and SEM analysis of the e-PTFE and titanium membranes in guided tissue regeneration. *J. Biomed. Mater. Res. B Appl. Biomater.* **2009**, *91*, 772–779. [CrossRef]
28. Engelke, W.; Deccó, O.; Cura, A.C.; Borie, E.; Beltrán, V. Rigid occlusive titanium barriers for alveolar bone augmentation: Two reports with 24-month follow-up. *Int. J. Clin. Exp. Med.* **2014**, *7*, 1160–1165.
29. Beltrán, V.; Engelke, W.; Fuentes, R.; Decco, O.; Prieto, R.; Wilckens, M.; Borie, E.; Beltran, V.; Engelke, W.; Fuentes, R.; et al. Bone augmentation with occlusive barriers and cortical particulate allograft in transverse maxillary defects: A pilot study. *Int. J. Morphol.* **2014**, *32*, 364–368. [CrossRef]
30. Beltrán, V.; Matthijs, A.; Borie, E.; Fuentes, R.; Valdivia-Gandur, I.; Engelke, W. Bone healing in transverse maxillary defects with different surgical procedures using anorganic bovine bone in humans. *Int. J. Morphol.* **2013**, *31*, 75–81. [CrossRef]
31. Gaggl, A.; Schultes, G. Titanium foil-guided tissue regeneration in the treatment of periimplant bone defects. *Implant Dent.* **1999**, *8*, 368–375. [CrossRef] [PubMed]
32. Moher, D.; Liberati, A.; Tetzlaff, J.; Altman, D.G. PRISMA Group. Preferred reporting items for systematic reviews and meta-analyses: The PRISMA statement. *PLoS Med.* **2009**, *6*, e1000097. [CrossRef] [PubMed]

33. Ebell, M.H.; Siwek, J.; Weiss, B.D.; Woolf, S.H.; Susman, J.; Ewigman, B.; Bowman, M. Strenght of recommendation taxonomy (SORT): A patient-centered approach to grading evidence in the medical literature. *Am. Fam. Phys.* **2004**, *69*, 548–556.
34. Sterne, J.A.C.; Savović, J.; Page, M.J.; Elbers, R.G.; Blencowe, N.S.; Boutron, I. RoB 2: A revised tool for assessing risk of bias in randomised trials. *BMJ* **2019**, *366*, l4898. [CrossRef] [PubMed]
35. Sterne, J.A.; Hernán, M.A.; Reeves, B.C.; Savović, J.; Berkman, N.D.; Viswanathan, M. ROBINS-1: A tool for assessing risk of bias in non-randomised studies of interventions. *BMJ* **2016**, *355*, i4919. [CrossRef] [PubMed]
36. Vrielinck, L.; Sun, Y.; Schepers, S.; Politis, C.; Slycke, S.V.; Agbaje, J.O. Osseous reconstruction using an occlusive titanium membrane following marginal mandibulectomy: Proof of principle. *J. Craniofac. Surg.* **2014**, *25*, 1112–1114. [CrossRef] [PubMed]
37. Khanna, R.; Khanna, R.; Pardhe, N.D.; Srivastava, N.; Bajpai, M.; Gupta, S. Pute titanium membrane (Ultra-Ti®) in the treatment of periodontal osseous defects: A split-mouth comparative study. *J. Clin. Diagn. Res.* **2016**, *10*, ZC47–ZC51.
38. Pinho, M.N.; Roriz, V.L.M.; Novaes, A.-B.; Taba, M.; Grisi, M.F.M.; de Souza, S.L.S.; Palioto, D.B. Titanium membranes in prevention of alveolar collapse after tooth extraction. *Implant Dent.* **2006**, *15*, 53–61. [CrossRef]
39. Watzinger, F.; Luksch, J.; Millesi, W.; Schopper, C.; Neugebauer, J.; Moser, D.; Ewers, R. Guided bone regeneration with titanium membranes: A clinical study. *Br. J. Oral Maxillofac. Surg.* **2000**, *38*, 312–315. [CrossRef]
40. Cucchi, A.; Vignudelli, E.; Napolitano, A.; Marchetti, C.; Corinaldesi, G. Evaluation of complication rates and vertical bone gain after guided bone regeneration with non-resorbable membranes versus titanium meses and resorbable membranes. A randomized clinical trial. *Clin. Implant Dent. Relat. Res.* **2017**, *19*, 821–832. [CrossRef]
41. Urban, I.A.; Montero, E.; Monje, A.; Sanz-Sánchez, I. Effectiveness of vertical ridge augmentation interventions: A systematic review and meta-analysis. *J. Clin. Periodontol.* **2019**, *46*, 319–339. [CrossRef] [PubMed]
42. Wessing, B.; Lettner, S.; Zechner, W. Guided bone regeneration with collagen membranes and particulate graft materials: A systematic review and meta-analysis. *Int. J. Oral Maxillodac. Implants* **2018**, *33*, 87–100. [CrossRef] [PubMed]
43. Urban, I.A.; Nagursky, H.; Lozada, J.L.; Nagy, K. Horizontal risge augmentation with a collagen membrane and a combination of particulated autogenous bone and anorganic bovine bone-derived mineral: A prospective case series in 25 patients. *Int. J. Periodontics Restor. Dent.* **2013**, *33*, 299–307. [CrossRef] [PubMed]
44. Meloni, S.M.; Jovanovic, S.A.; Urban, I.; Baldoni, E.; Pisano, M.; Tallarico, M. Horizontal ridge augmentation using GBR with a native collagen membrane and 1:1 ratio of particulate xenograft and autologous bone: A 3-year after final loading prospective clinical study. *Clin. Implant Dent. Relat. Res.* **2019**, *21*, 669–677. [CrossRef]
45. Moraschini, V.; Poubel, L.A.; Ferreira, V.F.C.; Barboza, E.S.P. Evaluation of survival and success rates of dental implants reported in longitudinal studies with a follow-up period of at least 10 years: A systematic review. *Int. J. Oral Maxillofac. Surg.* **2015**, *44*, 377–388. [CrossRef]

Publisher's Note: MDPI stays neutral with regard to jurisdictional claims in published maps and institutional affiliations.

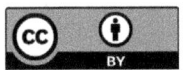

© 2020 by the authors. Licensee MDPI, Basel, Switzerland. This article is an open access article distributed under the terms and conditions of the Creative Commons Attribution (CC BY) license (http://creativecommons.org/licenses/by/4.0/).

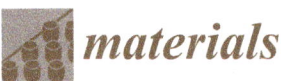

Article

Topological, Mechanical and Biological Properties of Ti6Al4V Scaffolds for Bone Tissue Regeneration Fabricated with Reused Powders via Electron Beam Melting

Maria Laura Gatto [1,*], Riccardo Groppo [2], Nora Bloise [3,4], Lorenzo Fassina [5], Livia Visai [3,4], Manuela Galati [6], Luca Iuliano [6] and Paolo Mengucci [1]

1. Department SIMAU, Università Politecnica delle Marche, Via Brecce Bianche 12, 60131 Ancona, Italy; p.mengucci@univpm.it
2. Department of Engineering "Enzo Ferrari", Università di Modena e Reggio Emilia, 41121 Modena, Italy; riccardo.groppo@unimore.it
3. Department of Molecular Medicine, Centre for Health Technologies (CHT), INSTM UdR of Pavia, University of Pavia, 27100 Pavia, Italy; nora.bloise@unipv.it (N.B.); livia.visai@unipv.it (L.V.)
4. Department of Occupational Medicine, Toxicology and Environmental Risks, ICS Maugeri, IRCCS, 27100 Pavia, Italy
5. Department of Electrical, Computer and Biomedical Engineering, Centre for Health Technologies (CHT), University of Pavia, Via Ferrata 5, 27100 Pavia, Italy; lorenzo.fassina@unipv.it
6. Department of Management and Production Engineering (DIGEP), Politecnico di Torino, 10129 Torino, Italy; manuela.galati@polito.it (M.G.); luca.iuliano@polito.it (L.I.)
* Correspondence: m.l.gatto@pm.univpm.it; Tel.: +39-071-2204751

Citation: Gatto, M.L.; Groppo, R.; Bloise, N.; Fassina, L.; Visai, L.; Galati, M.; Iuliano, L.; Mengucci, P. Topological, Mechanical and Biological Properties of Ti6Al4V Scaffolds for Bone Tissue Regeneration Fabricated with Reused Powders via Electron Beam Melting. *Materials* 2021, *14*, 224. https://doi.org/10.3390/ma14010224

Received: 25 November 2020
Accepted: 29 December 2020
Published: 5 January 2021

Publisher's Note: MDPI stays neutral with regard to jurisdictional claims in published maps and institutional affiliations.

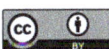

Copyright: © 2021 by the authors. Licensee MDPI, Basel, Switzerland. This article is an open access article distributed under the terms and conditions of the Creative Commons Attribution (CC BY) license (https://creativecommons.org/licenses/by/4.0/).

Abstract: Cellularized scaffold is emerging as the preferred solution for tissue regeneration and restoration of damaged functionalities. However, the high cost of preclinical studies creates a gap between investigation and the device market for the biomedical industry. In this work, bone-tailored scaffolds based on the Ti6Al4V alloy manufactured by electron beam melting (EBM) technology with reused powder were investigated, aiming to overcome issues connected to the high cost of preclinical studies. Two different elementary unit cell scaffold geometries, namely diamond (DO) and rhombic dodecahedron (RD), were adopted, while surface functionalization was performed by coating scaffolds with single layers of polycaprolactone (PCL) or with mixture of polycaprolactone and 20 wt.% hydroxyapatite (PCL/HA). The mechanical and biological performances of the produced scaffolds were investigated, and the results were compared to software simulation and experimental evidence available in literature. Good mechanical properties and a favorable environment for cell growth were obtained for all combinations of scaffold geometry and surface functionalization. In conclusion, powder recycling provides a viable practice for the biomedical industry to strongly reduce preclinical costs without altering biomechanical performance.

Keywords: titanium implants; additive manufacturing; reused powder; unit cell topology; tissue engineering; mechanical properties; stem cells; surface functionalization

1. Introduction

Recently, an approach to bone tissue regeneration based on cellularized-scaffold implantation was used to overcome the risks connected to bone grafts when self-healing fails [1].

The focal point of scaffolds for bone tissue regeneration is unit cell topology which influences mechanical and biological performance [1]. Suitable mechanical properties are required in load-bearing applications while suitable mass transport properties are necessary for biological activities [2]. Both these features relate to porosity, pore size and pore interconnectivity, that in turn are determined by scaffold elementary unit cell geometry. Therefore, scaffold design must be balanced to allow nutrients and oxygen supply, metabolic waste removal, cell penetration and reduction of stress shielding to prevent mechanical failure [3,4].

Two main elementary unit cell geometries for the scaffold are proposed in the literature: (a) diagonal symmetrical and (b) midline symmetrical. Finite element analysis (FEA) [5] showed that a porous structure with midline symmetry exhibited superior compressive performances than diagonal symmetry, while the opposite trend was observed in the case of torsion. Therefore, rhombic dodecahedron (RD) unit cell geometry (midline symmetrical) is well suited for load-bearing implants, while diamond (DO) unit cell geometry (diagonal symmetrical) is preferable for implants subjected to torsional forces. In addition, numerical analysis by computational fluid dynamics (CFD) [6] has demonstrated that DO shows advantages in implant fixation (greater tortuosity and larger aperture), cell growth environment (more appropriate adhesion areas), and tissue regeneration (due to regular mechanical stimulation), while RD shows a superior mass transport performance (higher flow velocity value). Therefore, DO and RD elementary unit cells are valid alternatives for bone tissue regeneration.

Accurate control of the anatomical shape, size and topology of the scaffold's elementary unit cell can be efficiently obtained by additive manufacturing (AM) technology alternatives to traditional subtractive methods. Typically, AM processes for metal alloys consist of melting powders through an energy source (laser or electron beam) in a layer-by-layer process, according to a CAD file [7,8]. Laser-manufactured parts show lower surface roughness in comparison to electron beam melting (EBM) products, that generally exhibit residual stresses and gas contamination. Laser-melting technology is widely used for dental implants [9,10], while EBM is commonly employed in a patient's customized bone implants [11,12].

Titanium alloys have an elastic modulus in the range 50–118 GPa, closer to natural cortical bone (10–30 GPa) than any other widely investigated alloy for permanent implant, such as cobalt chromium (240 GPa) and stainless steel (216 GPa) [13]. However, the difference in elastic modulus between cortical bone and titanium alloys leads to stress shielding with reabsorption of the unstressed bone portion and consequent risk of implant failure [14].

A combination of EBM technology and Ti6Al4V alloy has been investigated by Popov et al. [11], that produced biomedical patient-specific implants for clavicle, mandibular bone, foot osteotomy and hip. In the reported clinical cases, EBM revealed a reduction of time in operation and patient recovery.

Despite the key advantages of combining EBM technology with Ti-based alloys, only a small percentage of tissue engineering research in this field achieves clinical application, due to the high cost of preclinical studies. To overcome this gap, Martinez–Marquez et al. [15] proposed a step model to ensure the cost-effectiveness of customized scaffolds. In particular, they proposed material feedstock recycling as the first step in cost reduction. Material feedstock in EBM processes can affect up to 31% of the cost of built parts [16]. Therefore, recycling Ti6Al4V metal powder represents an affordable solution to reduce waste and save costs [17]. However, powder reuse means repeated preheating steps and prolonged thermal treatments in a vacuum during the EBM process that can induce changes in the reused powder, in terms of chemical composition, morphology and physical properties [18]. In Ti6Al4V alloy thermal cycling due to powder reuse induces variations in particle size distribution and oxygen uptake that can lead it to exceed the $O < 0.2$ wt.% condition required by ASTM F2924-14 [19]. Oxygen stabilizes the α-Ti phase which pins dislocation during part deformation. Thus, with powder reuse, ultimate yield strength slightly increases, while ductility decreases [18,20,21].

In addition to elementary unit cell geometry and scaffold production technology, the engineering aspect to be improved for implant success is surface functionalization, which must fulfill scaffold–bone interface requirements. The most common functionalization treatment is coating the scaffold's surface with a layer of biocompatible material or a combination of biocompatible compounds [22–24]. Surface coating plays a double role: (a) avoids the release of toxic ions [3,4,25,26] and (b) improves implant osteointegration.

Currently, the researchers' interest is focused on synthetic bioresorbable and biocompatible polymers such as polylactide (PLA), polycaprolactone (PCL) and polyglycolide (PGA) [27]. Among them, PCL is the most promising due to slow degradation time (>24 months) with respect to PLA (12–16 months) and PGA (6–12 months) [28]. However, to overcome the PCL drawbacks concerning structural (elevated hydrophobicity) and biological aspects (poor bioactivity and low cell adhesion), PCL is usually combined with ceramic materials such as hydroxyapatite (HA). HA shows excellent biocompatibility, bioactivity and osteoconductive properties, allowing enhanced bone formation and implant-site recovery [29,30].

In this paper, the elementary unit cell geometry, surface functionalization, mechanical properties and biological response of scaffolds based on Ti6Al4V alloy, produced with a mixture of reused and virgin new powders by the EBM technology, were considered for bone tissue regeneration. The aim of the work is to fabricate suitable scaffolds for in vivo perspectives starting from industrial EBM process based on cost and waste reduction in order to overcome issues connected to the high costs of preclinical studies. Starting from reused powder blended with virgin new powder as the raw material of the EBM process, scaffolds with DO and RD elementary unit cell geometry were produced. After production, scaffolds were submitted to topological and mechanical characterization to compare their performances with the experimental and simulated results reported in literature [5] for identical structures (same alloy composition, production technology and elementary unit cell geometries). Afterwards, scaffolds were coated with a single layer of PCL or PCL/HA for surface functionalization and then submitted to biological tests. Human mesenchymal stem cell cultures for 24 h and 4 days were used as a fast check of the scaffold's biological response. The role of unremoved residual powder in the scaffold core on mechanical and biological behavior was also considered. Results evidenced mechanical and biological performance of scaffolds produced by EBM industrial methods fully comparable to the literature data from scaffolds produced by virgin new powder, thus providing an indication for viable industrial processes for cost reduction of preclinical studies.

2. Materials and Methods
2.1. Material

Scaffolds were produced using Arcam Ti6Al4V powder. The raw material was a mixture of Arcam powder in recycled and virgin new conditions blended in unknown proportions. In this paper, from now on, the blended raw powder is indicated as P1, while the virgin new powder, used as reference, is indicated as P2. As provided by the manufacturer (Arcam website [31]), the virgin new powder P2 has a particle size in the range 45–106 µm, density 2.47 g/cm^3 and the nominal chemical composition reported in Table 1.

Table 1. Nominal chemical composition (wt.%) of the Arcam Ti6Al4V powder in virgin new condition (P2).

Al	V	C	Fe	O	N	H	Ti
6.0	4.0	0.03	0.1	0.1	0.01	<0.003	Bal.

2.2. Scaffold Geometry

The scaffolds' local geometries adopted in this study are schematically shown in Figure 1. Scaffolds were designed using Magics 21.0 in diamond (DO, Figure 1A) and rhombic dodecahedron (RD, Figure 1B) elementary unit cell. Scaffold volume, independently on elementary unit cell geometry, corresponds to a cube 1 cm side length.

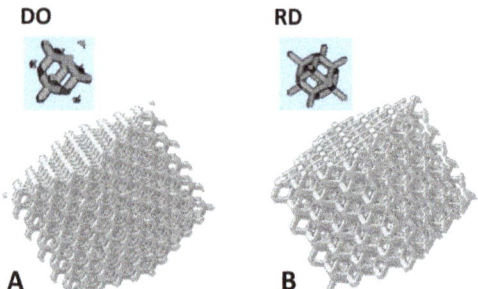

Figure 1. Schematics of the scaffolds' elementary unit cell geometry: (**A**) diamond (DO) and (**B**) rhombic dodecahedron (RD).

Nominal porosity and strut size are reported in Table 2 for diagonal symmetrical (DO) and midline symmetrical (RD) elementary unit cells. Theoretical porosity is constant (80%) for both geometries, while strut size changes on the basis of pore size and interconnectivity.

Table 2. CAD values of porosity and strut size for DO and RD geometries.

Geometry	Porosity (%)	Strut Size (μm)
DO	80	420
RD	80	460

2.3. Scaffold Manufacturing

Scaffolds were additively manufactured using Arcam A2X electron beam melting (EBM) system. The entire procedure was carried out in a vacuum with the powder bed heated to 750 °C before the production process to induce partial sintering of powder particles. Sintering improves powder thermal conductivity and mechanical strength, thus allowing production of parts with a reduced number of supports or even without any supporting structure [32]. Processing parameters are reported in Table 3. After production and cooling, scaffolds were cleaned by Ti6Al4V ELI powder blasting at 4 bar pressure.

Table 3. Arcam A2X printing parameters.

Printing Parameters	Outer Contour	Inner Contour
Maximum beam current (mA)	3	3
Focus offset (mA)	0	0
Speed (mm/s)	450	470
Offset (mm)	0.13	
Number of perimeters	1	1

2.4. Scaffold Porosity and Residual Powder Volume

After powder blasting, some unremoved residual powder was still present in the inner central part of the scaffold. Residual powder was visible by visual inspection. Observations carried out by optical (Nikon OPTIPHOT-100, Tokyo, Japan) and scanning electron microscopy confirmed the presence of residual powder that partially and sometimes totally occluded pores in the scaffold core. The unremoved residual powder was partially sintered during scaffold production and could not be removed even after repeated blasting processes.

Scaffold porosity resulting from the production process was experimentally obtained by X-ray computed tomography (XCT) (Bruker Skyscan 1174 system, Kontich, Belgium) measurements performed on a slice cut from a scaffold external part, free of residual powder. The external slice total volume was 160 mm^3.

The total volume of residual powder was estimated from experimental measurement of scaffold mass by using precision balance and five weighing operations. The mass of residual powder (m_{pw}) was obtained from Equation (1):

$$m_s = m_{Ti} + m_{pw} \qquad (1)$$

where m_s is scaffold mass, m_{Ti} mass of struts calculated from porosity data and alloy nominal density (ρ_{Ti} = 4.43 g/cm^3) and m_{pw} total mass of unremoved residual powder. Residual powder volume (V_{pw}) was calculated from residual powder density $\rho_{pw} = 0.68$ $\rho_{Ti} = 3.012$ g/cm^3, as suggested by Tolochko et al. [33].

In order to check distribution of residual powder and presence of porosity occlusions in the scaffold core, scaffolds were cut by diamond blade at half height (about 0.5 cm below the upper scaffold surface). After acetone cleaning in ultrasonic system followed by air jetting, the scaffold was observed by scanning electron microscope.

2.5. Surface Functionalization

Surface functionalization was performed by coating the scaffold with a single layer of: (a) polycaprolactone (PCL) or (b) a mixture of polycaprolactone and 20% hydroxyapatite (PCL/HA). The coating operation was carried out by manually dipping the scaffold in the bath solution for 20 s, followed by air drying. The solvent used in the bath solution was tetrahydrofuran (THF, CH_2Cl_2), selected after C. Bordes et al. [34]. Chemical grade powders of polycaprolactone (PCL, Eurocoating S.p.a.) and hydroxyapatite (HA, Boc Sciences, Inc., Shirley, NY, USA) were used as solutes. The bath solution was obtained by gradually melting PCL and PCL/HA powders in THF solvent under magnetic stirring at room temperature.

2.6. Morphological, Structural and Mechanical Characterization

Morphological characterization of blended powder (P1) and reference virgin powder (P2) as well as of the DO and RD scaffolds was carried out by Zeiss Supra 40 field emission scanning electron microscope (FESEM) (Carl Zeiss AG, Oberkochen, Germany) equipped with Bruker Z200 energy dispersive microanalysis (EDS) (Billerica, MA, USA) and Tescan Vega 3 scanning electron microscope (SEM) (Brno, Czech Republic) equipped with EDAX Elements EDS system. Starting from FESEM images, powder mean grain size was evaluated by ImageJ software (version 1.52a, NIH, Bethesda, MD, USA [35]).

Scaffolds in DO and RD geometries were morphologically characterized by 3D light microscopy (3D LM) and FESEM observations.

Scaffold porosity was experimentally obtained by XCT analysis carried out in Bruker Skyscan 1174 system at V = 40 kV, I = 800 µA with Cu-Kα radiation source, pixel size 13.8 µm, rotation step 0.2°, total rotation angle 360°, exposure time per projection 8 s, aluminum filter (1 mm) for optimization of X-ray energy transmission. Projections were processed by SkyScan reconstruction program NRecon, collecting stacks of cross-sectional slices generated with the following settings: misalignment compensation = −3, smoothing = 3, ring artefacts reduction = 5, beam hardening correction = 8%. The 3D reconstructions of DO and RD slices were carried out by VG Studio MAX 1.2 software (Volume Graphics, Heidelberg, Germany).

Structural information from powders and scaffolds were obtained by X-ray diffraction (XRD), while EDS microanalysis was used to estimate chemical composition.

A Bruker D8 Advance diffractometer operating at V = 40 kV and I = 40 mA, with Cu-Kα radiation, in the angular range 2θ = 34°–43° was used for XRD measurements. Pattern analysis was carried out by DIFFRAC.EVA software package including ICDD—PDF 2 license for search/match analysis. Shape analysis of XRD peaks was carried out by OriginPro (version 8.5) software package.

EDS analysis was carried out by a Bruker Z200 microanalysis system installed in a Zeiss Supra 40 FESEM. Chemical composition by EDS were obtained by averaging data taken from three different sample areas observed at same magnification (1000×). Results are reported as average value (AV) and standard deviation (SD) calculated from the three measurements.

Topographic maps were obtained by Nikon LV 150 Confovis Microscope (Tokyo, Japan). Scaffold roughness parameters were measured from topographic maps, according to ISO 25178-603 [36].

Mechanical performance of uncoated scaffold was investigated by uniaxial compressive tests carried out in Instron 5567 system (5 kN load cell, 0.5 mm/min speed) (Norwood, MA, USA) in accordance with the standard ISO 13314:2011 [37]. For each scaffold geometry, four cubic samples $10 \times 10 \times 10$ mm^3 were tested. The results of compressive tests are plotted as a stress–strain curve from which were calculated: (a) maximum stress value at first peak, assumed as compression strength, after Li et al. [5], (b) Young modulus and (c) compressive strength at 40% strain. Mechanical parameters estimated from stress–strain curves allowed the comparison of results obtained in this work to literature data.

2.7. Biological Characterization

2.7.1. Cell Culture Conditions

Human mesenchymal stem cells derived from bone marrow were isolated and phenotypically analyzed to assess their mesenchymal properties according to the International Society for Cellular Therapy by a method previously described [38,39]. The study was conducted in accordance with the Institution Review Board of Fondazione IRCCS Policlinico San Matteo and the University of Pavia (2011). Written informed consent was obtained from all participants enrolled in the study. Cells used in all experiments were mainly at passage 4–5.

Cells were grown at 37 °C in 5% CO_2 humidified atmosphere, maintained in low-glucose DMEM (Dulbecco's modified Eagle's) supplemented with 10% FBS, 1% glutamine, 1% penicillin-streptomycin and amphotericin B (Lonza Group Ltd., Basel, Switzerland).

Before cell seeding, the scaffold was sterilized in an autoclave (Vapor Matic 770) at 120 °C for 20 min, washed with phosphate-buffered saline (PBS 1X), while coated scaffolds were sterilized by immersing in 70% ethanol bath for 20 min. Subsequent scaffolds were placed inside a standard 24-well-plate (Corning Inc., Corning, NY, USA), washed several times with sterile distillated water followed by PBS 1X and finally dried under ultraviolet light exposure for 40 min in order to prevent contamination. A cell suspension of 5×10^4 was placed on the top of each scaffold. After 0.5 h of incubation, 1.3 mL of culture medium was added to the scaffold covering. The hMSC seeded and cultured on tissue culture plates (TCPS) wells were inserted as control.

2.7.2. Cell Viability Assay

Cell viability on different scaffolds was estimated by using resazurin-based assay (TOX8-1KT Sigma Aldrich, St. Louis, MO, USA) after 1 and 4 days of incubation, as previously reported [40]. According to manufacturer instructions, resazurin solution (Sigma-Aldrich) was added in 1:10 ratio with respect to culture volume to each well plate, and incubated for 3 h at 37 °C in 5% CO_2. At the end of incubation time, absorbance was measured at 570 and 600 nm wavelengths using a microplate reader (Bio-Rad Laboratories, Hercules, CA, USA). Each biological experiment was performed in triplicate and in at least three separate tests. Results were expressed as mean value ± standard deviation. Statistical analysis of hMSC viability data at 24 h and 4 days was performed using the GraphPad Prism (version 5.00 for Windows, GraphPad Software, San Diego, CA, USA) software package. Two-way ANOVA analysis was carried out to check the influence of geometry and surface treatments on cell viability at 24 h and 4 days, separately. Since two-way ANOVA analysis did not provide any significant results, t-tests were performed for DO and RD scaffold geometries on the following parameters: uncoated, PCL coated and PCL/HA coated scaffolds and vice versa, for both the cell viability times. Statistical significance was analyzed at: $p < 0.05$ *.

2.7.3. Focal Adhesion Kinase—Enzyme-Linked Immunosorbent Assay

The activation of the Focal Adhesion Kinase (FAK) was measured by human phospho-FAK enzyme-linked immunosorbent assay (ELISA) kit (Human Phospho-FAK (Y397) and Total FAK ELISA, RayBiotech, Inc., Peachtree Corners, GA, USA). After 24 h from seeding, cell-seeded samples were washed extensively with sterile PBS to remove culture medium and lysed with ice-cold lysis buffer (50 mM Tris pH 7.5, 50 mM NaCl, 5 mM ethylenediaminetetraacetic acid, 0.1% Triton, and 1 mM sodium orthovanadate) for 30 min on ice. Afterwards, lysates were centrifuged at 13,000 rpm for 15 min at 4 °C and supernatants were analyzed by ELISA kit in accordance with manufacturer's instructions. Data were expressed as mean value with standard deviation. Statistical analysis was performed using two-way ANOVA, to understand if geometry and surface treatments have statistically significative effects on the phospho-FAK on the total FAK signal. The software package used was GraphPad Prism (version 5.00 for Windows, GraphPad Software, San Diego, CA, USA) and differences were considered significant for $p < 0.05$ *. A graph was obtained normalizing the phospho-FAK on the total FAK signal.

2.7.4. FESEM Observation

After 24 h and 4 days of incubation, cell seeded onto scaffolds were treated as previously described [41]. The specimens were fixed with 2.5% (v/v) glutaraldehyde solution in 0.1 M Na-cacodylate buffer (pH = 7.2) for 1 h at 4 °C, washed with Na-cacodylate buffer and then dehydrated at room temperature in ethanol gradient series up to 100%. Samples were frozen for at least one day and then lyophilized 6 h to complete dehydration. Finally, scaffolds were sputter-coated with gold and observed by FESEM.

3. Results

3.1. Structural and Morphological Characterization of Powders

FESEM observation allowed the morphology of the raw blended powder P1 to be compared to the reference virgin new powder P2 (Figure 2). Spherically shaped particles were visible in both P1 (Figure 2A) and P2 (Figure 2B). However, particle aggregation was clearly visible in P1 (Figure 2A), due to joint neck formation at the particle contact points, caused by the heating and cooling cycle for powder reuse.

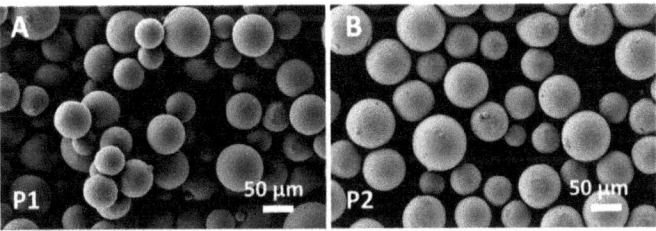

Figure 2. FESEM images of powders: (**A**) blended P1 and (**B**) virgin new P2.

The virgin new powder P2 (Figure 2B) is formed of spherical particles with small satellites and a size in the range of 40–110 μm in agreement with the values provided by the manufacturer. The blended powder P1 (Figure 2A) was also formed of spherical particles with a few residual satellites and a size in the range of 50–130 μm. Aggregation of spherical particles with neck formation was evident in P1 (Figure 2A).

The experimental chemical composition obtained by EDS analysis of P1 and P2 powders is reported in Table 4. Within experimental uncertainties, both powders had similar average chemical composition.

Table 4. Chemical composition (wt.%) of P1 and P2 powders obtained by EDS analysis. AV—average value, SD—standard deviation.

Element	P1 (wt.%)		P2 (wt.%)	
	AV	SD	AV	SD
Al	5.8	0.2	6.1	0.4
Ti	90.60	0.14	90.5	0.2
V	3.60	0.11	3.4	0.2

XRD patterns of powders are reported in Figure 3. Peak position of α-Ti (ICDD file n. 44-1294) and β-Ti (ICDD file n. 44-1288) phases are indicated by full dots and full squares, respectively.

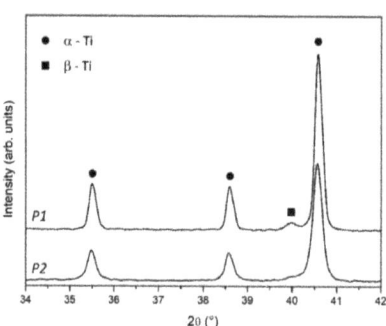

Figure 3. XRD patterns of P1 and P2 powders. Full dot—α-Ti, full square—β-Ti.

Powders are mainly formed of α-Ti with a small contribution of β-Ti, which is more evident in P1, due to the recycled part of the blended powder.

3.2. Scaffold Characterization

3.2.1. Geometry

The structure of the scaffold's top surface as well as the scaffold's inner structure were observed by FESEM and SEM, results are reported in Figures 4 and 5. Morphology of the scaffold's top surface is shown in Figure 4A for DO and Figure 4B for RD, while Figure 5A,B report the scaffold's inner structure.

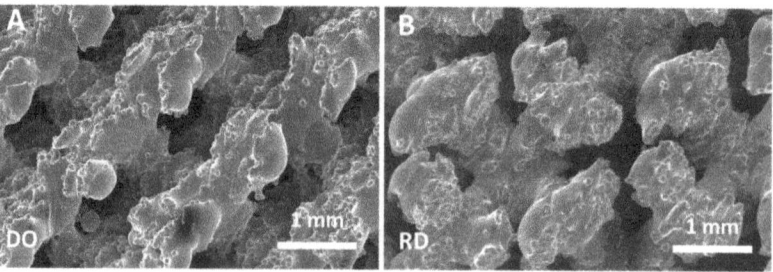

Figure 4. FESEM images of the scaffold's top surface: (**A**) DO geometry, (**B**) RD geometry.

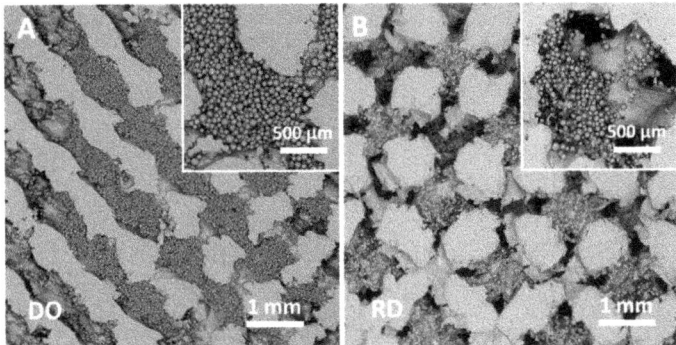

Figure 5. SEM images of the scaffold's inner structure: (**A**) DO geometry, (**B**) RD geometry. Insets show the same area of sample at higher magnification.

Independently of geometry (DO or RD), the top surface of the scaffold is formed of partially melted particles (Figure 4A,B) with well interconnected open pores.

The scaffold's inner structure showed pores partially filled with unmelted and neck connected powder particles (Figure 5A,B).

Images in Figure 5 were taken in the central part (core) of the cut scaffold at the same magnification for comparison. High density residual powder in DO geometry (Figure 5A) with total occlusion of most pores was clearly evident. In contrast, RD geometry (Figure 5B) had pores only partially occluded. It is worth noting that SEM observations of the peripheric regions, far from the scaffold core, show open pores free from residual powder.

3.2.2. Porosity and Residual Powder Volume

XCT measurements carried out on scaffold slices free from residual powder provided identical scaffold porosity values for all geometries, within experimental uncertainties. From porosity values, the total mass of struts (m_{Ti}) and total volume of residual powder were obtained, according to Equation (1). The results are summarized in Table 5 for the scaffold geometries investigated.

Table 5. Experimental values resulting from XCT analysis and calculated values of residual powder weight (m_{pw}) and volume (V_{pw}). m_s—total scaffold mass; V_s—total scaffold volume; m_{Ti}—total mass of struts; V_{Ti}—total volume of struts; m_{pw}—total mass of residual powder; V_{pw}—total volume of residual powder.

Geometry	Porosity (%)	m_s (g)	V_s (cm^3)	m_{Ti} (g)	V_{Ti} (cm^3)	m_{pw} (g)	V_{pw} (cm^3)
DO	63	1.94	1	1.64	0.37	0.30	0.0996
RD	63	1.81	1	1.64	0.37	0.17	0.0564

From the data in Table 5, it was evident that the amount of residual powder inside the scaffold strongly depended on geometry, with DO containing about double the quantity of residual powder compared to RD. The relative density ($\rho = 1 - p$), where p is the scaffold porosity, as defined by Zhou et al. [42], could be also estimated from data in Table 5. For both geometries, the relative density ρ result was 37%.

3.2.3. Structural and Chemical Characterization

Experimental chemical composition of the scaffolds obtained by EDS analysis was almost the same for both DO and RD geometries, the results are reported in Table 6. It is worth noting that the average chemical composition of the scaffold showed a slight decrease of vanadium with respect to the experimental composition of P1 and P2 powders (Table 4).

Table 6. Chemical composition of scaffold obtained by EDS analysis. AV—average value, SD—standard deviation.

Element	Scaffold (wt. %)	
	AV	SD
Al	6.0	0.5
Ti	91.7	0.7
V	2.4	0.2

Figure 6 shows XRD patterns of DO and RD scaffolds. The patterns reported the peaks of α-Ti (ICDD file n. 44-1294) and β-Ti (ICDD file n. 44-1288) phases as full dots and full squares, respectively. Scaffolds showed low intensity and broad diffraction peaks suggested low crystallization. Residual stresses and/or variations in crystalline state of scaffolds could be responsible for the slight angular peak shift visible in Figure 6.

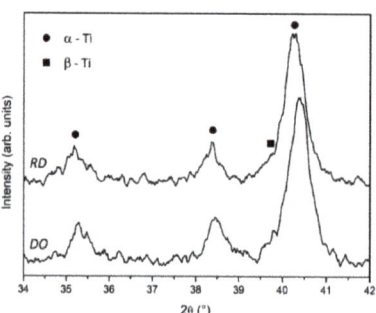

Figure 6. XRD patterns of DO and RD scaffolds. Full dot—α-Ti, full square—β-Ti.

3.2.4. Mechanical Tests

Compression tests carried out on scaffolds provided the mechanical behavior shown in Figure 7 for DO and RD geometries. The gradual collapse of scaffold elementary unit cells arranged on the scaffold layers was clearly evident in the DO curve, up to 40% reduction of initial scaffold height, which corresponded to a displacement of 4 mm.

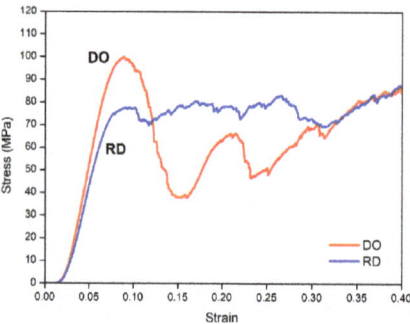

Figure 7. Mechanical behavior of scaffolds under compression for DO and RD geometries.

In the RD curve the gradual collapse of scaffold elementary unit cells was less evident, although compaction occurred at about the same value of compression on initial height.

On compression, scaffolds showed a "barrel" phenomenon during layer compaction, with mechanically different behaviors along the x, y and z directions.

Maximum stress value at first peak was assumed as compression strength, after Li et al. [5].

Stress–strain curves in Figure 7 also allowed the calculation of Young modulus and compressive strength at 40%. Results are summarized in Table 7 with values obtained by Li et al. [5] and Ahmadi et al. [43] for comparison. Table 7 also shows reference values for cortical bone. It is worth underlining that the values of porosity and relative density reported in Table 7 for this work referred only to struts without any contribution from residual powder. Therefore, all values in Table 7 can be reliably compared.

Table 7. Experimental results obtained from the compression tests compared to the results obtained by Li et al. [5] and Ahmadi et al. [43] with the same scaffold geometries, and reference values for cortical bone.

Reference	Porosity (%)		Relative Density (%)		Young Modulus (GPa)		Compression Strength (MPa)		Compression Strength at 40% (MPa)	
	DO	RD	DO	RD	DO	RD	DO	RD	DO	RD
This work	63	63	37	37	1.949 ± 0.001	1.622 ± 0.001	99	78	86	88
Li et al. [5]	70	70	30	30	2.59 ± 0.13	4.89 ± 0.05	88 ± 5	174 ± 4		
Ahmadi et al. [43]	80	72	20	28			45	80	30	70
Cortical bone					3.9–11.7				80	

3.2.5. Surface Functionalization

SEM observations in cross-section of PCL and PCL/HA coatings are shown in Figure 8. DO and RD scaffolds coated with PCL are reported in Figure 8A,B, respectively, while DO and RD scaffolds coated with PCL/HA are shown in Figure 8C,D for comparison. In SEM images the coatings appeared brighter than the metal struts of scaffold, continuous and well-adhered to the scaffold's top surface as well as to surface of inner struts, when the coating penetrated inside the scaffold. Coating reduces scaffold surface roughness resulting in a smoothing effect leading to thickness variation of coating from a few tens of microns up to about 1 mm. The coating on the top surface always exhibits a porous structure due to solvent evaporation (inset in Figure 8C), as already reported by Abdal-hay et al. [44].

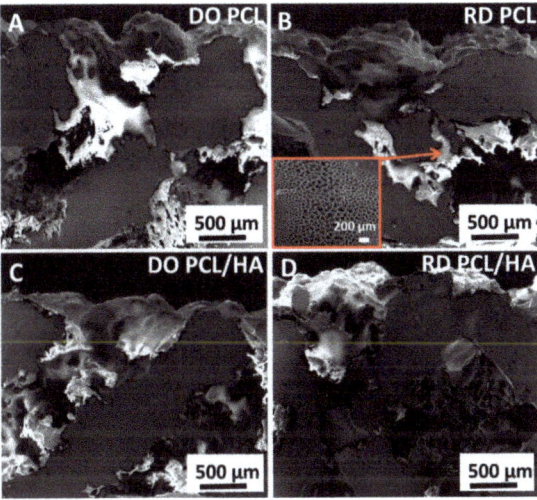

Figure 8. Micrographs of DO and RD scaffold coated with (**A,B**) PCL and (**C,D**) PCL/HA.

3.2.6. Surface Roughness

Top surface roughness maps of uncoated and coated scaffolds are reported in Figure 9 for comparison. From the roughness maps the roughness parameters of both scaffold geometries in uncoated and coated conditions were derived. The scaffold roughness parameters that estimated statistical distribution of height values along z axis, are listed in Table 8, with: Ra—average surface roughness, mean value of absolute distances in the roughness profile; Ssk—surface skewness, symmetry of roughness profile with respect to the mean line; Sku—surface kurtosis, sharpness of roughness profile; Sp—surface peak, maximum height of roughness profile from the mean line; Sv—surface valley, maximum depth of roughness profile from the mean line. Average surface roughness (Ra) shows the same trend for DO and RD, higher values for uncoated scaffolds and a slight decrease for PCL and PCL/HA coated scaffolds. All scaffolds, except for the DO uncoated condition that has valley predominance (Ssk < 0), show predominance of peaks in the roughness profile (Ssk > 0), with higher values of maximum peak height (Sp) and maximum valley depth (Sv) for the RD uncoated condition. Sharpness of roughness profile (Sku) is higher for PCL than for PCL/HA coating regardless of scaffold cell geometry.

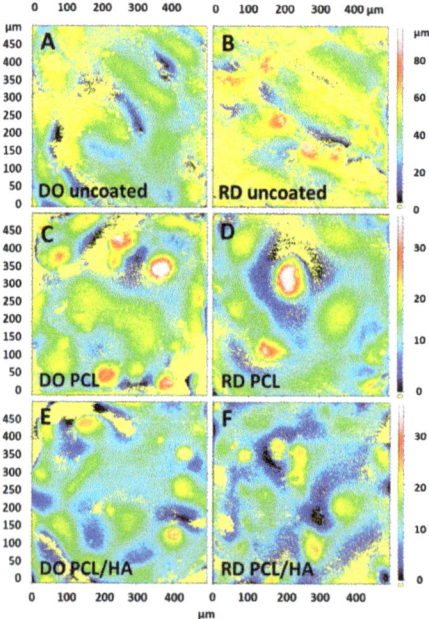

Figure 9. Roughness maps of DO and RD (**A,B**) uncoated, (**C,D**) coated with PCL and (**E,F**) with PCL/HA.

Table 8. Roughness parameters estimated from roughness maps.

Parameters	DO			RD		
	Uncoated	PCL	PCL/HA	Uncoated	PCL	PCL/HA
Ra (μm)	6.5	3.9	2.8	10	3.5	3.27
Ssk	−0.8	0.7	0.13	0.4	1.14	0.5
Sku	4.3	5.4	4.1	4.0	7.13	3.6
Sp (μm)	2.9	3.8	2.1	9.1	3.26	2.7
Sv (μm)	5.8	2.18	1.7	9.8	1.5	1.6

3.3. Scaffold Interaction with hMSCs

In order to evaluate scaffold interaction with hMSCs, all groups were examined for cell viability, morphology and activation of the FAK protein typically involved in the cell adhesion process.

Tests of cell viability in Figure 10 were carried out on DO and RD scaffolds in uncoated and coated condition, after 24 h (Figure 10A) and 4 days of incubation (Figure 10B). Data were normalized on the control (TCPS) and are reported as percentage values.

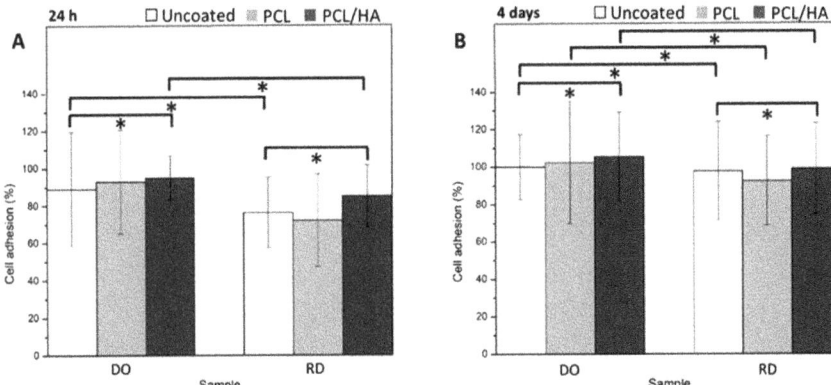

Figure 10. Cell viability at (**A**) 24 h and (**B**) 4 days on DO and RD uncoated, coated with PCL and with PCL/HA—$p < 0.05$ *.

The results of SEM observations performed in the same experimental setup on DO and RD scaffolds in uncoated and coated conditions after 24 h and 4 days of cell incubation are reported in Figure 11. After 24 h incubation, the cell distribution in the uncoated scaffolds are shown in Figure 11A,B for the DO and RD geometry, respectively. Images of the DO and RD scaffolds coated with PCL are shown in Figure 11C,D, respectively. Images of the DO and RD scaffolds coated with PCL/HA are shown in Figure 11E,F, respectively. In all scaffold conditions (coated and uncoated) and geometries (DO and RD), effective hMSCs presence was evidenced, while cell morphology suggested that after 24 h incubation, cells were in the spreading phase on the scaffold surface.

After 4 days incubation cell number had increased, with cells starting to colonize scaffold inner layers. Although, in DO and RD uncoated condition (Figure 11G,H) cells were clearly visible on the scaffold surface, they were not visible on the top surface of the coated scaffolds. In order to observe cell colonization of the scaffold inner part, coated scaffolds with PCL and PCL/HA were cut at 2 mm depth from the top surface and then observed by SEM. In the scaffold's deeper layers, SEM observations clearly evidenced cells in spreading phase independently of scaffold geometry (DO or RD) and coating type (PCL or PCL/HA). The results of SEM observations of the coated scaffold inner region are reported in Figure 11I,J for DO and RD coated with PCL, and in Figure 11K,L for DO and RD coated with PCL/HA.

ELISA assay analysis of FAK phosphorylation in hMSCs revealed that P-FAK was highly upregulated in cells grown on DO compared with cells grown on RD, indicating activation of FAK signaling by geometry cues (Figure 12).

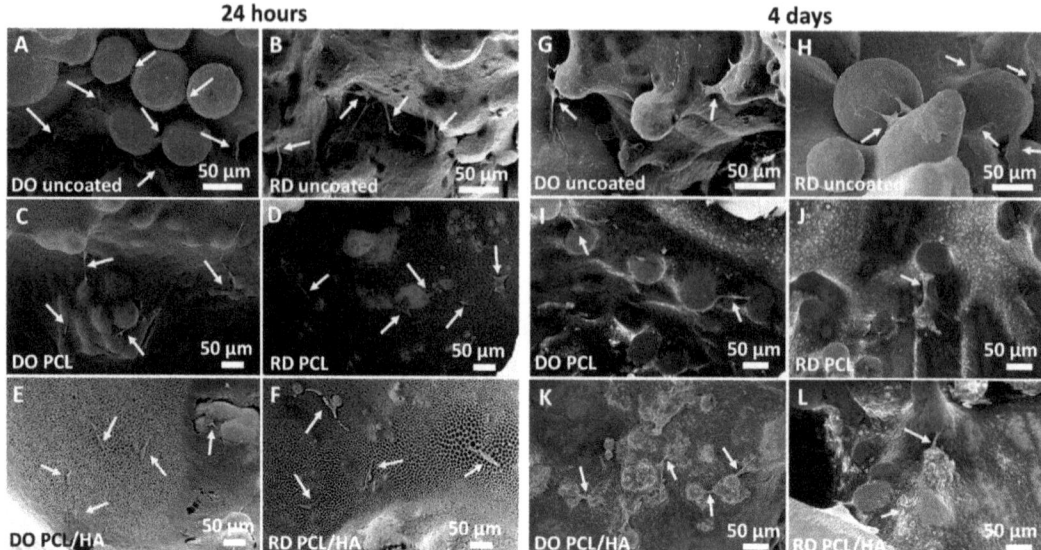

Figure 11. hMSCs after 24 h of incubation on DO and RD (**A,B**) uncoated, (**C,D**) coated with PCL and (**E,F**) with PCL/HA and hMSCs after 4 days of incubation on DO and RD (**G,H**) uncoated, (**I,J**) coated with PCL and with (**K,L**) PCL/HA. The hMSCs are indicated by the arrows.

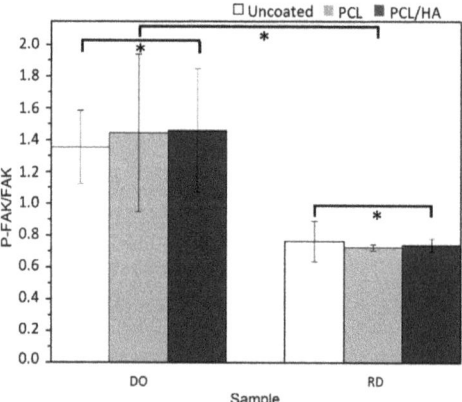

Figure 12. The activation level of FAK was measured by ELISA assay after 24h of incubation onto the different scaffolds. Bar graphs show P-FAK values normalized on the total FAK—$p < 0.05$ *.

4. Discussion

The ideal scaffold for tissue regeneration must: (a) support the normal cellular activity without producing any harmful effect (biocompatibility), (b) allow cells to adhere, proliferate and form extracellular matrix on its pore and surface, (c) allow formation of blood vessels to support the transport of oxygen, nutrients and waste products. Therefore, obtaining an ideal scaffold means taking control of any aspect of the production chain starting from the selection of raw materials and production technology to the design of pore shape, size and interconnectivity. Furthermore, cell viability tests allow the checking of material biocompatibility and cell colonization of the produced scaffolds. Therefore, in the perspective of tissue regeneration, biological characterization is as essential as mechanical and structural characterization.

In this study, cell viability tests were used as a fast check of biological response concerning scaffold pore topology and surface functionalization coating. For this reason, viability tests were stopped after only 4 days of culture, even before stem cell differentiation.

The raw material used to fabricate the scaffolds was Arcam Ti6Al4V powder blended in an unknown proportion with the same powder after several recycles. Blending recycled powder used in previous EBM processes with virgin new powder is common practice in the additive manufacturing industry to reduce costs and waste [17]. Although the chemical composition (Table 4) and lattice structure (Figure 3) of the raw powder (P1) were almost unaltered with respect to the virgin new powder (P2), in agreement with Alamos et al. [45], SEM images clearly showed particle aggregation through neck formation in P1 (Figure 2A).

Powder sintering occurring during the preheating and melting steps of the EBM process led to the formation of necks between particles (Figure 2A), that were responsible for powder aggregation. Although aggregation increased powder strength [32], aggregated particles remained entrapped in the pores of scaffold core (Figure 5) with consequences on scaffold topology-connected performance and mechanical properties.

The amount of residual powder inside the scaffold depended on geometry as evident in Figure 5 and Table 5. In particular, DO geometry, which had more intricate pore pathway for the release of unmelted powder entrapped inside the scaffold [6], contained about 76% more residual powder than RD (Table 5).

The most important geometrical features in DO and RD geometries such as pore size, strut size and porosity were investigated by Li et al. [46] using software analysis. All these parameters not only affect biological performance but also play a central role in mechanical properties [5].

Li et al. [5,46] investigated scaffold produced from virgin new powder with the same unit cell geometries (DO and RD) of our scaffolds that were produced with the blended P1 powder described above. Therefore, results obtained by Li et al. from software simulation [46] and mechanical tests [5] were taken here as reference and compared with our results in Table 7.

In particular, Li et al. [5] estimated a porosity value around 70% for both DO and RD unit cell geometry (Table 7). In our case, the porosity experimental value was 63% for both geometries (Table 7). Discrepancies between software calculated (Table 2) and experimental values were fully due to the EBM manufacturing technique. In particular, the EBM processing parameters reported in Table 3 allowed scaffold to be obtained with a strut size much larger (ranging from 800 to 1000 μm for both DO and RD geometries) than the nominal CAD values listed in Table 2. This reduced scaffold porosity to 63% against the expected 80% of CAD calculation (Table 2). Nevertheless, the struts were fully dense without pores or lack of fusion defects (Figure 5).

The EBM process occurs in vacuum, thus avoiding any oxygen contamination that could modify the chemical composition and physical properties of the powder, even after reuse [32]. However, the melting process in EBM can induce compositional variations in the final parts with respect to the metal powder. In our case, this event was confirmed by EDS analysis of scaffolds whose average chemical composition (Table 6) showed slight decrease of vanadium with respect to the alloy's nominal composition (Table 1) and the experimental composition of the blended powder (Table 4).

XRD analysis of P1 and P2 powders (Figure 3) clearly showed the joint presence of α-Ti and β-Ti phases in both specimens. The peak intensity in the patterns evidenced better crystallization and higher β-Ti content in P1, due to the recycled part of blended raw powder. XRD patterns of scaffolds (Figure 6) confirmed the joint presence of α-Ti and β-Ti phases suggesting that the vanadium decrease measured by EDS was incapable of deeply changing the alloy's microstructure. Nevertheless, comparing the XRD patterns of powders (Figure 3) and scaffolds (Figure 6) a markedly reduced crystallinity and possible residual stresses in scaffolds could be argued.

During the melting step of the EBM process, the electron beam provides enough energy to induce localized powder melting. However, in regions adjacent to the melted zone, the powder temperature does not reach the melting value so that large numbers of spherical titanium particles remain partially bonded to the walls of the melted pool, giving rise to the surface morphology reported in Figure 4. Studies on surface roughness of EBM implants identified Ra = 24.9 µm as the upper limit value for positive effects on cell proliferation and differentiation [47]. Roughness values of the scaffold surface reported in Table 8 are well below this limit, even in uncoated condition, confirming that scaffolds manufactured with the EBM parameters reported in Table 3 meet the needs of scaffold−host tissue interface for bone regeneration. Moreover, surface functionalization coating further decreases average surface roughness (Table 8). Recent studies demonstrated beneficial effects in several biomedical applications of as-fabricated rippled surfaces in EBM processed alloys [48,49].

Concerning additional topology-connected performances of scaffolds, it is worth noting that the DO geometry generally provides a more suitable structure for cell vitality than RD, both at 24 h and 4 days. Metabolic protein quantification confirms the better biological response of DO against RD. Quantification of P-FAK on total FAK (Figure 12), being the phosphorylation of FAK, the activator signal of the cell adhesion pathway, is indicative of a gentler environment for cell adhesion. Regardless of the percentage of viable cells present in scaffolds, a higher value of P-FAK/FAK of DO geometry corresponds to a greater number of viable cells attached to the scaffold. Therefore, since cell adhesion is a regulator of cellular proliferation, migration and differentiation [50], this result suggests a better biological response of the DO unit cell geometry against RD, in perfect agreement with the numerical analysis by Li et al. [6].

Further improvement in cell adhesion and proliferation was obtained by coating the scaffold surface with a single layer of PCL or PCL/HA. For both scaffold geometries (DO and RD) surface coating enhanced cell viability at 24 h and 4 days, especially in the presence of HA (Figure 10). The PCL coating, with or without HA, promoted enhancement of P-FAK activation independently of the scaffold geometry (DO or RD).

Coatings (Figure 8) adhered to the substrate in varying thickness according to the surface topography developed by partially melted powder particles. Independently of coating type (PCL or PCL/HA), a porous structure formed on the coating surface due to solvent evaporation (inset in Figure 8B). This porous structure promoted nutrient diffusion and osteointegration, thus supporting cell differentiation and proliferation [44]. The coating changed the morphology and chemical composition of the scaffold surface, thus improving further surface biofunctions [18]. Moreover, coating reduced the surface roughness, PCL/HA had the lowest Ra value (Table 8) and improved the biological behavior of stem cells (Figure 10B). SEM observations at 4 days incubation showed an absence of stem cells on the scaffold's coated surface, suggesting penetration of hMSCs inside the scaffold (Figure 11). Therefore, the investigated coatings enhanced cell penetration into the scaffold, with PCL/HA showing better performance due to lower surface roughness.

In terms of mechanical behavior under uniaxial compressive testing (Figure 7) scaffold unit cell geometry seemed to be the most influencing parameter, although powder aggregation effects in the scaffold core must be considered. Stress–strain curves shown in Figure 7 for DO and RD unit cell geometry exhibited a general shape in agreement with the results in literature for the same cell topology [5,43]. The DO curve grew rapidly up to maximum stress value, corresponding to the compression strength, then large oscillations due to collapse of unit cells under compressive load followed. The collapse mechanism was clearly described by Ahmadi et al. [43] and Del Guercio et al. [51] In contrast, the RD curve after its first rise showed small oscillations around the same average stress value (Figure 7), in agreement with the results in literature [5,43]. However, contrary to the results in literature, DO and RD curves in Figure 7 reached the same stress value in the final part of the curve at high strain values. The two curves were completely superimposed above 35% strain, when the unit cells were all collapsed, and the scaffold structure arrived at compaction (Figure 7). Ahmadi et al. [43] reported the trend of compression strength and yield stress as a function of relative density for DO and RD geometries, showing that for relative density below 25% the two curves were superimposed, while for higher values RD always exhibited higher mechanical properties against DO. Ahmadi et al. [43] attributes the lower mechanical properties of DO to the unit cell geometry which is relatively simple and different struts provide only limited support to each other during compression. The relative density of our scaffolds, obtained by experimental calculation of porosity from XCT analysis, was 37% with compression strength of RD (78 MPa) lower than DO (99 MPa), as reported in Table 7. Generally, the mechanical behavior of our scaffolds strongly differed from the results of Li et al. [5] and Ahmadi et al. [43] for similar structures (Table 7). In particular, the large size of struts (ranging from 800 to 1000 µm) in our scaffolds determined the elastic behavior (Young modulus) and compression strength of DO and RD geometries (Table 7). Following Ahmadi et al. [43], the more complex unit cell geometry (RD) exhibited lower elastic properties (Table 7), while absolute values of Young modulus were always lower than the values from Li et al. [5] for similar cell geometries with lower strut size and lower relative density (Table 7). Therefore, higher strut size gives rise to stiffer structures with different behaviors for different unit cell geometries. In our case, both strut size and the absence of structural defects inside the struts (Figure 5) were responsible for higher compression strength of DO with respect to RD (Table 7).

On compression, in the simpler DO geometry failure of a single strut caused collapse of an entire elementary unit cell, then producing the large oscillations visible in the DO curve in Figure 7. As the collapse of elementary unit cells occurred from outside to inside during compression, the first part of the stress–strain curve (Figure 7) was not influenced by the residual powder stored in the scaffold core (Figure 5). However, when all external elementary unit cells had collapsed, elementary unit cells in the scaffold core that were partially filled with sintered residual powder, started to deform. On collapse of core elementary unit cells, the scaffold's mechanical properties became dependent on sintered residual powder, which increased compressive stress and stress on struts in the longitudinal direction perpendicular to the compressive force. In this way, differences in mechanical properties linked to different elementary unit cell geometry vanished, overruled by the presence of residual powder, so stress–strain curves of DO and RD unit cells coincided. It is worth noting that the compression strength at 40% of our scaffolds is very close to the experimental value of cortical bone (Table 7), suggesting that the presence of residual sintered powder did not deteriorate the mechanical performance of the scaffolds.

5. Conclusions

In biomedical industries, the high cost of device preclinical studies generates a gap between investigation and device commercialization. The aim of this study is to fill the gap by checking the feasibility of cost saving processes based on EBM technology. Starting from a mixture of reused and virgin new powders, as commonly done in industrial practice, scaffolds with diamond (DO) and rhombic dodecahedron (RD) elementary unit cells were produced and surface functionalized from the perspective of tissue regeneration applications. Surface functionalization was carried out by coating the scaffold with either PCL or PCL/HA layers. The feasibility of our industrial approach was verified by comparing scaffold biomechanical performance with standard preclinical studies in literature.

The main results obtained can be summarized as follows:

- EBM technology is suitable for the production of porous structures with controlled topology and well-defined unit cell geometry showing appropriate biological performance and surface characteristics for in vivo perspectives. Low surface roughness typical of the EBM process promotes hMSC proliferation, while the partially sintered residual powder in the scaffold's core is responsible for the porosity mismatch between experimental and CAD design values;
- The mechanical performance of the scaffold is mainly influenced by elementary unit cell geometry. The presence of residual powder becomes evident for compression

values outside the range of in vivo use of the device and tends to cancel out the differences between geometries. In general, the compression behavior of the scaffolds is quite similar to natural bone tissue and follows trends reported in literature, although strut size and the absence of structural defects inside the struts are responsible for the higher compression strength of DO against RD;
- Short-term cell viability and metabolic protein quantification identifies DO as a better biological environment than RD, in agreement with literature-reported numerical simulations. After 4 days incubation, hMSCs start to penetrate inside the scaffold, favored by adherent, continuous and protective layers of PCL and PCL/HA.

From the above results it is evident that powder recycling represents a convenient industrial practice applicable to the manufacture of biomedical devices to heavily reduce preclinical costs without altering biomechanical performance.

Author Contributions: M.L.G.: conceptualization, methodology, writing—original draft preparation, R.G.: data curation, N.B.: investigation, L.F.: validation, L.V.: resources, M.G.: investigation, software, L.I.: resources, P.M.: supervision, formal analysis, writing—reviewing and editing. All authors have read and agreed to the published version of the manuscript.

Funding: This research received no external funding.

Institutional Review Board Statement: Not applicable.

Informed Consent Statement: Not applicable.

Data Availability Statement: Data sharing not applicable.

Acknowledgments: Nora Bloise and Livia Visai acknowledge the grant of the Italian Ministry of Education, University and Research (MIUR) to the Department of Molecular Medicine of the University of Pavia under the initiative "Dipartimenti di Eccellenza (2018–2022)".

Conflicts of Interest: The authors declare no conflict of interest.

References

1. Ho-Shui-Ling, A.; Bolander, J.; Rustom, L.E.; Johnson, A.W.; Luyten, F.P.; Picart, C. Bone Regeneration Strategies: Engineered Scaffolds, Bioactive Molecules and Stem Cells Current Stage and Future Perspectives. *Biomaterials* **2018**, *180*, 143–162. [CrossRef] [PubMed]
2. Wu, S.; Liu, X.; Yeung, K.W.K.; Liu, C.; Yang, X. Biomimetic Porous Scaffolds for Bone Tissue Engineering. *Mater. Sci. Eng. R Rep.* **2014**, *80*, 1–36. [CrossRef]
3. Wang, X.; Xu, S.; Zhou, S.; Xu, W.; Leary, M.; Choong, P.; Qian, M.; Brandt, M.; Xie, Y.M. Topological Design and Additive Manufacturing of Porous Metals for Bone Scaffolds and Orthopaedic Implants: A Review. *Biomaterials* **2016**, *83*, 127–141. [CrossRef]
4. Wubneh, A.; Tsekoura, E.K.; Ayranci, C.; Uludağ, H. Current State of Fabrication Technologies and Materials for Bone Tissue Engineering. *Acta Biomater.* **2018**, *80*, 1–30. [CrossRef] [PubMed]
5. Li, J.; Chen, D.; Zhang, Y.; Yao, Y.; Mo, Z.; Wang, L.; Fan, Y. Diagonal-Symmetrical and Midline-Symmetrical Unit Cells with Same Porosity for Bone Implant: Mechanical Properties Evaluation. *J. Bionic Eng.* **2019**, *16*, 468–479. [CrossRef]
6. Li, J.; Chen, D.; Fan, Y. Evaluation and Prediction of Mass Transport Properties for Porous Implant with Different Unit Cells: A Numerical Study. *BioMed Res. Int.* **2019**, *2019*, 3610785. [CrossRef]
7. Barucca, G.; Santecchia, E.; Majni, G.; Girardin, E.; Bassoli, E.; Denti, L.; Gatto, A.; Iuliano, L.; Moskalewicz, T.; Mengucci, P. Structural Characterization of Biomedical Co–Cr–Mo Components Produced by Direct Metal Laser Sintering. *Mater. Sci. Eng. C* **2015**, *48*, 263–269. [CrossRef]
8. Mengucci, P.; Gatto, A.; Bassoli, E.; Denti, L.; Fiori, F.; Girardin, E.; Bastianoni, P.; Rutkowski, B.; Czyrska-Filemonowicz, A.; Barucca, G. Effects of Build Orientation and Element Partitioning on Microstructure and Mechanical Properties of Biomedical Ti-6Al-4V Alloy Produced by Laser Sintering. *J. Mech. Behav. Biomed. Mater.* **2017**, *71*, 1–9. [CrossRef]
9. Mengucci, P.; Barucca, G.; Gatto, A.; Bassoli, E.; Denti, L.; Fiori, F.; Girardin, E.; Bastianoni, P.; Rutkowski, B.; Czyrska-Filemonowicz, A. Effects of Thermal Treatments on Microstructure and Mechanical Properties of a Co–Cr–Mo–W Biomedical Alloy Produced by Laser Sintering. *J. Mech. Behav. Biomed. Mater.* **2016**, *60*, 106–117. [CrossRef]
10. Santecchia, E.; Gatto, A.; Bassoli, E.; Denti, L.; Rutkowski, B.; Mengucci, P.; Barucca, G. Precipitates Formation and Evolution in a Co-Based Alloy Produced by Powder Bed Fusion. *J. Alloys Compd.* **2019**, *797*, 652–658. [CrossRef]
11. Popov, V.V. Design and 3D-Printing of Titanium Bone Implants: Brief Review of Approach and Clinical Cases. *Biomed. Eng. Lett.* **2018**, *8*, 337–344. [CrossRef] [PubMed]

12. Calignano, F.; Galati, M.; Iuliano, L.; Minetola, P. Design of Additively Manufactured Structures for Biomedical Applications: A Review of the Additive Manufacturing Processes Applied to the Biomedical Sector. *J. Healthc. Eng.* **2019**, *2019*, 9748212. [CrossRef]
13. Stewart, C.; Akhavan, B.; Wise, S.G.; Bilek, M.M.M. A Review of Biomimetic Surface Functionalization for Bone-Integrating Orthopedic Implants: Mechanisms, Current Approaches, and Future Directions. *Prog. Mater. Sci.* **2019**, *106*, 100588. [CrossRef]
14. Yuan, L.; Ding, S.; Wen, C. Additive Manufacturing Technology for Porous Metal Implant Applications and Triple Minimal Surface Structures: A Review. *Bioact. Mater.* **2019**, *4*, 56–70. [CrossRef] [PubMed]
15. Martinez-Marquez, D.; Mirnajafizadeh, A.; Carty, C.P.; Stewart, R.A. Application of Quality by Design for 3D Printed Bone Prostheses and Scaffolds. *PLoS ONE* **2018**, *13*, e0195291. [CrossRef]
16. Powell, D.; Rennie, A.E.W.; Geekie, L.; Burns, N. Understanding Powder Degradation in Metal Additive Manufacturing to Allow the Upcycling of Recycled Powders. *J. Clean. Prod.* **2020**, *268*, 122077. [CrossRef]
17. Chandrasekar, S.; Coble, J.B.; Yoder, S.; Nandwana, P.; Dehoff, R.R.; Paquit, V.C.; Babu, S.S. Investigating the Effect of Metal Powder Recycling in Electron Beam Powder Bed Fusion Using Process Log Data. *Addit. Manuf.* **2020**, *32*, 100994. [CrossRef]
18. Tang, H.P.; Qian, M.; Liu, N.; Zhang, X.Z.; Yang, G.Y.; Wang, J. Effect of Powder Reuse Times on Additive Manufacturing of Ti-6Al-4V by Selective Electron Beam Melting. *JOM* **2015**, *67*, 555–563. [CrossRef]
19. ASTM. *ASTM F2924-14, Standard Specification for Additive Manufacturing Titanium-6 Aluminum-4 Vanadium with Powder Bed Fusion*; ASTM: West Conshohocken, PA, USA, 2014.
20. Ghods, S.; Schultz, E.; Wisdom, C.; Schur, R.; Pahuja, R.; Montelione, A.; Arola, D.; Ramulu, M. Electron Beam Additive Manufacturing of Ti6Al4V: Evolution of Powder Morphology and Part Microstructure with Powder Reuse. *Materialia* **2020**, *9*, 100631. [CrossRef]
21. Liu, S.; Shin, Y.C. Additive Manufacturing of Ti6Al4V Alloy: A Review. *Mater. Des.* **2019**, *164*, 107552. [CrossRef]
22. Jia, B.; Yang, H.; Han, Y.; Zhang, Z.; Qu, X.; Zhuang, Y.; Wu, Q.; Zheng, Y.; Dai, K. In Vitro and in Vivo Studies of Zn-Mn Biodegradable Metals Designed for Orthopedic Applications. *Acta Biomater.* **2020**, *108*, 358–372. [CrossRef] [PubMed]
23. Liu, X.; Sun, J.; Zhou, F.; Yang, Y.; Chang, R.; Qiu, K.; Pu, Z.; Li, L.; Zheng, Y. Micro-Alloying with Mn in Zn–Mg Alloy for Future Biodegradable Metals Application. *Mater. Des.* **2016**, *94*, 95–104. [CrossRef]
24. Shuai, C.; Wang, B.; Bin, S.; Peng, S.; Gao, C. TiO_2-Induced In Situ Reaction in Graphene Oxide-Reinforced AZ61 Biocomposites to Enhance the Interfacial Bonding. *ACS Appl. Mater. Interfaces* **2020**, *12*, 23464–23473. [CrossRef] [PubMed]
25. Su, Y.; Cockerill, I.; Zheng, Y.; Tang, L.; Qin, Y.-X.; Zhu, D. Biofunctionalization of Metallic Implants by Calcium Phosphate Coatings. *Bioact. Mater.* **2019**, *4*, 196–206. [CrossRef] [PubMed]
26. Kaur, M.; Singh, K. Review on Titanium and Titanium Based Alloys as Biomaterials for Orthopaedic Applications. *Mater. Sci. Eng. C* **2019**, *102*, 844–862. [CrossRef] [PubMed]
27. Kajzer, W.; Jaworska, J.; Jelonek, K.; Szewczenko, J.; Kajzer, A.; Nowińska, K.; Hercog, A.; Kaczmarek, M.; Kasperczyk, J. Corrosion Resistance of Ti6Al4V Alloy Coated with Caprolactone-Based Biodegradable Polymeric Coatings. *Eksploat. Niezawodn. Maint. Reliab.* **2017**, *20*, 30–38. [CrossRef]
28. Nair, L.S.; Laurencin, C.T. Biodegradable Polymers as Biomaterials. *Prog. Polym. Sci.* **2007**, *32*, 762–798. [CrossRef]
29. Hajiali, F.; Tajbakhsh, S.; Shojaei, A. Fabrication and Properties of Polycaprolactone Composites Containing Calcium Phosphate-Based Ceramics and Bioactive Glasses in Bone Tissue Engineering: A Review. *Polym. Rev.* **2018**, *58*, 164–207. [CrossRef]
30. Mohd Yusoff, M.F.; Abdul Kadir, M.R.; Iqbal, N.; Hassan, M.A.; Hussain, R. Dipcoating of Poly (ε-Caprolactone)/Hydroxyapatite Composite Coating on Ti6Al4V for Enhanced Corrosion Protection. *Surf. Coat. Technol.* **2014**, *245*, 102–107. [CrossRef]
31. Official Web-Site of Arcam EBM AB, Machines Manufacturer. Available online: http://www.arcam.com (accessed on 20 November 2020).
32. Galati, M.; Iuliano, L. A Literature Review of Powder-Based Electron Beam Melting Focusing on Numerical Simulations. *Addit. Manuf.* **2018**, *19*, 1–20. [CrossRef]
33. Tolochko, N.K.; Arshinov, M.K.; Gusarov, A.V.; Titov, V.I.; Laoui, T.; Froyen, L. Mechanisms of Selective Laser Sintering and Heat Transfer in Ti Powder. *Rapid Prototyp. J.* **2003**, *9*, 314–326. [CrossRef]
34. Bordes, C.; Fréville, V.; Ruffin, E.; Marote, P.; Gauvrit, J.Y.; Briançon, S.; Lantéri, P. Determination of Poly(ε-Caprolactone) Solubility Parameters: Application to Solvent Substitution in a Microencapsulation Process. *Int. J. Pharm.* **2010**, *383*, 236–243. [CrossRef]
35. Rasband, W.S. *ImageJ*; National Institutes of Health: Bethesda, MD, USA, 2016. Available online: http://imagej.nih.gov/ij/ (accessed on 20 November 2020).
36. ISO. *ISO 25178-603:2013, Geometrical Product Specifications (GPS)—Surface Texture: Areal—Part 603: Nominal Characteristics of Non-Contact (Phase-Shifting Interferometric Microscopy) Instruments*; International Organization for Standardization: Geneva, Switzerland, 2013.
37. ISO. *ISO 13314:2011: Mechanical Testing of Metals—Ductility Testing—Compression Test for Porous and Cellular Metals*; International Organization for Standardization (ISO): Geneva, Switzerland, 2011.
38. Bernardo, M.E.; Avanzini, M.A.; Perotti, C.; Cometa, A.M.; Moretta, A.; Lenta, E.; Del Fante, C.; Novara, F.; de Silvestri, A.; Amendola, G.; et al. Optimization of in Vitro Expansion of Human Multipotent Mesenchymal Stromal Cells for Cell-Therapy Approaches: Further Insights in the Search for a Fetal Calf Serum Substitute. *J. Cell. Physiol.* **2007**, *211*, 121–130. [CrossRef]

39. Ceccarelli, G.; Bloise, N.; Mantelli, M.; Gastaldi, G.; Fassina, L.; De Angelis, M.G.C.; Ferrari, D.; Imbriani, M.; Visai, L. A Comparative Analysis of the In Vitro Effects of Pulsed Electromagnetic Field Treatment on Osteogenic Differentiation of Two Different Mesenchymal Cell Lineages. *BioRes. Open Access* **2013**, *2*, 283–294. [CrossRef]
40. Cristofaro, F.; Gigli, M.; Bloise, N.; Chen, H.; Bruni, G.; Munari, A.; Moroni, L.; Lotti, N.; Visai, L. Influence of Nanofiber Chemistry and Orientation of Biodegradable Poly(Butylene Succinate)-Based Scaffolds on Osteoblast Differentiation for Bone Tissue Regeneration. *Nanoscale* **2018**, *10*. [CrossRef]
41. Bloise, N.; Patrucco, A.; Bruni, G.; Montagna, G.; Caringella, R.; Fassina, L.; Tonin, C.; Visai, L. In Vitro Production of Calcified Bone Matrix onto Wool Keratin Scaffolds via Osteogenic Factors and Electromagnetic Stimulus. *Materials* **2020**, *13*, 3052. [CrossRef]
42. Zhou, D.; Gao, Y.; Lai, M.; Li, H.; Yuan, B.; Zhu, M. Fabrication of NiTi Shape Memory Alloys with Graded Porosity to Imitate Human Long-Bone Structure. *J. Bionic Eng.* **2015**, *12*, 575–582. [CrossRef]
43. Ahmadi, S.; Yavari, S.; Wauthle, R.; Pouran, B.; Schrooten, J.; Weinans, H.; Zadpoor, A. Additively Manufactured Open-Cell Porous Biomaterials Made from Six Different Space-Filling Unit Cells: The Mechanical and Morphological Properties. *Materials* **2015**, *8*, 1871–1896. [CrossRef]
44. Abdal-hay, A.; Amna, T.; Lim, J.K. Biocorrosion and Osteoconductivity of PCL/NHAp Composite Porous Film-Based Coating of Magnesium Alloy. *Solid State Sci.* **2013**, *18*, 131–140. [CrossRef]
45. Alamos, F.J.; Schiltz, J.; Kozlovsky, K.; Attardo, R.; Tomonto, C.; Pelletiers, T.; Schmid, S.R. Effect of Powder Reuse on Mechanical Properties of Ti-6Al-4V Produced through Selective Laser Melting. *Int. J. Refract. Met. Hard Mater.* **2020**, *91*, 105273. [CrossRef]
46. Li, J.; Chen, D.; Luan, H.; Yan, W.; Fan, Y. Mechanical Performance of Porous Implant with Different Unit Cells. *J. Mech. Med. Biol.* **2017**, *17*, 1750101. [CrossRef]
47. Trevisan, F.; Calignano, F.; Aversa, A.; Marchese, G.; Lombardi, M.; Biamino, S.; Ugues, D.; Manfredi, D. Additive Manufacturing of Titanium Alloys in the Biomedical Field: Processes, Properties and Applications. *J. Appl. Biomater. Funct. Mater.* **2018**, *16*, 57–67. [CrossRef] [PubMed]
48. Nune, K.C.; Li, S.; Misra, R.D.K. Advancements in Three-Dimensional Titanium Alloy Mesh Scaffolds Fabricated by Electron Beam Melting for Biomedical Devices: Mechanical and Biological Aspects. *Sci. China Mater.* **2018**, *61*, 455–474. [CrossRef]
49. Gong, X.; Anderson, T.; Chou, K. Review on Powder-Based Electron Beam Additive Manufacturing Technology. *Manuf. Rev.* **2014**, *1*, 2. [CrossRef]
50. Xia, L.; Xie, Y.; Fang, B.; Wang, X.; Lin, K. In Situ Modulation of Crystallinity and Nano-Structures to Enhance the Stability and Osseointegration of Hydroxyapatite Coatings on Ti-6Al-4V Implants. *Chem. Eng. J.* **2018**, *347*, 711–720. [CrossRef]
51. Del Guercio, G.; Galati, M.; Saboori, A. Innovative Approach to Evaluate the Mechanical Performance of Ti–6Al–4V Lattice Structures Produced by Electron Beam Melting Process. *Met. Mater. Int.* **2020**. [CrossRef]

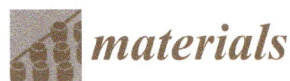

Article

Histomorphometric Evaluation of Peri-Implant Bone Response to Intravenous Administration of Zoledronate (Zometa®) in an Osteoporotic Rat Model

Amani M. Basudan [1], Marwa Y. Shaheen [1], Abdurahman A. Niazy [2], Jeroen J. J. P. van den Beucken [3], John A. Jansen [3] and Hamdan S. Alghamdi [1,*]

1. Department of Periodontics and Community Dentistry, College of Dentistry, King Saud University, Riyadh 11451, Saudi Arabia; abasudan@ksu.edu.sa (A.M.B.); mashaheen@ksu.edu.sa (M.Y.S.)
2. Department of Oral Medicine and Diagnostic Sciences, College of Dentistry, King Saud University, Riyadh 11451, Saudi Arabia; aaniazy@ksu.edu.sa
3. Department of Dentistry-Biomaterials, Radboudumc, 6500HB Nijmegen, The Netherlands; Jeroen.vandenBeucken@radboudumc.nl (J.J.J.P.v.d.B.); John.Jansen@radboudumc.nl (J.A.J.)
* Correspondence: dalghamdi@ksu.edu.sa

Received: 20 October 2020; Accepted: 18 November 2020; Published: 20 November 2020

Abstract: We evaluated the response to peri-implant bone placed in the femoral condyle of osteoporotic rats, following intravenous zoledronate (ZOL) treatment in three settings: pre-implantation (ZOL-Pre), post-implantation (ZOL-Post), and pre- + post-implantation (ZOL-Pre+Post). Twenty-four female Wistar rats were ovariectomized (OVX). After 12 weeks, the rats received titanium implants in the right femoral condyle. ZOL (0.04 mg/kg, weekly) was administered to six rats 4 weeks pre-implantation and was stopped at implant placement. To another six rats, ZOL was given post-implantation and continued for 6 weeks. Additional six rats received ZOL treatment pre- and post-implantation. Control animals received weekly saline intravenous injections. At 6 weeks post-implantation, samples were retrieved for histological evaluation of the percentage of bone area (%BA) and of the percentage of bone-to-implant contact (%BIC). BA% for ZOL-Pre (29.6% ± 9.0%) and ZOL-Post (27.9% ± 5.6%) rats were significantly increased compared to that of the controls (17.3% ± 3.9%, $p < 0.05$). In contrast, ZOL-Pre+Post rats (20.4% ± 5.0%) showed similar BA% compared to Saline controls ($p = 0.731$). BIC% revealed a significant increase for ZOL-Post (65.8% ± 16.9%) and ZOL-Pre+Post (68.3% ± 10.0%) rats compared with that of Saline controls (43.3% ± 9.6%, $p < 0.05$), while ZOL-Pre rats (55.6% ± 19%) showed a BIC% comparable to that of Saline controls ($p = 0.408$). Our results suggest that receiving intravenous ZOL treatment before or after implant placement enhances peri-implant bone responses in terms of bone area. However, the effect of different ZOL treatment regimens on BIC% was found to be inconclusive.

Keywords: dental implants; osseointegration; osteoporosis; zoledronate; animal model

1. Introduction

The worldwide use of dental implants is still increasing, as these fixtures offer many advantages above the more conventional prosthetic reconstruction of lost teeth [1]. This is also because of improved long-term prognosis thanks to innovations in implant design [2]. Overall, the success of dental implants is attributed to their ability to integrate well in living bone (i.e., osseointegration) [3]. However, bone–implant integration can be challenging in compromised conditions, like in the absence of sufficient bone mass and density. Such a condition is frequently diagnosed in older adults and is called osteopenia [4]. Osteopenia is an initial condition that can develop into osteoporosis and is characterized by a reduction in bone density below a standard score compared to healthy young adults [5]. Especially, women are at higher risk for osteopenia as a consequence of menopausal estrogen deficiency [6]. Osteopenia makes bones weaker, which results in a higher risk of fractures and delayed bone healing [7]. Consequently, it can be hypothesized that dental implants installed in patients suffering from osteopenia are more prone to failure. Currently, there is no consensus regarding the effect of osteoporosis on the survival rate of dental implants [8,9]. Clinically, some studies observed significantly higher implant failure in patients with osteoporosis [10,11], while other studies could not associate osteoporosis with increased implant loss [12,13]. An explanation for this discrepancy can be the used selection criteria for inclusion or exclusion of patients in the various clinical studies, the wide variation in implant types, and the administration of different drugs [9]. Therefore, it is recommended that standardized experiments are performed to elaborate further on this topic and clarify this matter. The present study is part of a series of experiments, which were designed to fill in the lack of knowledge about the relationship between osteoporosis and bone–dental implant response.

The pharmaceutical treatment of osteoporosis includes the use of a wide range of drugs (e.g., bisphosphonates, statins, drugs for estrogen replacement therapy (ERT), calcitonin, parathyroid hormone, and calcium supplements) as well as various routes of administration (i.e., oral or systemic) [14]. Besides being used to decrease fracture risk in osteoporotic patients, these drugs have also been suggested to support bone formation around dental implants [14,15]. The data of these preclinical studies generally indicated that the application of systemic bisphosphonate treatment has a positive effect on implant osseointegration [16]. Bisphosphonates (BPs) are a class of drugs capable of mediating bone metabolism and reducing bone turnover [17]. BPs exhibit antiresorptive effects by reducing osteoclastic recruitment and activity [18]. Moreover, BPs have been reported to stimulate the function of osteoblasts [19,20]. A recent systematic review by Gelazius et al. examined the effect of bisphosphonates on dental implant placement procedure, and the results showed no significant implant success rate difference in intravenously and orally medicated groups. Moreover, patients treated with intravenous bisphosphonates seemed to have a higher chance of developing implant-related osteonecrosis of the jaw, and implant placement in patients treated intraorally could be considered safe with precautions [21]. One of the most potent BPs is zoledronate (ZOL), which is characterized by long-term retention in bone tissues compared to other BPs [22,23]. ZOL is primarily administrated intravenously (IV) to avoid gastrointestinal adverse effects associated with oral administration of BPs [24,25]. ZOL has been shown to favor the bone–implant response [26–28]. It is also well documented that ZOL has possible side effects, as it may cause initial influenza-like illness associated with the first infusion. Renal failure has been noted in patients with cancer after repetitive high-dose ZOL infusions. Moreover, osteonecrosis of the jaw after tooth extraction has been recorded as a result of the systemic administration of ZOL [29]. However, the effect of the timing of drug administration, i.e., before and/or after placing dental implants, is not clear [14]. Considering all this, we hypothesized that an initial treatment targeting an osteopenic bone condition before implant installation would be more favorable for implant–bone integration compared to a treatment started after implant placement.

Therefore, the purpose of the present study was to evaluate the bone response to titanium implants placed in osteoporotic rats treated with intravenous ZOL at three different times (pre-implantation, post-implantation, and pre- and post-implantation) compared to non-treated controls.

2. Materials and Methods

2.1. Ovariectomy Rat Model

All animal experiments in the present study were in accordance to the guidelines (national and international) for animal care and conformed to the ARRIVE guidelines. The Animal Ethics Committee at King Saud University, Saudi Arabia, approved the present study (No. 4/67/389683). Twenty-four female Wistar rats (weight of ~250 g) were used. The animals were housed in standardized rat cages (4–5 animals per cage) maintained in a laboratory environment with controlled temperature (22–24 °C) and humidity (45–55%) and 12 hourly light and dark cycles. All animals had ad libitum access to a standard rat chow diet and water. All rats were subjected to bilateral ovariectomy (OVX) procedures under general anesthesia (GA) to induce an osteoporotic condition as previously described [30].

2.2. Sample Number Estimation

The power analysis of sample size was done using the formula ($n1 = n2 = n3 = 1 + 2 \times c(s/d)^2$). Standard deviation (s) was 12.5, effect size (d) was 15, C was 7.85 (resulting from $1-\beta = 0.8$ and $\alpha = 0.05$). The final result was 24 rats (one implant per rat).

2.3. Implantation Procedures and Study Groups

At 12 weeks post-ovariectomy, a sterile condition was applied for the implantation surgery. A single intraperitoneal injection of 0.2 mg/kg xylazine (Chanazine, Chanelle Pharmaceutical, Galway, Ireland) and 0.5 mg/kg ketamine hydrochloride (Ketamine, Pharmazeutische Praparate, Gießen, Germany) was used for general anesthesia. Then, the right rat's leg was shaved and disinfected using 10% Povidone–iodine (Alphadin, MedicScience Life Care Pvt. Ltd., Haryana, India). An incision was made over the knee joint to expose the femoral condyle. Then, we drilled a small hole (1.5 mm in diameter and 8 mm in depth) using surgical burs and a rotary handpiece along with saline irrigation. Then, a commercially available mini-implant (Unitek™ TADs, 3M Oral Care, St Paul, MN, USA, diameter, 1.8 mm, length, 8 mm) was placed in the prepared hole (1 implant per rat). Finally, the skin was sutured with 4-0 resorbable sutures (VICRYL® Polyglactin 910, Ethicon, Johnson & Johnson, New Brunswick, NJ, USA). For the anti-osteoporotic treatment, a ZOL injection (Zometa® 4 mg, Novartis, Basel, Switzerland) was prepared and administered intravenously via the tail vein, as described previously [26]. For the experiment, rats were divided into four equal groups (n = 6 rats per group):

1. ZOL-Pre: weekly ZOL administration (0.04 mg/kg body weight) in the 4 weeks prior to implant placement [31].
2. ZOL-Post: weekly ZOL administration in the 6 weeks from implant placement until the end of the study (=6 weeks) [14].
3. ZOL-Pre+Post: weekly ZOL administration from 4 weeks prior to implant placement until the end of the study (=10 weeks).
4. Saline: weekly intravenous injection with 1 mL saline from 4 weeks prior to implant placement until the end of the study; this group was considered the non-treated control.

2.4. Animal Euthanasia and Specimen Retrieval

All rats were euthanized with CO_2 after 6 weeks of healing. The bone specimens were retrieved and fixed in 10% formalin for 2 days. Then, the samples were kept in 70% ethanol for histological preparation.

2.5. Histological and Histomorphometric Examination

First, the bone samples were dehydrated in ethyl alcohol from 70% to 100%, then embedded in poly(methylmethacrylate) (pMMA) resin. Thereafter, longitudinal sections (10 μm thick) were prepared using a microtome and stained with methylene blue and basic fuchsin. A light microscope (Aperio ImageScope, Leica Biosystems, Buffalo Grove, IL, USA) was used for their observation. Histologic observations were performed by two examiners (AB & JJ). Using the Aperio ScanScope (Aperio ImageScope, Leica Biosystems, Buffalo Grove, IL, USA) image extraction tool, individual histology images were extracted in 25% jpg format. An image analysis software (IMAGE-J 1.4, National Institute of Health, Bethesda, MD, USA) was used to perform blinded histomorphometric measurements for three histological sections per implant (at ×20 objective magnification). The color hue and saturation of bone tissues were selected and standardized to red, while the other tissues were in yellow. Then, bone area (BA%) was measured in a region of interest (ROI) on both sides of the implant, i.e., a rectangular box (1 mm width, 4 mm length) that started at the 2nd top implant thread

(Figure 1). Bone-to-implant contact (BIC%) was assessed by manually measuring the relative length of bone tissue in direct contact with the implant. The measurements from both sides of the implant in three different sections were averaged and used for statistical analysis.

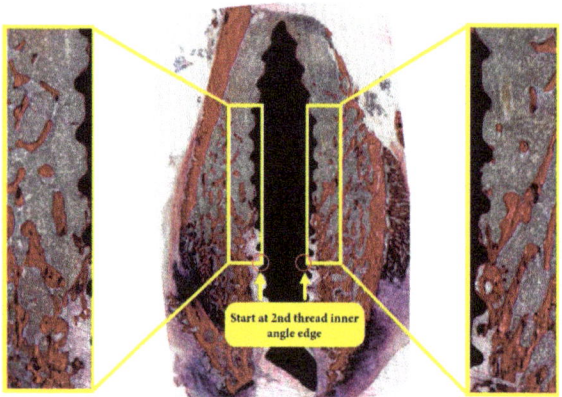

Figure 1. Sequence of representative histological sections (stained with methylene blue and basic fuchsin) showing the region of interest (ROI) for the measurement of bone area (BA%) and bone-to-implant contact (BIC%): from the left and right sides of the implant (yellow box).

2.6. Statistical Analysis

SPSS Statistical Program (Version 26, IBM, USA) was used to perform the descriptive statistics of BA% and BIC%, as mean and standard deviation (SD). Comparisons between test and saline groups were performed using one-way analysis of variance (ANOVA) with Dunnett post-hoc test, with statistical significance of $p < 0.05$.

3. Results

3.1. Rat Model

Animals in all groups showed no clinical complications or infections post-implantation. Table 1 summarizes the number of implants placed and retrieved and the numbers of sections used for histomorphometric analyses.

Table 1. Summary of implants placed and submitted to histological evaluation. ZOL, zoledronate.

Groups	Osteoporotic Condition		
	No. Placed Implants	No. Used Implants	No. Histological Sections
ZOL-Pre	6	5 *	15
ZOL-Post	6	6 #	18
ZOL-Pre+Post	6	6	18
Saline	6	5 *	14

* Two implants failed (no osseointegration); # Three implants had bicortical penetration of cortical layers. ZOL-Pre, ZOL administration prior to implant placement, ZOL-Post, ZOL administration after implant placement, ZOL-Pre+Post, ZOL administration prior and after implant placement (see text for details).

3.2. Histological Evaluation

Saline controls: light microscopical examination of the histological sections revealed that the bone of the femoral condyle had an osteopenic appearance, which was characterized by the presence of a limited amount of bone trabeculae as well as a wide spacing between the bone trabeculae (Figure 2A). Bone marrow was present between the bone trabeculae and in the areas where bone was completely lacking. The bone looked very mature and lacked substantial remodeling activity. Only occasionally, osteoclasts were observed, which were in tight contact with the bone trabeculae. Although very limitedly, bone trabeculae did make contact with the implant surface (Figure 2A,B). The majority of the contact sites was at the tip of the screw thread. On the other hand, all implants were covered for a significant part of their surface with a very thin layer of bone (Figure 2B). The bone was in close contact with the implant surface without intervening fibrous tissue layers. Again, the remodeling activity of the deposited bone was very limited, and no active layer of osteoblasts was observed.

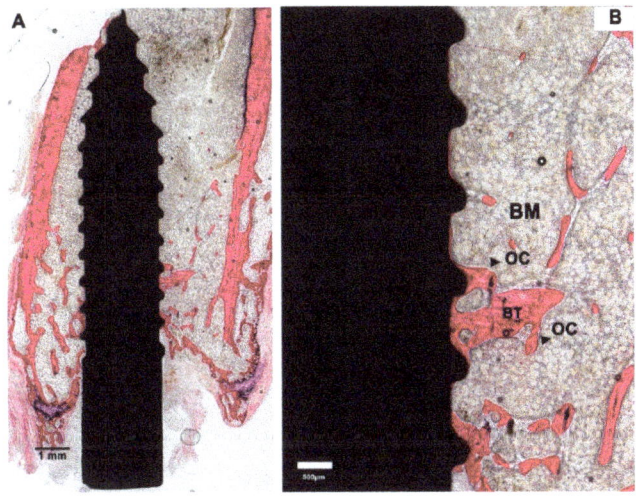

Figure 2. Histological sections of an implant in the saline group (control). (**A**). Low-magnification image showing a limited amount of bone formation. (**B**). Representative histological images at higher magnification showing osteoclast-like cells (OC) on the surface of the bone trabeculae (BT). Bone marrow (BM) was present between the bone trabeculae and in the areas where bone was lacking. Between the tips of the screw threads, a thin layer of bone is visible on the implant surface.

ZOL-Pre: examination of the histological sections suggested that the amount of bone in the femoral condyle as well as surrounding the implant was increased compared to Saline controls (Figure 3A). This increase was very evident in three of the six specimens but was more limited in the other three specimens. Strikingly, the remodeling activity of the bone was very low (Figure 3B). Also, the major part of the implant surface was covered with a thin layer of bone, but bone formation was not very active, as no layer of osteoblasts nor osteoid was observed. One of the specimens was considered a failure (Figure 4), as about 75% of the implant was not in direct contact with bone and was surrounded by a wide gap with a width of approximately 0.1–0.2 mm. This gap was filled with fibrous tissue, but no inflammatory reaction was observed.

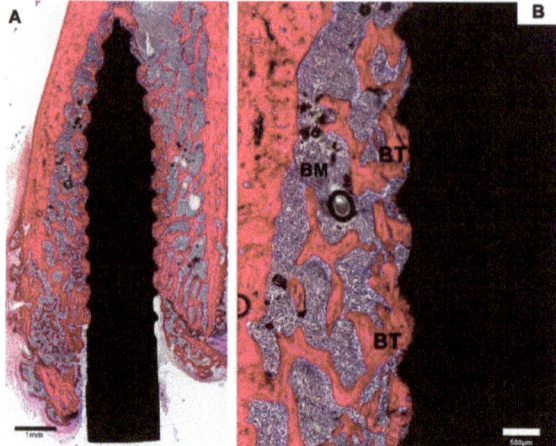

Figure 3. Representative histological images of an implant in the ZOL-Pre study group. (**A**). Low-magnification image showing bone trabeculae surrounding most of the implant. (**B**). Higher magnification revealed that bone was in tight contact with the majority of the implant surface.

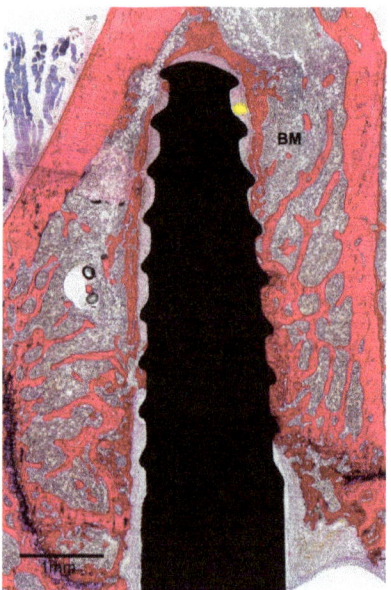

Figure 4. Histological image showing a "failed" implant. The implant was surrounded by a wide space filled with fibrous tissue (yellow star).

ZOL-Post: a light-microscope assessment indicated features largely similar to those observed in ZOL-Pre rats. The bone amount in the femoral condyle and around the implants was larger compared to that of Saline controls and appeared very similar to that observed in ZOL-Pre rats (Figure 5). Remodeling activity of the bone was not obvious. Trabecular bone was in contact with the implant surface in all retrieved specimens, and a thin layer of bone was present on all implant surfaces (Figure 5).

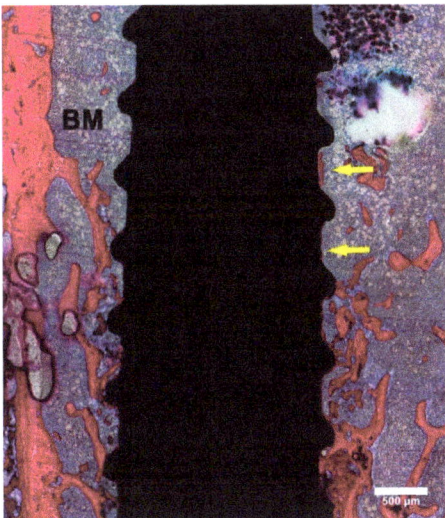

Figure 5. Light micrograph of a specimen of the ZOL-Post study group. Trabecular bone appears in contact with the implant surface, and a thin layer of bone covers part of the implant surface (yellow arrows).

ZOL-Pre+Post: histological images suggested enhanced bone formation in the femoral condyle. In contrast to ZOL-Pre and ZOL-Post rats, the increase was mainly seen at the crestal side of the implant and extended about halfway up the implant length (Figure 6A). Areas that were not occupied by bone trabeculae were filled with bone marrow. Trabecular bone was in contact with the implant surface, and bone remodeling activity was low. A thin layer of bone was covering major areas of all implants and bone was also deposited in areas where no trabecular bone was present (Figure 6B).

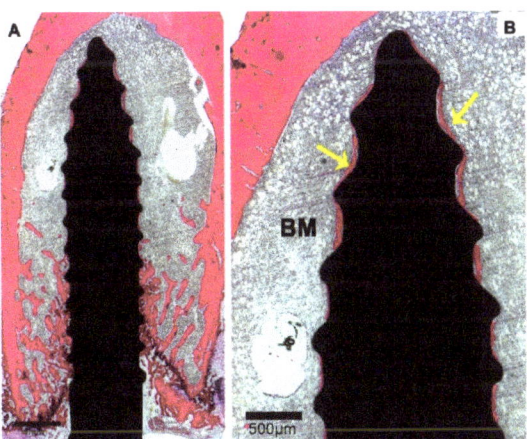

Figure 6. Low- and high-magnification images of a specimen of the ZOL-Pre+Post group. (**A**) Low-magnification image showing that bone formation mainly occurred at the crestal side of the implant and extended about halfway up the implant length. (**B**) High magnification revealed that a thin layer of bone covered the implant surface (yellow arrows).

3.3. Histomorphometric Evaluation

Both BA% and BIC% were determined and are shown in Table 2. One specimen in Saline controls was excluded from the histomorphometric analysis, as the histological sections did deviate too much from a section plane parallel to the longitudinal axis, which made proper measurements impossible. Further, the failed specimen of the ZOL-Pre group was excluded from the measurements. Data showed a mean BA% of 29.6% ± 9.0% for ZOL-Pre, 27.9% ± 5.6% for the ZOL-Post, 20.4% ± 5.0% for ZOL-Pre+Post, and 17.3% ± 3.9% for Saline controls. The results of the repeated measures analysis of variance with Dunnett's multiple comparison test revealed that BA% for ZOL-Pre and ZOL-Post was significantly higher compared to that of Saline controls ($p = 0.013$ and 0.025, respectively, Figure 7A). In contrast, ZOL-Pre+Post rats showed similar BA% compared to that of Saline controls ($p = 0.731$). BIC% values were 55.6% ± 19.0% for ZOL-Pre, 65.8% ± 16.9% for ZOL-Post, 68.3% ± 10.0% for ZOL-Pre+Post, and 43.3% ± 9.6% for Saline controls. Statistical testing revealed a significant difference for ZOL-Post and ZOL-Pre+Post with respect to Saline controls ($p = 0.049$ and 0.027 resp), while ZOL-Pre showed a BIC% comparable to that of Saline controls ($p = 0.408$, Figure 7B).

Table 2. Mean and standard deviation (SD) for BA% and BIC% in the different study groups.

Study Groups	ZOL-Pre	ZOL-Post	ZOL-Pre+Post	Saline
Bone area (BA%) (Mean ± SD)	29.6 ± 9.0	27.9 ± 5.6	20.4 ± 5.0	17.3 ± 3.9
Bone–implant contact (BIC%) (Mean ± SD)	55.6 ± 19.0	65.8 ± 16.9	68.3 ± 10.0	43.3 ± 9.6

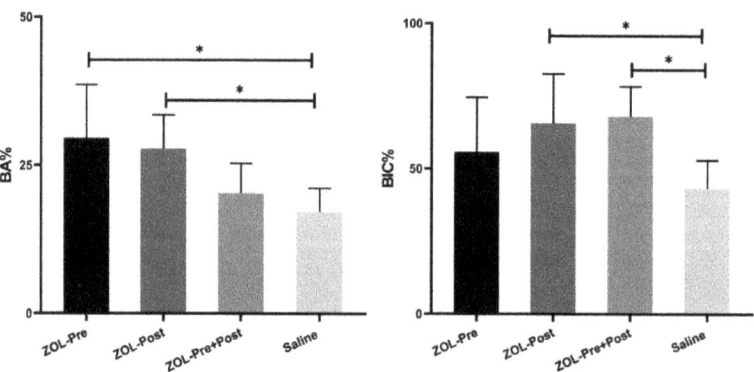

Figure 7. Bar chart with mean and standard deviation for (**A**) BA% and (**B**) BIC% in all study groups. (* indicates $p < 0.05$).

4. Discussion

In the present study, the peri-implant bone response was compared in OVX rats, which were treated with ZOL (0.04 mg/kg, once a week) via intravenous infusion at three different times: pre-implantation, post-implantation, and pre+post-implantation; rats receiving weekly saline injections served as controls. Both bone area (BA%) and bone–implant contact (BIC%) were histomorphometrically evaluated. In comparison to saline controls, the pre- and post-implantation ZOL treatment showed a significant gain of BA% ($p < 0.05$). Additionally, BIC% data showed a significant difference when comparing post-implantation and pre+post-implantation ZOL-treated rats to saline controls ($p < 0.05$).

One of the treatment approaches for osteopenia/osteoporosis is the systemic administration of ZOL [24,25,32,33]. ZOL has been shown to (1) effectively suppress the recruitment and function of osteoclastic cells that cause bone resorption [22,32] and (2) have a positive effect on bone formation by stimulating osteoblasts, in comparison to other BPs [34]. Moreover, several studies reported that ZOl has a greater impact and stronger effects on osseointegration than other BPs [28,35]. Therefore, ZOL is considered a potent bisphosphonate, whose effectiveness has been confirmed in several clinical trials involving osteoporotic patients [36]. The recommended administration option of ZOL for treating osteoporosis is by once-yearly intravenous infusion of 5 mg [37].

Although bisphosphonates have a relatively good safety record and are tolerated by the majority of patients, these drugs are reported to be associated with several side effects. For instance, the most notable adverse drug reaction associated with oral bisphosphonates is upper gastrointestinal discomfort, which may include heartburn, indigestion, esophageal erosion, and esophageal ulcer [38]. In order to avoid these reactions, drugs should be administered with a full glass of water in the morning on an empty stomach 30 min prior to a meal or other medications (60 min for ibandronate). Additionally, patients should remain upright for at least 30 min post-dose to prevent esophageal irritation. Osteonecrosis of the jaw is another complication detected in patients receiving prolonged intravenous bisphosphonate therapy, especially ZOL, who undergo invasive dental procedures, such as tooth extractions and implant placement. Physicians should consider either discontinuation or a drug holiday when the risks of use outweigh the benefits [38].

Considering the above-mentioned observations, we intended to examine in the current experimental animal study the effect of ZOL administration on bone formation around dental implants installed in osteoporotic bone. Although a wide variety of animal models is available, ovariectomized rats are well established to closely simulate osteopenia/osteoporotic bone conditions and the response to pharmacological therapy observed in humans [39]. As such, we utilized ovariectomized rats to study whether systemic ZOL administration before and/or after implant placement improves the peri-implant bone response.

Our study design for evaluating the peri-implant bone response in osteoporotic animals is distinct from previous studies, which focused on testing the effect of ZOL administration only post-implantation. Our aim was to test different clinical scenarios, as can occur in patients with postmenopausal osteopenia requiring dental implant installation. For example, August et al. [40] observed in a retrospective manner that postmenopausal women with an osteopenia-like condition in their maxilla showed a significant failure rate (13.6%) of installed dental implants compared to healthy women (6.3%, $p = 0.039$) if they did not receive anti-osteoporotic therapy before implant surgery. Consequently, we decided to investigate the effect of three ZOL administration regimens related to the moment of implant installation. A key aim was to determine whether post-implantation continuation of the administration of ZOL would be more beneficial in comparison with only pre- or post-implantation drug administration. A delay in the delivery of ZOL to the implant site was hypothesized to have less pharmacological benefit than pre-implantation ZOL binding to the target site. In addition, prolonged ZOL administration was supposed to better "treat" the diseased bone at the implant site. In a continuous approach, the preoperative administration of ZOL has to control the unbalanced bone metabolism, while the postoperative administration of ZOL has to enhance bone–implant healing [22].

However, the above-mentioned hypothesized effect of a continuous approach was not proven. In contrast, an improvement in BA% around the implants was observed for the intravenous administration of ZOL to OVX rats for only 4 weeks pre-implantation or only post-implantation. However, no favorable effect was seen for the continued administration, which led to a BA% comparable to that non-treated osteoporotic rats. The beneficial effect of only pre- or post-implantation administration of ZOL on BA% corroborates other studies. For example, Yoshioka at al. [41] demonstrated that systemic administration of ZOL in osteoporotic ovariectomized rats resulted in increased bone formation after 4 weeks. Another study assessed the effect of simultaneous insertion of titanium implants and systemic treatment with ZOL in osteoporotic and sham-operated rabbits [42].

They found that ZOL treatment significantly increased the BA% in the osteoporotic rabbits 3 months after surgery. Additionally, Bobyn et al. [43] examined the effect of an intravenous injection of ZOL (0.1 mg/kg) post-implantation in a dog model and reported that ZOL increased peri-implant bone formation by twofold compared to non-treated controls [43]. Cardemil et al. revealed that a systemic single dose of ZOL in ovariectomized animals improved bone-to-implant contact [31]. Recently, He et al. [29] reviewed the literature and described 10 preclinical studies that confirmed a possible effect of systemic ZOL administration on implant osseointegration. Consequently, the conclusion seems justified that intravenous ZOL can improve implant osseointegration in osteoporotic animals.

On the other hand, the pre+post-implantation ZOL treatment of osteoporotic rats did not favor BA% increase. An explanation for this finding can be related to the applied doses of ZOL. The effect of nitrogen-containing BPs, like ZOL, on osteoclasts is known to be depending on dose and dose frequency [44]. In addition, it has to be remarked that the concentration of ZOL in the plasma after intravenous administration reduces rapidly due to the fast adsorption of the ZOL onto the bone surface [45]. In line with this, the efficacy of ZOL dosage was investigated in a clinical study involving patients suffering from Paget's disease [46]. The data of this study indicated that doses above 200 g had a reduced therapeutic effect.

As mentioned earlier, the recommended treatment approach for osteoporosis is a once-yearly intravenous infusion of ZOL. In our study, ZOL was administered once weekly for a period of 10 weeks. Therefore, it cannot be excluded that this dosing was too high, resulting in a decreased effect on bone formation. In view of this, it is recommended to determine the alkaline phosphatase (ALP) level in the blood serum of the rats in future studies. This will provide information about the therapeutic effect of ZOL in an osteoporotic condition.

The measurements of BIC% showed a significantly higher BIC% in rats receiving post- and pre+post-implantation ZOL treatment compared to saline controls. These data are inconclusive, and their relevance is not evident. These inconsistent observations can be explained by a low remodeling activity of the trabecular bone surrounding the implant bed in all treatment scenarios. How this interferes with bone formation at the implant interface remains elusive. In combination with the relatively short implantation time, it can be assumed that the bone present at the implant surface was mainly already existing bone and not newly deposited bone. In this condition, BIC% represents just the amount of bone present during implant installation. This explanation is in agreement with other studies, which suggested that a follow-up time of 6 weeks is too short, and more than 8 weeks of observation are necessary to detect a possible effect of pharmacological drugs on the interfacial implant–bone response [29,47].

Additionally, implant location as well seems to have a significant effect on the results. For instance, Cardemil et al. studied the different biological reactions of the tibia and the mandible in rats, both in response to ovariectomy and in response to the ZOL treatment. They reported an increase of BIC in the tibia, whereas the opposite occurred in the mandible [31]. This variation can be attributed to different turnover rates and density in different bones [48].

Finally, a comment has to be made regarding the experimental conditions of the current study. Some authors noticed that a high calcium diet may reverse the condition of osteopenia in ovariectomized animals [49]. In our model, OVX rats were fed a standard diet with a considerable amount of calcium. This was done with the purpose of mimicking the human clinical situation: human osteoporotic patients are not given a specific diet but are recommended to eat healthily and include sufficient amounts of dairy products as well as vitamin D-containing food in their meals daily. Nevertheless, the standard diet may have influenced the effect of ZOL on the osteoporotic-like bone in the present study.

5. Conclusions

Under the current experimental conditions, our results suggest that receiving intravenous ZOL treatment before or after implant placement enhances peri-implant bone responses in terms of bone area. However, the effect of different ZOL treatment regimens on BIC% was found to be inconclusive.

Further, the following recommendations can be made for future studies dealing with implant installation in osteoporotic animals and co-administration of anti-osteoporotic drugs: (1) allow an implantation time longer than 8 weeks and (2) determine ALP blood serum levels to assess the therapeutic efficacy of the anti-osteoporotic drugs.

Author Contributions: Conceptualization, A.M.B., M.Y.S., A.A.N., J.J.J.P.v.d.B., J.A.J. and H.S.A.; data curation, A.M.B.; formal analysis, M.Y.S.; funding acquisition, H.S.A.; investigation, A.M.B. and M.Y.S.; methodology, A.M.B., M.Y.S., A.A.N., J.J.J.P.v.d.B. and H.S.A.; project administration, A.A.N.; resources, A.A.N. and J.J.J.P.v.d.B.; validation, J.J.J.P.v.d.B. and J.A.J.; visualization, J.A.J.; writing—original draft, A.M.B.; writing—review and editing, J.J.J.P.v.d.B., J.A.J. and H.S.A. All authors have read and agreed to the published version of the manuscript.

Funding: The authors extend their appreciation to the Deanship of Scientific Research at King Saud University for funding this work through research group No (RG-1439-026).

Acknowledgments: The authors are grateful to the technical support of Vincent Cuijpers, Martijn Martens, Natasja van Dijk in histological preparation and sectioning. The authors are also grateful to Mary Grace Baysa Vigilla and Anne Rhodanne Nicole Lambarte for their support during animal experimental procedures. Finally, the authors would like to thank Terrence Sumague for his assistance during the histomorphometric measurements.

Conflicts of Interest: The authors declare that they have no known competing financial interests or personal relationships that could have appeared to influence the work reported in this paper.

References

1. Alghamdi, H.S.; Jansen, J.A. The development and future of dental implants. *Dent. Mater. J.* **2020**, *39*, 167–172. [CrossRef] [PubMed]
2. Ducommun, J.; El Kholy, K.; Rahman, L.; Schimmel, M.; Chappuis, V.; Buser, D. Analysis of trends in implant therapy at a surgical specialty clinic: Patient pool, indications, surgical procedures, and rate of early failures—A 15-year retrospective analysis. *Clin. Oral Implant. Res.* **2019**, *30*, 1097–1106. [CrossRef] [PubMed]
3. Albrektsson, T.; Brånemark, P.-I.; Hansson, H.-A.; Lindström, J. Osseointegrated Titanium Implants:Requirements for Ensuring a Long-Lasting, Direct Bone-to-Implant Anchorage in Man. *Acta Orthop. Scand.* **1981**, *52*, 155–170. [CrossRef]
4. Wright, N.C.; Looker, A.C.; Saag, K.G.; Curtis, J.R.; Delzell, E.S.; Randall, S.; Dawson-Hughes, B. The Recent Prevalence of Osteoporosis and Low Bone Mass in the United States Based on Bone Mineral Density at the Femoral Neck or Lumbar Spine. *J. Bone Miner. Res.* **2014**, *29*, 2520–2526. [CrossRef] [PubMed]
5. Bone Mass Measurement: What the Numbers Mean. NIH Osteoporosis and Related Bone Diseases—National Resource Center. 2018. Available online: https://www.bones.nih.gov/health-info/bone/bone-health/bone-mass-measure (accessed on 10 November 2020).
6. Begum, R.A.; Ali, L.; Akter, J.; Takahashi, O.; Fukui, T.; Rahman, M. Osteopenia and osteoporosis among 16–65 year old women attending outpatient clinics. *J. Community Health* **2014**, *39*, 1071–1076. [CrossRef] [PubMed]
7. Pang, J.; Ye, M.; Gu, X.; Cao, Y.; Zheng, Y.; Guo, H.; Zhao, Y.; Zhan, H.; Shi, Y. Ovariectomy-Induced Osteopenia Influences the Middle and Late Periods of Bone Healing in a Mouse Femoral Osteotomy Model. *Rejuvenation Res.* **2015**, *18*, 356–365. [CrossRef]
8. Chen, H.; Liu, N.; Xu, X.; Qu, X.; Lu, E. Smoking, Radiotherapy, Diabetes and Osteoporosis as Risk Factors for Dental Implant Failure: A Meta-Analysis. *PLoS ONE* **2013**, *8*, e71955. [CrossRef]
9. De Medeiros, F.; Kudo, G.; Leme, B.; Saraiva, P.; Verri, F.; Honório, H.; Pellizzer, E.; Santiago, J.F. Dental implants in patients with osteoporosis: A systematic review with meta-analysis. *Int. J. Oral Maxillofac. Surg.* **2018**, *47*, 480–491. [CrossRef]
10. Trullenque-Eriksson, A.; Guisado-Moya, B. Retrospective Long-term Evaluation of Dental Implants in Totally and Partially Edentulous Patients. Part, I. *Implant. Dent.* **2014**, *23*, 732–737. [CrossRef]
11. Alsaadi, G.; Quirynen, M.; Komárek, A.; Van Steenberghe, D. Impact of local and systemic factors on the incidence of oral implant failures, up to abutment connection. *J. Clin. Periodontol.* **2007**, *34*, 610–617. [CrossRef]

12. Temmerman, A.; Rasmusson, L.; Kubler, A.C.; Thor, A.; Quirynen, M. An open, prospective, non-randomized, controlled, multicentre study to evaluate the clinical outcome of implant treatment in women over 60 years of age with osteoporosis/osteopenia: 1-year results. *Clin. Oral Implant. Res.* **2017**, *28*, 95–102. [CrossRef] [PubMed]
13. Amorim, M.A.L.; Takayama, L.; Jorgetti, V.; Pereira, R.M.R. Comparative study of axial and femoral bone mineral density and parameters of mandibular bone quality in patients receiving dental implants. *Osteoporos. Int.* **2007**, *18*, 703–709. [CrossRef] [PubMed]
14. Basudan, A.M.; Shaheen, M.; De Vries, R.B.; Beucken, J.J.J.P.V.D.; Jansen, J.A.; Alghamdi, H.S. Antiosteoporotic Drugs to Promote Bone Regeneration Related to Titanium Implants: A Systematic Review and Meta-Analysis. *Tissue Eng. Part B Rev.* **2019**, *25*, 89–99. [CrossRef] [PubMed]
15. Alghamdi, H.S.; Jansen, J.A. Bone Regeneration Associated with Nontherapeutic and Therapeutic Surface Coatings for Dental Implants in Osteoporosis. *Tissue Eng. Part B Rev.* **2013**, *19*, 233–253. [CrossRef]
16. Cattalini, J.P.; Boccaccini, A.R.; Lucangioli, S.; Mouriño, V. Bisphosphonate-Based Strategies for Bone Tissue Engineering and Orthopedic Implants. *Tissue Eng. Part B Rev.* **2012**, *18*, 323–340. [CrossRef]
17. Fuchs, R.K.; Faillace, M.E.; Allen, M.R.; Phipps, R.J.; Miller, L.M.; Burr, D. Bisphosphonates do not alter the rate of secondary mineralization. *Bone* **2011**, *49*, 701–705. [CrossRef]
18. Aspenberg, P. Bisphosphonates and implants. *Acta Orthop.* **2009**, *80*, 119–123. [CrossRef]
19. Plotkin, L.I.; Lezcano, V.; Thostenson, J.; Weinstein, R.S.; Manolagas, S.C.; Bellido, T. Connexin 43 Is Required for the Anti-Apoptotic Effect of Bisphosphonates on Osteocytes and Osteoblasts In Vivo. *J. Bone Miner. Res.* **2008**, *23*, 1712–1721. [CrossRef]
20. Hu, L.; Wen, Y.; Xu, J.; Wu, T.; Zhang, C.; Wang, J.; Du, J.; Wang, S. Pretreatment with Bisphosphonate Enhances Osteogenesis of Bone Marrow Mesenchymal Stem Cells. *Stem Cells Dev.* **2017**, *26*, 123–132. [CrossRef]
21. Gelažius, R.; Poskevicius, L.; Sakavicius, D.; Grimuta, V.; Juodzbalys, G. Dental Implant Placement in Patients on Bisphosphonate Therapy: A Systematic Review. *J. Oral Maxillofac. Res.* **2018**, *9*, e1. [CrossRef]
22. Caraglia, M.; Marra, M.; Naviglio, S.; Botti, G.; Addeo, R.; Abbruzzese, A. Zoledronic acid: An unending tale for an antiresorptive agent. *Expert Opin. Pharmacother.* **2009**, *11*, 141–154. [CrossRef] [PubMed]
23. Papapoulos, S.E. Bisphosphonates: How do they work? *Best Pr. Res. Clin. Endocrinol. Metab.* **2008**, *22*, 831–847. [CrossRef] [PubMed]
24. Maricic, M. The role of zoledronic acid in the management of osteoporosis. *Clin. Rheumatol.* **2010**, *29*, 1079–1084. [CrossRef] [PubMed]
25. Sunyecz, J.A. Zoledronic acid infusion for prevention and treatment of osteoporosis. *Int. J. Women's Health* **2010**, *2*, 353–360. [CrossRef]
26. Ying, G.; Bo, L.; Yanjun, J.; Lina, W.; Binquan, W. Effect of a local, one time, low-dose injection of zoledronic acid on titanium implant osseointegration in ovariectomized rats. *Arch. Med Sci.* **2016**, *12*, 941–949. [CrossRef]
27. Dikicier, E.; Karacayli, U.; Dikicier, S.; Günaydın, Y. Effect of systemic administered zoledronic acid on osseointegration of a titanium implant in ovariectomized rats. *J. Cranio Maxillofac. Surg.* **2014**, *42*, 1106–1111. [CrossRef]
28. Chen, B.; Li, Y.; Yang, X.; Xu, H.; Xie, D. Zoledronic acid enhances bone-implant osseointegration more than alendronate and strontium ranelate in ovariectomized rats. *Osteoporos. Int.* **2013**, *24*, 2115–2121. [CrossRef]
29. He, Y.; Bao, W.; Wu, X.-D.; Huang, W.; Chen, H.; Li, Z. Effects of Systemic or Local Administration of Zoledronate on Implant Osseointegration: A Preclinical Meta-Analysis. *BioMed Res. Int.* **2019**, *2019*, 1–10. [CrossRef]
30. Alghamdi, H.S.; Beucken, J.J.J.P.V.D.; Jansen, J.A. Osteoporotic Rat Models for Evaluation of Osseointegration of Bone Implants. *Tissue Eng. Part C Methods* **2014**, *20*, 493–505. [CrossRef]
31. Cardemil, C.; Omar, O.; Norlindh, B.; Wexell, C.L.; Thomsen, P. The effects of a systemic single dose of zoledronic acid on post-implantation bone remodelling and inflammation in an ovariectomised rat model. *Biomaterials* **2013**, *34*, 1546–1561. [CrossRef]
32. Liu, M.; Guo, L.; Pei, Y.; Li, N.; Jin, M.; Ma, L.; Liu, Y.; Sun, B.; Li, C. Efficacy of zoledronic acid in treatment of osteoporosis in men and women-a meta-analysis. *Int. J. Clin. Exp. Med.* **2015**, *8*, 3855–3861. [PubMed]
33. Hegde, V.V.; Jo, J.E.; Andreopoulou, P.; Lane, J.M. Effect of osteoporosis medications on fracture healing. *Osteoporos. Int.* **2016**, *27*, 861–871. [CrossRef] [PubMed]

34. Pan, B.; To, L.B.; Farrugia, A.N.; Findlay, D.M.; Green, J.; Gronthos, S.; Evdokiou, A.; Lynch, K.; Atkins, G.J.; Zannettino, A.C.W. The nitrogen-containing bisphosphonate, zoledronic acid, increases mineralisation of human bone-derived cells in vitro. *Bone* **2004**, *34*, 112–123. [CrossRef]
35. Basso, F.G.; Pansani, T.N.; Soares, D.G.; Cardoso, L.M.; Hebling, J.; Costa, C.A.D.S. Influence of bisphosphonates on the adherence and metabolism of epithelial cells and gingival fibroblasts to titanium surfaces. *Clin. Oral Investig.* **2017**, *22*, 893–900. [CrossRef] [PubMed]
36. Reid, D.M.; Devogelaer, J.-P.; Saag, K.; Roux, C.; Lau, C.-S.; Reginster, J.; Papanastasiou, P.; Ferreira, A.; Hartl, F.; Fashola, T.; et al. Zoledronic acid and risedronate in the prevention and treatment of glucocorticoid-induced osteoporosis (HORIZON): A multicentre, double-blind, double-dummy, randomised controlled trial. *Lancet* **2009**, *373*, 1253–1263. [CrossRef]
37. Novartis Pharmaceuticals, Aclasta Product Information. 2020. Available online: http://guildlink.com.au/gc/ws/nv/pi.cfm?product=nvpaclin11115 (accessed on 18 November 2020).
38. Tu, K.N.; Lie, J.D.; Wan, C.K.V.; Cameron, M.; Austel, A.G.; Nguyen, J.K.; Van, K.; Hyun, D. Osteoporosis: A Review of Treatment Options. *Pharm. Ther.* **2018**, *43*, 92–104.
39. Lelovas, P.P.; Xanthos, T.T.; Thoma, S.E.; Lyritis, G.P.; Dontas, I.A. The Laboratory Rat as an Animal Model for Osteoporosis Research. *Comp. Med.* **2008**, *58*, 424–430. [PubMed]
40. August, M.; Chung, K.; Chang, Y.; Glowacki, J. Influence of estrogen status on endosseous implant osseointegration. *J. Oral Maxillofac. Surg.* **2001**, *59*, 1285–1289. [CrossRef]
41. Yoshioka, Y.; Yamachika, E.; Nakanishi, M.; Ninomiya, T.; Nakatsuji, K.; Matsubara, M.; Moritani, N.; Kobayashi, Y.; Fujii, T.; Iida, S. Molecular alterations of newly formed mandibular bone caused by zoledronate. *Int. J. Oral Maxillofac. Surg.* **2018**, *47*, 1206–1213. [CrossRef]
42. Qi, M.; Hu, J.; Li, J.; Li, J.; Dong, W.; Feng, X.; Yu, J. Effect of zoledronic acid treatment on osseointegration and fixation of implants in autologous iliac bone grafts in ovariectomized rabbits. *Bone* **2012**, *50*, 119–127. [CrossRef]
43. Bobyn, J.D.; Hacking, S.A.; Krygier, J.J.; Harvey, E.J.; Little, D.G.; Tanzer, M. Zoledronic acid causes enhancement of bone growth into porous implants. *J. Bone Jt Surgery Br. Vol.* **2005**, *87*, 416–420. [CrossRef] [PubMed]
44. Fisher, J.E.; Rosenberg, E.; Santora, A.C.; Reszka, A.A. In Vitro and In Vivo Responses to High and Low Doses of Nitrogen-Containing Bisphosphonates Suggest Engagement of Different Mechanisms for Inhibition of Osteoclastic Bone Resorption. *Calcif. Tissue Int.* **2013**, *92*, 531–538. [CrossRef]
45. Lambrinoudaki, I.; Vlachou, S.; Galapi, F.; Papadimitriou, D.; Papadias, K. Once-yearly zoledronic acid in the prevention of osteoporotic bone fractures in postmenopausal women. *Clin. Interv. Aging* **2008**, *3*, 445–451. [CrossRef] [PubMed]
46. Bruggeman, R.W.G.; Weening, E.C. Zolendroninezuur als intraveneuze infusie een nieuwe behandelingslijn bij de ziekte van Paget. *Pharma Sel.* **2006**, *22*, 33–35.
47. Clokie, C.M.; Warshawsky, H. Morphologic and radioautographic studies of bone formation in relation to titanium implants using the rat tibia as a model. *Int. J. Oral Maxillofac. Implant.* **1995**, *10*, 155–165.
48. Khojasteh, A.; Dehghan, M.M.; Nazeman, P. Immediate implant placement following 1-year treatment with oral versus intravenous bisphosphonates: A histomorphometric canine study on peri-implant bone. *Clin. Oral Investig.* **2019**, *23*, 1803–1809. [CrossRef]
49. Minematsu, A.; Yoshimura, O.; Yotsuji, H.; Ichigo, H.; Takayanagi, K.; Kobayashi, R.; Hosoda, M.; Sasaki, H.; Maejima, H.; Matsuda, Y.; et al. The Effect of Low Calcium Diet on Bone in Ovariectomized Mice. *J. Jpn. Phys. Ther. Assoc.* **2000**, *3*, 13–16. [CrossRef]

Publisher's Note: MDPI stays neutral with regard to jurisdictional claims in published maps and institutional affiliations.

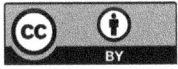

© 2020 by the authors. Licensee MDPI, Basel, Switzerland. This article is an open access article distributed under the terms and conditions of the Creative Commons Attribution (CC BY) license (http://creativecommons.org/licenses/by/4.0/).

Article

Histological and Histomorphometric Analyses of Bone Regeneration in Osteoporotic Rats Using a Xenograft Material

Marwa Y. Shaheen [1], Amani M. Basudan [1], Abdurahman A. Niazy [2], Jeroen J. J. P. van den Beucken [3], John A. Jansen [3] and Hamdan S. Alghamdi [1,*]

1. Department of Periodontics and Community Dentistry, College of Dentistry, King Saud University, P.O. Box 2455, Riyadh 11451, Saudi Arabia; mashaheen@ksu.edu.sa (M.Y.S.); abasudan@ksu.edu.sa (A.M.B.)
2. Department of Oral Medicine and Diagnostic Sciences, College of Dentistry, King Saud University, P.O. Box 2455, Riyadh 11451, Saudi Arabia; aaniazy@ksu.edu.sa
3. Department of Dentistry-Biomaterials, Radboudumc, P.O. Box 9101, 6500HB Nijmegen, The Netherlands; Jeroen.vandenBeucken@radboudumc.nl (J.J.J.P.v.d.B.); John.Jansen@radboudumc.nl (J.A.J.)
* Correspondence: dalghamdi@ksu.edu.sa

Abstract: We evaluated the effect of osteoporotic induction after eight weeks of initial healing of bone defects grafted with a xenograft material in a rat model. Bone defects were created in the femoral condyles of 16 female Wistar rats (one defect per rat). The defects were filled with bovine bone (Inter-Oss) granules. After eight weeks of bone healing, rats were randomly ovariectomized (OVX) or sham-operated (SHAM). At 14 weeks of bone healing, all animals were euthanized. Bone specimens were harvested and processed for histological and histomorphometric analyses to assess new bone formation (N-BF%), remaining bone graft (RBG%) and trabecular bone space (Tb.Sp%) within the defect area. After 14 weeks of bone healing, histological evaluation revealed a significant alteration in trabecular bone in OVX rats compared to SHAM rats. There was lower N-BF% in OVX rats ($22.5\% \pm 3.0\%$) compared to SHAM rats ($37.7\% \pm 7.9\%$; $p < 0.05$). Additionally, the RBG% was significantly lower in OVX ($23.7\% \pm 5.8\%$) compared to SHAM ($34.8\% \pm 9.6\%$; $p < 0.05$) rats. Finally, the Tb.Sp% was higher in OVX ($53.8\% \pm 7.7\%$) compared to SHAM ($27.5\% \pm 14.3\%$; $p < 0.05$) rats. In conclusion, within the limitations of this study, inducing an osteoporotic condition in a rat model negatively influenced bone regeneration in the created bone defect and grafted with a xenograft material.

Keywords: osteoporotic condition; animal model; xenograft; bone regeneration

1. Introduction

Dento-alveolar as well as cranio-facial bone defects can be the consequence of trauma by accidents or surgical interventions [1]. Several grafting approaches can be applied to successfully treat such bone defects [2]. Bone grafting involves using natural or synthetic bone substitutes to stimulate healing of bone through three different mechanisms: osteogenesis, osteoconduction and osteoinduction [3]. Osteogenesis is the formation of new bone by osteoblastic cells present within the graft material, osteoconduction is the ability to support the growth of bone over its surface and osteoinduction is the ability to induce differentiation of pluripotential stem cells from surrounding tissue to an osteoblastic phenotype [4]. For instance, autogenic bone grafting is considered the "gold standard", but it is associated with problems of availability and it needs a second surgical procedure [1,5]. In contrast, allograft obtained from bone bank is easily available but has a significant risk of disease transmission [2,6]. Therefore, xenograft and synthetic bone substitutes are the most commonly used graft materials in dental clinics [6]. Among them, anorganic bovine bone (e.g., Bio-Oss or similar products) is perhaps the most widely used and considered as reference material by notified bodies involved in medical device registration [7,8].

Several hard tissue alveolar ridge augmentation methods of implant therapy have been reported, including guided bone regeneration (GBR), maxillary sinus floor augmentation, vertical and/or lateral alveolar ridge augmentation and distraction. In the GBR method, barrier membrane is used [9]. A systematic review on the efficacy of barrier membranes on bone regeneration [10] showed that the use of such membranes would increase the amount of vertical augmented bone. Concerning vertical and/or lateral alveolar ridge augmentation, a Cochrane systematic review [11] showed that, although it is efficient to use a bone substitute (Bio-Oss) for horizontal bone augmentation, implants placed in bone augmented with Bio-Oss showed an increased failure rate, and the healing time was increased by three months compared with that of autogenous bone. Although the distraction technique costs more than GBR and bone grafting, it could shorten the treatment period, so this technique is effective for vertical ridge augmentation. However, the distraction technique is hard to apply to thin knife-edge bone. In any case, vertical augmentation techniques are associated with a higher complication rate [9]. Bone augmentation procedures are advanced surgical interventions. Growth factors that promote healing and regeneration are mostly used along with the grafting materials since there are multiple factors affecting the treatment outcomes. Growth factors used in dentistry are divided into platelet concentrates and recombinant growth factors. These agents are broadly used when bone-healing mechanisms are affected by the patient's medical conditions. Guided bone regeneration and autogenous block bone grafting are two of the well-documented and safely applicable augmentation techniques [12]. The recent Food and Drug Administration approval of recombinant human bone morphogenetic proteins (rhBMPs) has given clinicians an added treatment option for reconstructing localized and large jaw defects. Currently, several patients have been successfully treated with the combination of bone graft and rhBMP-2 and the results have been documented as predictable and safe by clinical and radiologic examinations follow-up. A systematic review on the rhBMP-2 application in craniomaxillofacial reconstruction defects evaluated the real efficacy and safety of BMPs [13]. According to the results, the use of different BMPs can positively influence the surgery. In addition, there are no statistically significant differences between the use of biomaterials added with BMP and not. The study data confirm the excellent documents about the possible combination of using substitute materials and growth factor for treating large and minor craniofacial bone defects [13].

Although anorganic bovine bone products perform well in healthy patients, limited information is available about their performance under compromised conditions, e.g. diabetes and osteoporosis [14]. In patients suffering from these systemic diseases, bone healing can be very unpredictable [15]. As demonstrated in previous studies, an osteoporotic condition may delay bone healing, increase resorption of bone materials and decrease the rate of bone ingrowth [16,17]. A common observation associated with osteoporosis is that the bone formation by osteoblasts is decreased. This is in part due to the lower proliferation/differentiation rate of mesenchymal stem cells (MSCs) into mature osteoblasts [18]. Suppression of MSCs in osteoporotic bone can be the consequence of a decreased synthesis of specific osteogenic-related factors [18]. Further, increased osteoclast activity is also commonly observed in osteoporotic bone [19].

Despite available knowledge on osteoporosis, its influence on bone regeneration in relation to bone grafting is still less understood. In addition, no information is available about how osteoporosis affects bone regeneration in grafted defects if osteoporosis onset is after graft installation.

The success of alveolar ridge bone augmentation treatment is associated first with their early integration, and then for their long-term performance on the maintenance of bone graft healing. Although there are several studies involving bone grafting healing in a well-established osteoporotic condition, information about the effect of altered bone metabolism on the bone grafting healing after establishment of bone grafting healing is scarce. While it is apparent that bone augmentation in osteoporotic patients has a risk of failure for new bone regeneration, it can be hypothesized that such alteration of bone metabolism developed after bone graft placement can also negatively affect bone regeneration [20].

However, there is no scientific literature reporting on the effect of distribution of bone metabolism on bone graft healing characteristics of already well-integrated bone graft.

Clinically, the mission of regenerative dentistry is restoring damaged alveolar bone in both healthy and medically compromised patients. The key step in alveolar bone regeneration is to stimulate a cascade of healing events, which can promote bone quantity and quality. Complications regarding bone regeneration in patients with systemic impaired bone metabolism (e.g., osteoporosis) represent a rapidly increasing clinical challenge.

In view of experimental procedures requiring osteoporotic conditions, several osteoporotic animal models have been described. For example, the ovariectomized (OVX) rat is commonly used model in osteoporosis-related research [16]. OVX animals exhibit loss of trabecular bone similar to humans. Furthermore, diminished trabecular bone morphology in the femoral condyle has been confirmed in OVX rats by histological examination [21]. Therefore, this OVX rat model seems appropriate to be used in studies dealing with the healing of a bone defect in relation to an osteoporotic condition.

The limitations of pre-clinical animal models should be mentioned: animal studies will only become more valid predictors of human reactions to exposures and treatments if there is both substantial improvement in their scientific methods and more systematic review of the animal literature as it evolves. Our research group published pre-clinical systematic review and meta-analysis aimed to systematically assess bone regeneration by using anti-osteoporotic drugs in adjunction with bone grafting [22]. Preclinical systematic reviews of data from preclinical literature are important for a number of reasons [23]. First, although systematic reviews are not bias free, their purpose is to reduce it by outlining transparent aims, objectives and methodology. This approach enables us to identify all of the published literature to answer a particular research question. In turn, this may highlight gaps in our knowledge which can be fulfilled by further preclinical experimentation, or it can help us avoid unnecessary replication which is unethical and of limited benefit. Systematic reviews of animal research, if they are used to inform the design of clinical trials, particularly with respect to appropriate drug dose, timing and other crucial aspects of the drug regimen, will further improve the predictability of animal research in human clinical trials and successful translational process [23].

However, there is a lack of evidence as to whether altered bone metabolism due to osteoporosis can affect bone regeneration related to bone-defect grafting. Differently, our study model was designed to replicate the effects of late-induced osteoporosis after the bone grafting procedure was performed. Considering all this, we hypothesized that an initial healing of bone-defect grafting would be affected due to metabolic bone alteration. Consequently, the purpose of this study was to utilize this animal model to investigate the effect of an osteoporotic condition on bone regeneration after initial healing of a bone defect using a xenograft material.

2. Materials and Methods

2.1. Experimental Animal Model

The present study was approved by the Animal Ethical Committee at King Saud University, College of Dentistry, Riyadh, Saudi Arabia (Approval No. 4/67/389683). All in-vivo experiments obeyed the guidelines (national and international) for animal care and conformed to the ARRIVE guidelines. The study sample comprised a total of 16 healthy female Wistar rats (age ~12 weeks and weighing around ~250 g). The animals were housed under veterinary supervision in standardized rat cages (4–5 animals per cage), maintained in a laboratory environment with controlled temperature (22 °C–24 °C), humidity (45–55%) and 12-h light and dark cycles. All the animals had ad libitum access to a standard rat chow diet and water.

2.2. Sample Size Calculation

The sample number estimation was calculated based on a power analysis using the following formula: $n1 = n2 = n3 = 1 + 2C(s/d)^2$. We assumed a standard deviation (s) of

12.5 and an effect size (d) of 15. C-value was fixed at 7.85 (resulting from 1-β = 0.8 and α = 0.05). According to these assumptions, 6 animals were included.

2.3. Experimental Surgical Procedures

All experimental surgical procedures were performed under general anesthesia (GA), by administering a single intraperitoneal injection comprising a combination of 0.2 mg/kg xylazine (Chanazine, Chanelle Pharmacuetical, Dublin, Ireland) and 0.5 mg/kg ketamine hydrochloride (Ketamine, Pharmazeutische Präparate, Giessen, Germany). Once the animal was anesthetized, the left leg was shaved and disinfected using Povidone-iodine 10% solution (Alphadin, MedicScience, Haryana, India). A longitudinal parapatellar skin incision, 2 cm in length, was made along the midline over the distal femoral condyle. The knee joint capsule was identified through blunt dissection of the skin flap and was incised longitudinally. The patellar ligament was elevated and retracted laterally for complete exposure of the knee joint and distal femoral condyle. Using surgical drills in a low-speed rotary drill along with saline irrigation as coolant, a cylindrical bone defect (3 mm in diameter and 3 mm in depth) paralleling the long axis of the femoral shaft was created in the intercondylar notch. Then, bone defect was filled with a xenograft material, anorganic cancellous bone graft granules, and particle size: 0.25–1 mm (InterOss®, SigmaGraft Inc., Fullerton, CA, USA) (Figure 1). After placement of the graft material, the soft tissue layers and skin were closed with VICRYL™ (4-0) polyglactin 910 resorbable sutures (Ethicon, Somerville, NJ, USA).

After 8 weeks of bone healing, rats were randomly ovariectomized (OVX) or sham-operated (SHAM) (Table 1), as previously described [21]. Six weeks later, animals were euthanized by CO_2-suffocation. Bone specimens were harvested and processed for histological and histomorphometric evaluation. The timelines of experimental design are described in Figure 2.

Table 1. Study groups, material and number of animals (n).

Study Groups	Material	Number of Animals (n)
SHAM	xenograft material (anorganic cancellous bone graft granules) InterOss®	n = 7
OVX	xenograft material (anorganic cancellous bone graft granules) InterOss®	n = 8

Ovariectomized (OVX)/Sham-operated (SHAM) as control.

2.4. Histological Specimen Preparation and Evaluation

Harvested bone specimens were fixed in 10% neutral buffered formalin solution. The samples were dehydrated in ascending concentrations of ethyl alcohol from 70% to 100% and subsequently embedded in poly-(methyl methacrylate) (pMMA) resin, prepared by mixing 600 mL of methyl methacrylate monomer (Acros Organics BVBA, Thermo Fisher Scientific, Geel, Belgium), 60 mL dibutyl phthalate (Merck KGaA, Darmstadt, Germany) and 1.25 g perkadox (AkzoNobel, Amersfoort, Utrecht, The Netherlands). After polymerization, ~10–15 µm thick serial transverse sections (perpendicular to long axis of femur) of the resin embedded specimens were made using a diamond-coated hard-tissue microtome (Leica®, Microsystems SP 1600, Nussloch, Germany). The first section of each specimen was made about 1 mm below the bone surface, and then sectioning was continued distally. All sections were stained with methylene blue and basic fuchsine, as described previously [24]. Three sections, at different levels, were selected for further histological assessment. Histological and histomorphometric evaluation were carried out using a light microscope (Aperio ImageScope, Leica Biosystems, Buffalo Grove, IL, USA). The histomorphometric analyses were done using a computer-based image analysis system (IMAGE-J 1.4, National Institute of Health, Bethesda, MD, USA). Blinded histomorphometric measurements were performed for the three selected histological sections per defect (at ×10 objective magnification). First, a circular region of interest (ROI) with a 3-mm diameter equal to the created defect was identified (Figure 3). Then, within this ROI, the amount of new bone formation (N-BF%), residual graft material (RBG%) and trabecular bone space (Tb.Sp%) were determined as area percentages.

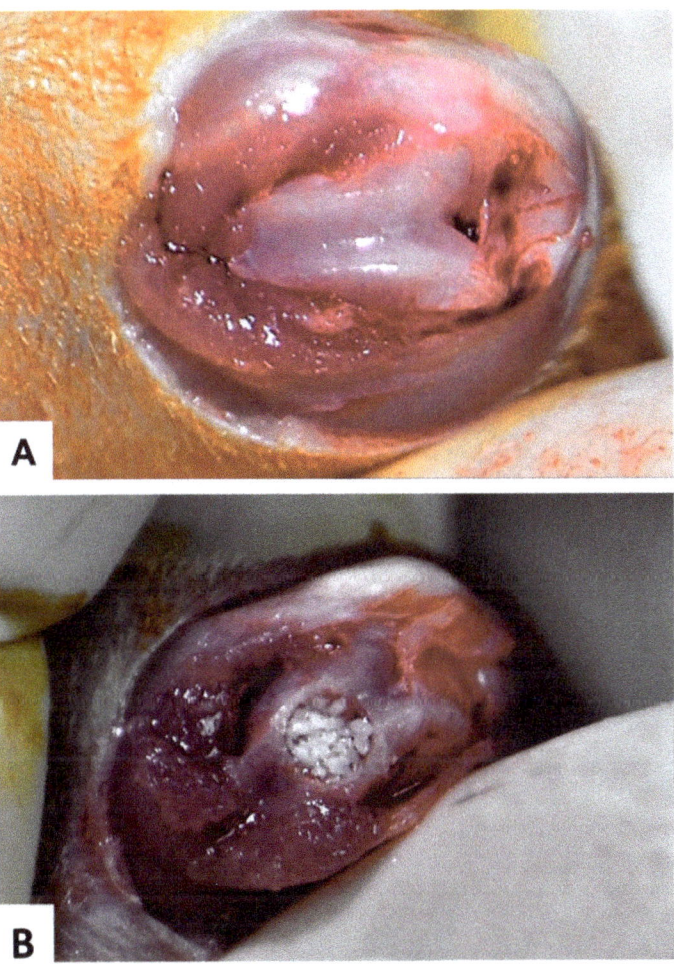

Figure 1. Pictures of the surgical procedure: (**A**) the femoral condyle exposed; and (**B**) bone defect filled with InterOss® material.

Experimental Groups and Time Schedules

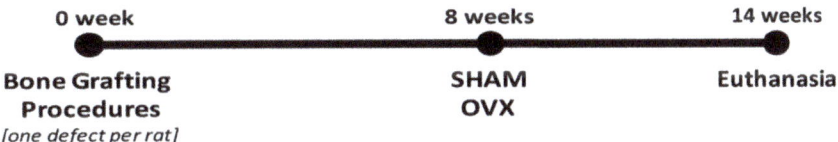

Figure 2. Experimental animal groups and timeline for surgical procedures and sacrifice in study animals.

A. 3mm ROI Creation

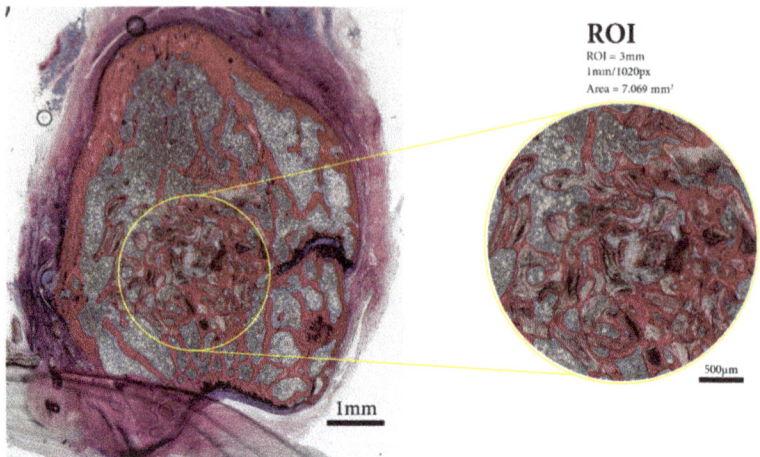

B. Measurement by ImageJ software

ANALYSIS 1: REGENERATED BONE   ANALYSIS 2: REMAINING BONE GRAFT

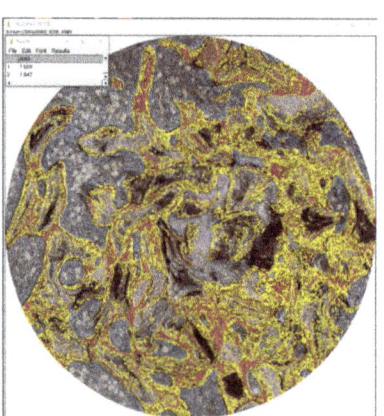 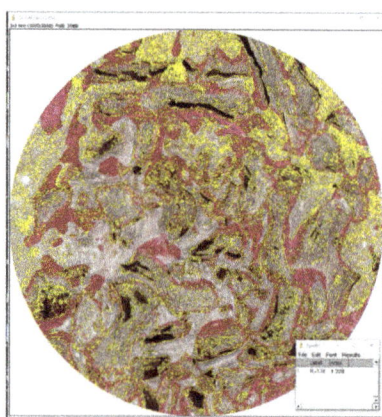

Figure 3. In the histological sections: (**A**) a 3-mm region of interest (ROI) was identified; and (**B**) quantitative measurements were then made to assess new bone formation (N-BF%), remaining bone graft (RBG%), and trabecular bone space (Tb.Sp%) using ImageJ software.

2.5. Statistical Analysis

All quantitative data were expressed as mean ± standard deviation (SD). Statistical analyses were performed using InStat Statistical Program (Version 3.05, GraphPad Software, San Diego, CA, USA). An unpaired Student's t-test was conducted to evaluate differences in the mean values between the two study groups. The level of significance was set at 95% ($p < 0.05$).

3. Results

3.1. Animal Observations

Postoperative healing was uneventful in all animals and no complications were observed after the bone grafting and ovariectomy surgeries, except one rat (from SHAM group) that died due to GA complications. Consequently, seven rats in the SHAM group and eight rats in the OVX group were finally examined.

3.2. Descriptive Histological Evaluation

Representative images of the histological sections are depicted in Figure 4. The histological sections of the OVX specimens revealed that the trabecular bone had an osteopenic appearance. The trabecular network was less dense and irregular compared to SHAM sections. At 14 weeks, images showed a higher trabecular number and less intertrabecular spacing for SHAM compared to OVX bone specimens. In between the bone trabeculae, bone marrow-like tissue was observed, characterized by the presence of mononuclear cells. As the bone tissue was stained pink, it could easily be discerned from the grafted InterOss® granules. More granules seemed to remain in the defects in the SHAM animals compared to OVX animals.

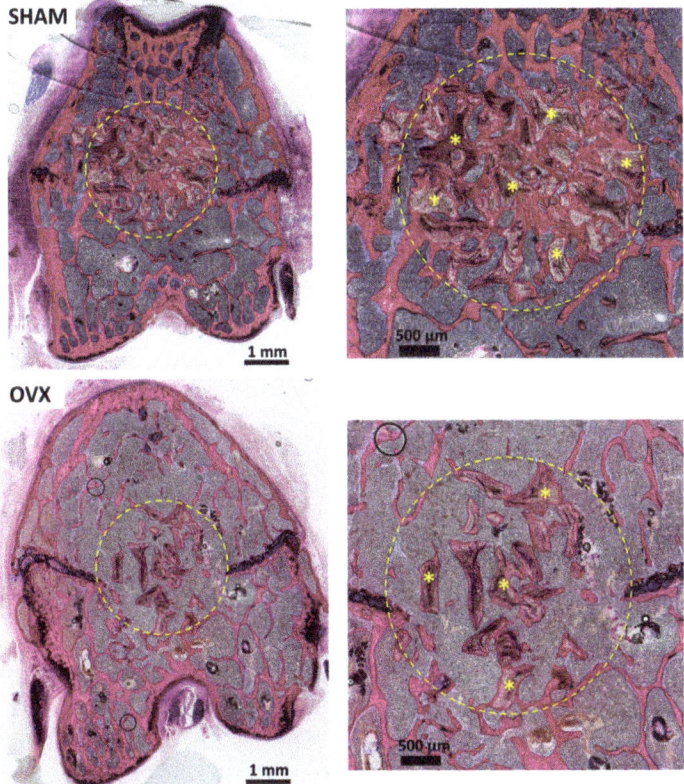

Figure 4. Representative histological images of pMMA sections: (**left**) for SHAM and OVX at 14 weeks post-implantation; and corresponding images at ×20 magnification (**right**). Methylene blue and basic fuchsin staining was performed. Within the ROI, images show the evident presence of new bone, remaining InterOss® material (yellow*) and trabecular bone space (Tb.Sp).

Higher magnification (Figure 5) revealed that the majority of the InterOss® granules in the SHAM specimens were surrounded by abundant new bone formation, which was in direct contact with the graft material. Further, bone bridging was observed between InterOss® granules. The grafted granules seemed to be completely covered by newly formed bone. High magnification images of the OVX specimen showed less newly formed bone in the osseous defects. The bone defect was for the major part filled with bone marrow-like tissue. The bone marrow-like tissue in the OVX rats contained more fat cells and less plasma cells compared to SHAM rats. Frequently, only a very superficial layer of bone was present on the surface of the granules. Occasionally, even no bone at all was seen covering the granules. Further, light micrographs showed the frequent presence of osteoclast-like cells at the interface between bone marrow-like tissue and granules (Figure 5). The images demonstrated also that some bone trabeculae in the OVX rats had an eroded appearance, which could be associated with the presence of osteoclast-like cells.

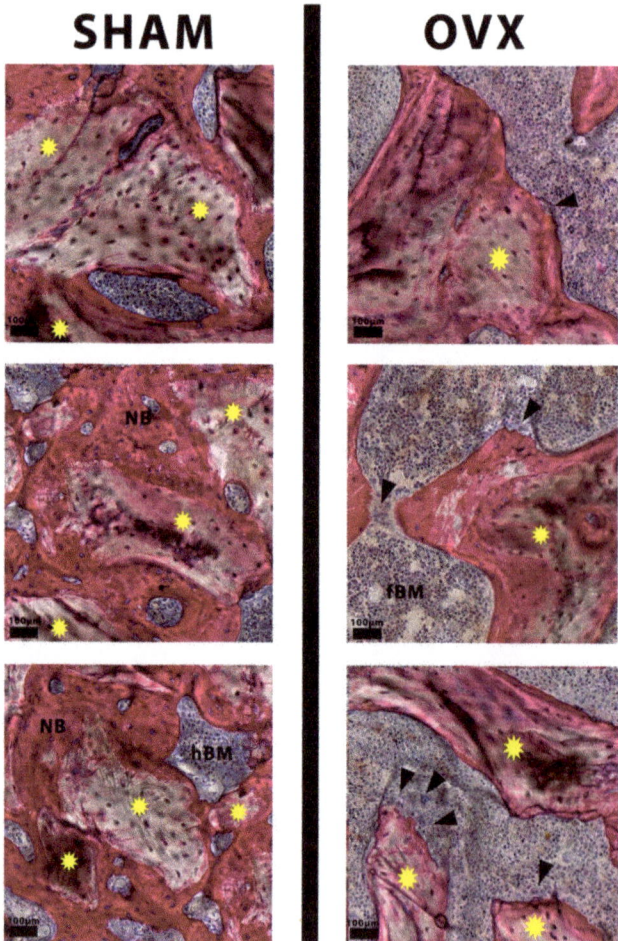

Figure 5. Representative histological images at higher magnification showing InterOss® granules (yellow stars) well integrated and completely covered with newly formed bone (NB) in SHAM rats (**left**). In OVX rats, eroded bone surface and osteoclast-like cells (black arrowheads) were present (**right**). Bone marrow-like tissue in OVX rats contained more fat cells (fBM) compared to the hypercellular bone marrow-like tissue (hBM) in the SHAM group.

3.3. Histomorphometric Evaluation

The results of the histomorphometric evaluation of osseous defects grafted with InterOss® granules are depicted in Table 2 and Figure 6. Data show a significantly decreased amount of new bone formation (N-BF%) in OVX rats compared to SHAM rats ($p < 0.05$). Additionally, the amount of remaining graft material (RBG%) was significantly lower in OVX compared to SHAM ($p < 0.05$). Finally, the mean of trabecular bone space (Tb.Sp%) was significantly higher in OVX compared to SHAM ($p < 0.05$).

Table 2. Quantitative histomorphometric data showing mean ± SD values for new bone formation (N-BF%), remaining bone graft (RBG%) and trabecular bone space (Tb.Sp%) in the two study groups.

	SHAM (*n* = 7)	OVX (*n* = 8)
New bone formation (N-BF%)	37.7 ± 7.9 *	22.5 ± 3.0
Remaining bone graft (RBG%)	34.8 ± 9.6 *	23.7 ± 5.8
Trabecular bone space (Tb.Sp%)	27.5 ± 14.3 *	53.8 ± 7.7

* indicates $p < 0.05$.

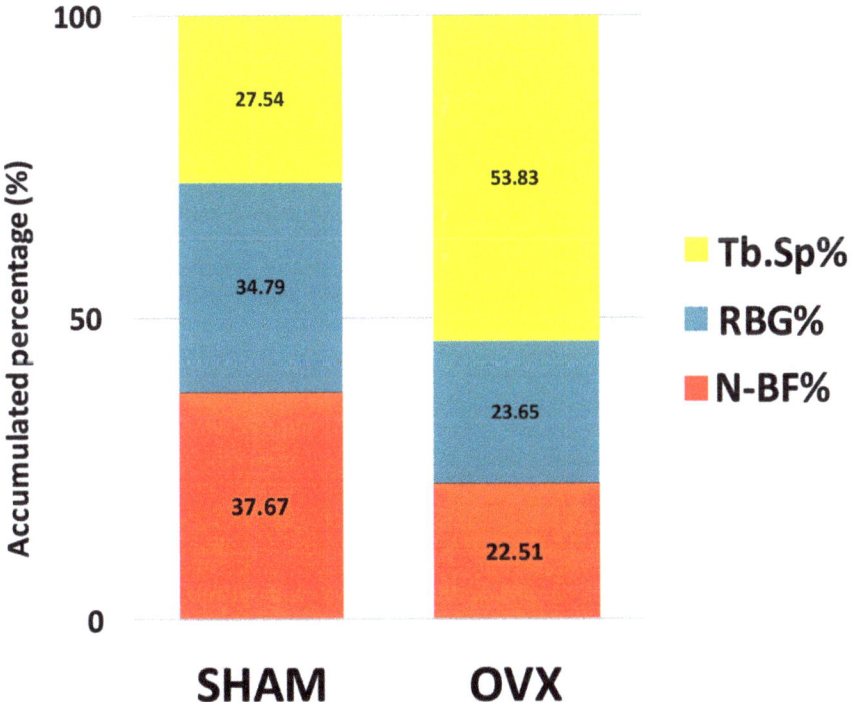

Figure 6. Histomorphometric evaluation of the mean volume fractions of new bone formation (N-BF%, red bar), remaining grafting material (RBG%, blue bar) and trabecular bone space (Tb.Sp%, yellow bar) occupying the defects after the 14 weeks of healing. Statistical analysis showed significant difference between SHAM and OVX for all parameters ($p < 0.05$).

4. Discussion

The present study aimed to evaluate the effect of inducing an osteoporotic condition after eight weeks of initial healing of bone defects grafted with xenograft in a rat model. The results reveal greater new bone formation within osseous defects in healthy compared to osteoporotic bone conditions. On the other hand, reduction in the remaining graft material was greater in the osteoporotic bone condition. In addition, osteoporotic bone showed larger areas of soft tissue/marrow space compared to healthy bone.

Clinically, deproteinized bovine bone graft material is extensively used to repair osseous defects [8]. Multiple human clinical studies have already been performed and long-term data regarding the outcome of bone grafting procedures have been reported. For instance, Piattelli et al. [7] conducted a histological analysis in 20 patients treated with Bio-Oss up to four years of bone healing. They concluded that anorganic bovine bone is osteoconductive and promotes the successful long-term outcome of bone grafting. In another study by Scarano et al. [25], bovine porous bone mineral for maxillary sinus augmentation was used and then dental implants installed. Histological results in an implant retrieved four years after insertion show direct contact between bone and implant without an interposition of the graft material particles. They concluded that that the slow resorption of the bovine graft particles did not jeopardize the osseointegration of the implant. Further, the results from a six-year randomized-controlled clinical trial with bovine bone material by Stavropoulos and Karring [26] show improvements in intrabony defect healing using radiographs and clinical assessment parameters.

Experiments performed with animal species such as rabbits, goats, sheep, dogs and rodents are often used to study bone regeneration. For mimicking osteoporotic bone conditions, rats were utilized in the present study to simulate alterations in bone regeneration following induced estrogen deficiency as in human. Although rats are small experimental animals and have a different bone formation and remodeling rate compared with humans, they are excellent preclinical models for studying osteoporotic changes as they closely emulate pharmaco-therapeutic response and allow studying the effect of estrogen depletion on the skeleton [27]. However, it has to be noticed that the preclinical model as used in the present study encounters several limitations that need to be solved in prospective studies. For instance, it has been noticed that ovariectomized rats have a faster bone turnover than patients with osteoporosis. Therefore, further in vivo studies can be suggested to validate the effect of osteoporosis on bone regeneration related to different bone substitutes. In addition, a larger animal model should be used to clarify the effect of osteoporosis with bone graft under challenged bone condition.

In animal models of experimental osteoporosis, the assessment of the biomaterial-mediated bone regeneration process in subcritical sized defects, considered established approaches relied on [28]. Despite the proven capability of the reported models, the usage of critical size defects, i.e., intraosseously established wounds that do not report spontaneous healing, has been considered the standard approach for the validation of translational bone regenerative strategies and output the intrinsic regenerative potential of the grafted bone. In the current study, the femoral condyle OVX rat model allowed examined bone regeneration in a 3-mm critical size defect. For instance, we recently published an in vivo experimental study using the same femoral condyle model of 3-mm critical size defect. The untreated (empty) defects did not heal without intervention, making the rat femoral condyle model a well-established and standardized critical size defect model highly useful for evaluating bone regeneration in healthy and osteoporotic bone [29].

The biological performance of deproteinized bovine bone grafts is widely investigated in preclinical studies using healthy animals [24,30–34]. These confirmed that bovine bone particles enhance bone regeneration, and its remnants can become integrated very well with the newly formed bone. In many histological studies, osteoblasts and osteoclasts were observed in conjunction with bovine bone particles as well as with the newly formed bone. Intimate contact between the implanted material and the newly formed bone was also commonly presented. For instance, van Houdt et al. [24] tested bovine bone (Bio-Oss) implanted in femoral condylar bone defects in rats. At 12 weeks, new bone formation in direct contact with the Bio-Oss granules was observed. The remaining Bio-Oss granules were completely covered by new bone. In line with those observations, histological analysis in the present study demonstrated similar findings in the SHAM (healthy) animals using InterOss® bone granules after 14 weeks of healing (Figure 5).

Beside the grafted material, the bone condition is the key factor affecting the graft healing and its integration with new bone [16,35,36]. In many clinical cases, the presence of osteoporosis is a major challenging condition in patients undergoing bone grafting surgery due to decreased capacity of bone regeneration [16,37]. In a retrospective analysis of 49 patients, an alveolar bone grafting procedure was impaired in 11 patients due to an unfavorable bone condition (i.e., osteopenia) [37]. This is primarily due to estrogen deficiency, which negatively influences the bone metabolism [38]. Estrogen deficiency causes an imbalance in osteoblastic/osteoclastic processes and results in an increased breakdown of bone and a reduced bone formation [39].

In previous preclinical studies, ovariectomized rats were used to evaluate qualitatively and quantitatively the influence of estrogen deficiency on bone grafting [40,41]. For example, Luize et al. [41] examined bone blocks to augment a mandibular defect in OVX rats. At 7, 14 and 28 days post-surgery, histological analysis showed a delay in the osteogenic activity and bone healing in OVX rats compared to SHAM rats. The majority of grafted materials in OVX animals appeared to be interspaced by fibrous tissue. Additionally, OVX rats exhibited significantly less new bone formation compared to SHAM rats. This result is in accordance with the present study.

In contrast, some other animal studies did not observe a significant effect in terms of new bone formation related to bone grafting in osteoporotic versus healthy animals [24,42–44]. This discrepancy might be due to differences in the experimental design, animal model, type of biomaterials, bone defects and evaluation periods. Therefore, it is difficult to establish direct correlations between these studies.

Despite the contradiction in previous studies, the present findings sustain an impaired regenerative potential of bone grafting in OVX animals. Differently, our study model was designed in such a way to replicate the effects of late-induced osteoporosis after the bone grafting procedure was performed. At 14 weeks of bone healing, the quality and quantity of bone formation (N-BF%) was significantly decreased in the osteoporotic rats, which indicates that bone formation in a bone defect can become compromised in an osteoporotic condition, as induced post-implantation. Nevertheless, the exact involved mechanism needs to be explored further in follow-up studies.

Previously, it has been reported that a deficiency in estrogen receptor (i.e., ER-α and ER-β) expression contributes negatively to the regenerative potential in osteoporotic bone [45]. Likewise, osteoblast-related gene expression (e.g., RUNX2, BMP2, COLLAGEN I and OSTEOCALCIN) were significantly decreased in OVX animals in relation to bone-biomaterial regeneration [30,46]. Further, the osteogenic differentiation of mesenchymal stem cells (MSCs) derived from osteoporotic bone was significantly altered [18]. This emphasizes the effect of intrinsic deficiencies in the regenerative capability of osteoporotic bone, particularly in the presence of bone biomaterials. Previous data also verify an increase of the adipogenic activation in the bone of OVX animals [46]. This seems to disrupt the normal osteogenic function within the bone tissue [26]. In agreement, we noticed more fat bone marrow with an hypocellular appearance in OVX rats compared to healthy control rats.

It is important to note that in the current study the amount of remaining graft material was significantly less in the osteoporotic bone conditions compared to healthy bone conditions. We suppose that this is caused by the observed increased presence of osteoclast-like cells around the graft granules in the OVX animals. In addition, we assume that the eroded surfaces of trabecular bone indicate hyperactivity of osteoclastic cells in osteoporotic bone compared to healthy bone. Usually, the remodeling of bone graft material occurs in multiple phases [46]. Bone graft resorption is initiated by the function of osteoclastic cells. Osteoclast activation is directly linked to osteoblast function [35]. The role of osteoclasts is not limited to the resorption of bone. They also have a significant impact on the local recruitment and bone-forming activity of osteoblasts via so-called cell–cell "crosstalk". Bone formation and resorption during remodeling have to be aligned carefully in a process that is called "coupling" [47]. Therefore, an imbalance of osteoclast/osteoblast activities in osteoporotic bone is connected with the decreased bone formation and increased rate of resorption, which limits the potential of bone-biomaterial incorporation, as observed in our study.

The performance of bone-biomaterials for bone defect augmentation showed limitation, in regard fast resorption rate, which correlated to high number osteoclast (resorbing) cells. One possible way to overcome the mentioned limitation incorporates biomaterial that showed lower number and activity of osteoclast cells. For instance, Westhauser et al. [48] showed that addition 45S5 bioactive glass to β-tricalcium phosphate might be a way to overcome the individual limitations of both materials by a combination of their respective strengths. They concluded that volume of combined materials during the 10-week implantation period remained almost unchanged correlating with significantly decreased physical presence and less pronounced genetic activity of bone-resorbing cell populations (TRAP+). Furthermore, the presence and activity of osteoclasts is highly dependent on the chemical composition of the bone substitute material and also influences osteoblast–osteoclast crosstalk and coupling [47]. The activity of osteoclastic bone resorption can be visualized by specific staining, i.e., tartrate-resistant acid phosphatase (TRAP) staining [30,49]. Decalcification of bone specimens is required for the application of TRAP staining. TRAP staining cannot be performed using pMMA embedding. However, in our study, we were limited to examining the activity of osteoclastic cells via their TRAP expression due to low number of available specimens to prepare decalcified sections. Consequently, osteoclasts could only be analyzed by histological appearance (i.e., relatively larger and multinucleated) at higher magnification (Figure 5). In addition, proper quantification of the number of osteoclasts was not feasible. This has to be considered as a limitation of our study design.

Although the OVX rat model is a well-established preclinical model for simulating osteoporotic bone conditions, differences among species and animal models size should be considered before transferring promising findings to clinical trials with human patients. Small animal models offer the easiest way to keep animals at low costs for longer time with a high reproduction rate. The offer of markers for laboratory use is the biggest in the market. On the other hand, clinical situation is far away. The results must be interpreted very carefully and often require further studies in larger animal models. Large animal models are as close to the clinical situation as a model can be. Organs, blood supply and common physiology are relatively close to humans. Disadvantages are high costs, high personal and work effort, limitation of follow-up period and availability of markers to study special histological issues [50].

In view of the above mentioned, it is very relevant to take care of the potential implication of impaired bone regeneration in osteoporotic conditions in relation to bone grafting procedures. In these situations, a solution can be the development of bone graft material that prospectively promotes the bone healing outcome.

5. Conclusions

Within the limitations of this study, inducing an osteoporotic condition in rats after initial healing of a bone graft material negatively influences bone regeneration in the created bone defect. Further investigations are needed to explore the clinical implications of these findings.

6. Impact Statement

Recently, increasing concerns have existed about the effect of bone diseases, such as osteoporosis, on bone regeneration. However, bone-grafting complications may occur in patients with compromised medical bone condition, e.g. osteoporosis, as bone healing in such patients can be challenged or impaired. This study assessed if altered bone metabolism due to osteoporosis affects bone regeneration related to bone-defect grafting using preclinical animal models. The results suggest that inducing an osteoporotic condition in rats after initial healing of a bone graft material negatively influences bone regeneration in the created bone defect.

Author Contributions: Conceptualization, M.Y.S., A.M.B., A.A.N., J.J.J.P.v.d.B., J.A.J. and H.S.A.; data curation, A.M.B.; formal analysis, M.Y.S.; funding acquisition, H.S.A.; investigation, M.Y.S., and A.M.B.; methodology, M.Y.S., A.M.B., A.A.N., J.J.J.P.v.d.B. and H.S.A.; project administration, A.A.N.; resources, A.A.N. and J.J.J.P.v.d.B.; validation, J.J.J.P.v.d.B. and J.A.J.; visualization, J.A.J.; writing—original draft, M.Y.S.; and writing—review and editing, J.J.J.P.v.d.B., J.A.J. and H.S.A. All authors have read and agreed to the published version of the manuscript.

Funding: The authors extend their appreciation to the Deanship of Scientific Research at King Saud University for funding this work through research group No (RG-1439-026).

Institutional Review Board Statement: The present study was approved by the Animal Ethical Committee at King Saud University, College of Dentistry, Riyadh, Saudi Arabia (Approval No. 4/67/389683). All in-vivo experiments obeyed the guidelines (national and international) for animal care and conformed to the ARRIVE guidelines.

Informed Consent Statement: Not applicable.

Data Availability Statement: Not applicable.

Acknowledgments: The authors are grateful to the technical support of Vincent Cuijpers, Martijn Martens and Natasja van Dijk in histological preparation and sectioning. The authors are also grateful to Mary Grace Baysa Vigilla and Rhodanne Nicole Lambarte for their support during animal experimental work. Finally, the authors thank Terrence Sumague for his assistance during the histomorphometric measurements.

Conflicts of Interest: The authors declare that they have no known competing financial interests or personal relationships that could have appeared to influence the work reported in this paper.

References

1. Brunsvold, M.A.; Mellonig, J.T. Bone grafts and periodontal regeneration. *Periodontol. 2000* **1993**, *1*, 80–91. [CrossRef] [PubMed]
2. Nasr, H.F.; Aichelmann-Reidy, M.E.; Yukna, R.A. Bone and bone substitutes. *Periodontol. 2000* **1999**, *19*, 74–86. [CrossRef] [PubMed]
3. Oryan, A.; Alidadi, S.; Moshiri, A.; Maffulli, N. Bone regenerative medicine: Classic options, novel strategies, and future directions. *J. Orthop. Surg. Res.* **2014**, *9*, 18. [CrossRef] [PubMed]
4. Cypher, T.J.; Grossman, J.P. Biological principles of bone graft healing. *J. Foot Ankle Surg.* **1996**, *35*, 413–417. [CrossRef]
5. Goulet, J.A.; Senunas, L.E.; DeSilva, G.L.; Greenfield, M.L. Autogenous iliac crest bone graft. Complications and functional assessment. *Clin. Orthop. Relat. Res.* **1997**, *339*, 76–81. [CrossRef]
6. Allegrini, S., Jr.; Koening, B., Jr.; Allegrini, M.R.; Yoshimoto, M.; Gedrange, T.; Fanghaenel, J.; Lipski, M. Alveolar ridge sockets preservation with bone grafting-review. *Ann. Acad. Med. Stetin* **2008**, *54*, 70–81.
7. Piattelli, M.; Favero, G.A.; Scarano, A.; Orsini, G.; Piattelli, A. Bone reactions to anorganic bovine bone (Bio-Oss) used in sinus augmentation procedures: A histologic long-term report of 20 cases in humans. *Int. J. Oral. Maxillofac Implant.* **1999**, *14*, 835–840.
8. Gazdag, A.R.; Lane, J.M.; Glaser, D.; Forster, R.A. Alternatives to autogenous bone graft: Efficacy and indications. *Jaaos-J. Am. Acad. Orthop. Surg.* **1995**, *3*, 1–8. [CrossRef]
9. Masaki, C.; Nakamoto, T.; Mukaibo, T.; Kondo, Y.; Hosokawa, R. Strategies for alveolar ridge reconstruction and preservation for implant therapy. *J. Prosthodont. Res.* **2015**, *59*, 220–228. [CrossRef]
10. Khojasteh, A.; Soheilifar, S.; Mohajerani, H.; Nowzari, H. The effectiveness of barrier membranes on bone regeneration in localized bony defects: A systematic review. *Int. J. Oral. Maxillofac. Implant.* **2013**, *28*, 1076–7089. [CrossRef]
11. Esposito, M.; Grusovin, M.G.; Felice, P.; Karatzopoulos, G.; Worthington, H.V.; Coulthard, P. The efficacy of horizontal and vertical bone augmentation procedures for dental implants-a Cochrane systematic review. *Eur. J. Oral Implant.* **2009**, *2*, 167–184.
12. Aytekin, M.; Arisan, V. Alveolar Ridge Augmentation Techniques in Implant Dentistry. In *Oral and Maxillofacial Surgery*; IntechOpen: London, UK, 2020.
13. Cicciù, M.; Fiorillo, L.; Cervino, G.; Habal, M.B. BMP Application as Grafting Materials for Bone Regeneration in the Craniofacial Surgery: Current Application and Future Directions by an RCT Analysis. *J. Craniofacial Surg.* **2020**. [CrossRef] [PubMed]
14. Dervis, E. Oral implications of osteoporosis. *Oral. Surg. Oral. Med. Oral. Pathol. Oral. Radiol. Endod.* **2005**, *100*, 349–356. [CrossRef] [PubMed]
15. Calciolari, E.; Mardas, N.; Dereka, X.; Kostomitsopoulos, N.; Petrie, A.; Donos, N. The effect of experimental osteoporosis on bone regeneration: Part 1, histology findings. *Clin. Oral. Implant. Res.* **2017**, *28*, e101–e110. [CrossRef] [PubMed]
16. Thompson, D.; Simmons, H.; Pirie, C.; Ke, H. FDA Guidelines and animal models for osteoporosis. *Bone* **1995**, *17*, S125–S133. [CrossRef]
17. Jiupeng, D.; Mengchun, Q.; Jianping, L.; Ming, Z.; Jinyuan, L.; Yongqiang, L.; Wei, D. Effect of local treatment with Zoledronate Acid on bone healing of Bio-oss bone graft and osseointegration of dental implants in osteoporotic rats. In Proceedings of the 2011 International Conference on Human Health and Biomedical Engineering, Jilin, China, 19–22 August 2011; pp. 973–976.

18. Benisch, P.; Schilling, T.; Klein-Hitpass, L.; Frey, S.N.P.; Seefried, L.; Raaijmakers, N.; Krug, M.; Regensburger, M.; Zeck, S.; Schinke, T. The transcriptional profile of mesenchymal stem cell populations in primary osteoporosis is distinct and shows overexpression of osteogenic inhibitors. *PLoS ONE* **2012**, *7*, e45142. [CrossRef]
19. Teitelbaum, S.L. Osteoclasts, integrins, and osteoporosis. *J. Bone Miner. Metab.* **2000**, *18*, 344. [CrossRef]
20. Jeffcoat, M. The association between osteoporosis and oral bone loss. *J. Periodontol.* **2005**, *76*, 2125–2132. [CrossRef]
21. Alghamdi, H.S.; van den Beucken, J.J.; Jansen, J.A. Osteoporotic rat models for evaluation of osseointegration of bone implants. *Tissue Eng. Part. C Methods* **2014**, *20*, 493–505. [CrossRef]
22. Shaheen, M.Y.; Basudan, A.M.; de Vries, R.B.; van den Beucken, J.J.; Jansen, J.A.; Alghamdi, H.S. Bone Regeneration Using Antiosteoporotic Drugs in Adjunction with Bone Grafting: A Meta-Analysis. *Tissue Eng. Part. B Rev.* **2019**, *25*, 500–509. [CrossRef]
23. Vesterinen, H.; Sena, E.; Egan, K.; Hirst, T.; Churolov, L.; Currie, G.; Antonic, A.; Howells, D.; Macleod, M. Meta-analysis of data from animal studies: A practical guide. *J. Neurosci. Methods* **2014**, *221*, 92–102. [CrossRef] [PubMed]
24. Van Houdt, C.I.A.; Ulrich, D.J.O.; Jansen, J.A.; van den Beucken, J. The performance of CPC/PLGA and Bio-Oss® for bone regeneration in healthy and osteoporotic rats. *J. Biomed. Mater. Res. B Appl. Biomater.* **2018**, *106*, 131–142. [CrossRef] [PubMed]
25. Scarano, A.; Pecora, G.; Piattelli, M.; Piattelli, A. Osseointegration in a sinus augmented with bovine porous bone mineral: Histological results in an implant retrieved 4 years after insertion. A case report. *J. Periodontol.* **2004**, *75*, 1161–1166. [CrossRef]
26. Stavropoulos, A.; Karring, T. Guided tissue regeneration combined with a deproteinized bovine bone mineral (Bio-Oss®) in the treatment of intrabony periodontal defects: 6-year results from a randomized-controlled clinical trial. *J. Clin. Periodontol.* **2010**, *37*, 200–210. [CrossRef] [PubMed]
27. Lelovas, P.P.; Xanthos, T.T.; Thoma, S.E.; Lyritis, G.P.; Dontas, I.A. The laboratory rat as an animal model for osteoporosis research. *Comp. Med.* **2008**, *58*, 424–430.
28. Durão, S.; Gomes, P.S.; Colaço, B.; Silva, J.; Fonseca, H.; Duarte, J.; Felino, A.; Fernandes, M.H. The biomaterial-mediated healing of critical size bone defects in the ovariectomized rat. *Osteoporos. Int.* **2014**, *25*, 1535–1545. [CrossRef] [PubMed]
29. Ahmed, A.G.; Awartani, F.A.; Niazy, A.A.; Jansen, J.A.; Alghamdi, H.S. A Combination of Biphasic Calcium Phosphate (Maxresorb®) and Hyaluronic Acid Gel (Hyadent®) for Repairing Osseous Defects in a Rat Model. *Appl. Sci.* **2020**, *10*, 1651. [CrossRef]
30. Van Houdt, C.I.; Tim, C.R.; Crovace, M.C.; Zanotto, E.D.; Peitl, O.; Ulrich, D.J.; Jansen, J.A.; Parizotto, N.A.; Renno, A.C.; van den Beucken, J.J. Bone regeneration and gene expression in bone defects under healthy and osteoporotic bone conditions using two commercially available bone graft substitutes. *Biomed. Mater.* **2015**, *10*, 035003. [CrossRef] [PubMed]
31. Jensen, S.S.; Aaboe, M.; Pinholt, E.M.; Hjorting-Hansen, E.; Melsen, F.; Ruyter, I.E. Tissue reaction and material characteristics of four bone substitutes. *Int. J. Oral Maxillofac Implant.* **1996**, *11*, 55–66.
32. Berglundh, T.; Lindhe, J. Healing around implants placed in bone defects treated with Bio-Oss. An experimental study in the dog. *Clin. Oral Implant. Res.* **1997**, *8*, 117–124. [CrossRef] [PubMed]
33. Pinholt, E.M.; Bang, G.; Haanaes, H.R. Alveolar ridge augmentation in rats by Bio-Oss. *Eur. J. Oral Sci.* **1991**, *99*, 154–161. [CrossRef] [PubMed]
34. Tapety, F.I.; Amizuka, N.; Uoshima, K.; Nomura, S.; Maeda, T. A histological evaluation of the involvement of Bio-Oss® in osteoblastic differentiation and matrix synthesis. *Clin. Oral Implant. Res.* **2004**, *15*, 315–324. [CrossRef] [PubMed]
35. Turner, A.S. Animal models of osteoporosis-necessity and limitations. *Eur Cell Mater.* **2001**, *1*, 13.
36. Sanfilippo, F.; Bianchi, A.E. Osteoporosis: The effect on maxillary bone resorption and therapeutic possibilities by means of implant prostheses-a literature review and clinical considerations. *Int. J. Periodontics Restor. Dent.* **2003**, *23*, 447–457. [CrossRef]
37. Blomqvist, J.E.; Alberius, P.; Isaksson, S.; Linde, A.; Hansson, B.-G.R. Factors in implant integration failure after bone grafting: An osteometric and endocrinologic matched analysis. *Int. J. Oral Maxillofac. Surg.* **1996**, *25*, 63–68. [CrossRef]
38. Khosla, S.; Oursler, M.J.; Monroe, D.G. Estrogen and the skeleton. *Trends Endocrinol. Metab.* **2012**, *23*, 576–581. [CrossRef] [PubMed]
39. Väänänen, H.K.; Härkönen, P.L. Estrogen and bone metabolism. *Maturitas* **1996**, *23*, S65–S69. [CrossRef]
40. Teófilo, J.M.; Brentegani, L.G.; Lamano-Carvalho, T.L. Bone healing in osteoporotic female rats following intra-alveolar grafting of bioactive glass. *Arch. Oral Biol.* **2004**, *49*, 755–762. [CrossRef]
41. Luize, D.S.; Bosco, A.F.; Bonfante, S.; de Almeida, J.M. Influence of ovariectomy on healing of autogenous bone block grafts in the mandible: A histomorphometric study in an aged rat model. *Int. J. Oral. Maxillofac. Implant.* **2008**, *23*, 207–214.
42. Hayashi, K.; Uenoyama, K.; Matsuguchi, N.; Nakagawa, S.; Sugioka, Y. The affinity of bone to hydroxyapatite and alumina in experimentally induced osteoporosis. *J. Arthroplast.* **1989**, *4*, 257–262. [CrossRef]
43. Hayashi, K.; Uenoyama, K.; Mashima, T.; Sugioka, Y. Remodelling of bone around hydroxyapatite and titanium in experimental osteoporosis. *Biomaterials* **1994**, *15*, 11–16. [CrossRef]
44. Fuegl, A.; Tangl, S.; Keibl, C.; Watzek, G.; Redl, H.; Gruber, R. The impact of ovariectomy and hyperglycemia on graft consolidation in rat calvaria. *Clin. Oral. Implant. Res.* **2011**, *22*, 524–529. [CrossRef] [PubMed]
45. He, Y.-X.; Zhang, G.; Pan, X.-H.; Liu, Z.; Zheng, L.-Z.; Chan, C.-W.; Lee, K.-M.; Cao, Y.-P.; Li, G.; Wei, L. Impaired bone healing pattern in mice with ovariectomy-induced osteoporosis: A drill-hole defect model. *Bone* **2011**, *48*, 1388–1400. [CrossRef]
46. Rolvien, T.; Barbeck, M.; Wenisch, S.; Amling, M.; Krause, M. Cellular mechanisms responsible for success and failure of bone substitute materials. *Int. J. Mol. Sci.* **2018**, *19*, 2893. [CrossRef] [PubMed]

47. Shiwaku, Y.; Neff, L.; Nagano, K.; Takeyama, K.-I.; de Bruijn, J.; Dard, M.; Gori, F.; Baron, R. The crosstalk between osteoclasts and osteoblasts is dependent upon the composition and structure of biphasic calcium phosphates. *PLoS ONE* **2015**, *10*, e0132903. [CrossRef]
48. Westhauser, F.; Essers, C.; Karadjian, M.; Reible, B.; Schmidmaier, G.; Hagmann, S.b.; Moghaddam, A. Supplementation with 45S5 Bioactive Glass Reduces In Vivo Resorption of the Œ≤-Tricalcium-Phosphate-Based Bone Substitute Material Vitoss. *Int. J. Mol. Sci.* **2019**, *20*, 4253. [CrossRef] [PubMed]
49. Oddie, G.; Schenk, G.; Angel, N.; Walsh, N.; Guddat, L.; De Jersey, J.; Cassady, A.; Hamilton, S.; Hume, D. Structure, function, and regulation of tartrate-resistant acid phosphatase. *Bone* **2000**, *27*, 575–584. [CrossRef]
50. Simon, F.; Oberhuber, A.; Schelzig, H. Advantages and Disadvantages of Different Animal Models for Studying Ischemia/Reperfusion Injury of the Spinal Cord. *Eur. J. Vasc. Endovasc. Surg.* **2015**, *49*, 744. [CrossRef]

MDPI
St. Alban-Anlage 66
4052 Basel
Switzerland
Tel. +41 61 683 77 34
Fax +41 61 302 89 18
www.mdpi.com

Materials Editorial Office
E-mail: materials@mdpi.com
www.mdpi.com/journal/materials

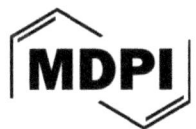

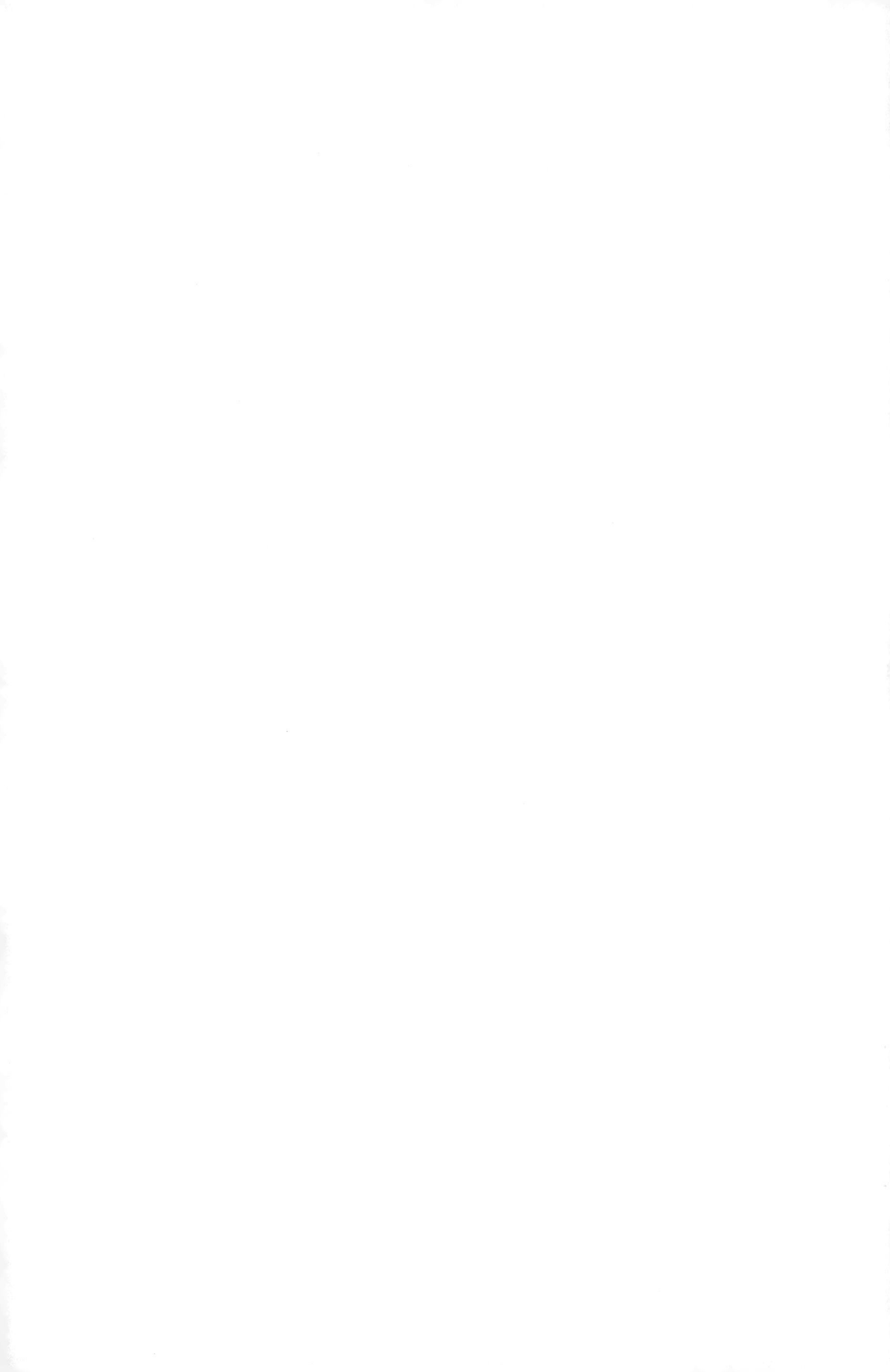

www.ingramcontent.com/pod-product-compliance
Lightning Source LLC
LaVergne TN
LVHW070430100526
838202LV00014B/1567